PHYSICAL EXAMINATION OF THE SURGICAL PATIENT

an introduction to clinical surgery

fourth edition

J. ENGLEBERT DUNPHY, M.D., F.A.C.S.

Professor of Surgery,
University of California School of Medicine,
San Francisco

THOMAS W. BOTSFORD, M.D., F.A.C.S.

Associate Professor of Surgery,
Harvard Medical School;
Surgeon, Peter Bent Brigham Hospital, Boston

1975 W. B. SAUNDERS COMPANY
Philadelphia • London • Toronto

W. B. Saunders Company: West Washington Square
Philadelphia, Pa 19105

12 Dyott Street
London, WC1A   1DB

833 Oxford Street
Toronto, Ontario M8Z 5T9, Canada

Library of Congress Cataloging in Publication Data

Dunphy, John Englebert, 1908–

Physical examination of the surgical patient.

Bibliography: p.

1. Diagnosis, Surgical.   I. Botsford, Thomas W., joint
author.   II. Title. [DNLM: 1. Diagnosis, Surgical.
WO141 D925p]

RD35.D78 1975   617'.075   74–4557

ISBN 0–7216–3267–X

Physical Examination of the Surgical Patient   ISBN   0–7216–3267–X

Last digit is the print number: 9   8   7   6   5   4   3   2   1

To

David Cheever, M.D.

and

John Homans, M.D.

who demonstrated the Art of Surgery
to many generations of Harvard Medical Students
on the wards of the Peter Bent Brigham Hospital,
this volume is affectionately dedicated

The Purpose:
> *To discover the presence and extent of injury or disease*

The Tools:
> *Eyes, ears, fingers, nose and brain*

The Maxim:
> *To discover the abnormal we must learn and know the normal*

"Learn to see, hear, feel, and smell and know that by practice alone you can become an expert"

William S. Thayer, M.D.

FOREWORD

Percussion and auscultation of the chest have dominated the teaching of physical diagnosis for over a century. In the interval between the development of the stethoscope in 1818 and the discovery of the roentgen ray in 1895, an acute sense of touch and of sound provided the astute physician with remarkable insight into the condition of his patient's heart and lungs. Because of the continuing satisfaction which comes from the high development of these methods, percussion and auscultation of the thorax still dominate the student's hours of instruction in bedside diagnosis, the most important of the clinical arts. Yet, in the actual practice of medicine and surgery the high development of the roentgenogram has permitted these two time-honored skills to recede to a position more truly reflecting their importance relative to the rest of the examination of the patient. In this book, Dr. Dunphy and Dr. Botsford have gathered together a guide to those important features of physical diagnosis which are not included in the conventional works on examination of the chest. These are the methods of observation, of palpation, of examination of external structures and internal viscera, and of deduction.

It is a pleasure to watch a skillful and merciful surgeon examining the abdomen of an acutely ill patient. The precision and perspicacity of his approach recall those of a skilled physician detecting the murmur of early mitral stenosis. Palpation of the acutely diseased abdomen, like the examination of an acutely injured patient, accurate detection of peripheral vascular disease, rectal examination, and pelvic examination, has been brought to a high degree of perfection by years of surgical practice. Indeed, these examinations have so often been associated with surgery that they are often referred to as "physical examination of the surgical patient," and indeed such is the title of this book.

Nevertheless, it is clearly of equal importance for the internist, the psychiatrist, or the neurologist to feel a small goiter or to observe the peripheral obliteration of pulses, which indicate a possible cause in the one instance of nervousness, or in the other of dementia. These are methods of bedside examination which every medical student should master, to prepare himself for whatever branch of medicine he enters as a career.

The authors have emphasized not only the detailed techniques of examination, but also the approach to the patient as an individual. It is in this wise that the student gradually develops that clinical acumen which later on will tell him so much about the patient, his disease, his educational and social status, his fears, his anxieties, and his adjustment to the medical environment in which he finds himself. It is this clinical sense which will lead the young doctor to think of his patient as a man away from home, not a hospital case.

This is a book of procedure, a book of technique. Yet it is misleading to discuss technique without at the same time discussing the diseases which the techniques reveal. The authors have steered a middle course, focusing on technique to the greatest extent, but discussing certain disease processes as they go, pointing out enough about the pathology or disordered physiology to give meaning to the physical signs encountered.

This book has been written as a simple informal statement of how to examine a patient and derive the most information by the simplest means. The authors' enthusiasm is infectious and will arouse in their students the same feeling of interest, curiosity, and ingenious perspicacity. Teachers of physical diagnosis will find this book a useful *vade mecum*. And patients will be better cared for by dint of this re-emphasis on the simple fundamentals of medicine and surgery. Student, teacher, and patient alike will stand in the authors' debt.

FRANCIS D. MOORE, M.D.

Boston, Massachusetts

PREFACE
to the 4th edition

As the subtitle implies, this book has been rewritten with a substantially revised orientation. The pathophysiology and more detailed descriptions of disease entities have been added to most chapters. This is in keeping with the one desirable trend in recent curricular changes, namely, an earlier introduction to clinical medicine with a simultaneous emphasis on the importance of the basic sciences.

Advances in our understanding of shock, respiratory insufficiency, vascular and cardiac disease, cancer, and pediatric surgery have also required major revisions.

It is hoped that this edition will serve as a valuable bridge between the basic sciences and clinical surgery, a stepping stone to the assumption of the responsibilities of a Senior Clinical Clerk as a member of the surgical team.

The reference bibliography has been supplemented by a suggested list of texts for advanced reading.

The authors are deeply appreciative of the major contributions made to this edition by Dr. Albert Starr, University of Oregon (cardiac surgery) and Drs. Alfred deLorimier, William Ehrenfeld, and Ronald Stoney, University of California, San Francisco (pediatric and vascular surgery). We are indebted to Dr. Nicholas E. O'Connor, Boston, for his contribution on frostbite.

Again, we thank our publishers for their patience and cooperation.

San Francisco, California   J. ENGELBERT DUNPHY
Boston, Massachusetts   THOMAS W. BOTSFORD

PREFACE
to the 1st edition

The complexities of modern medicine draw the attention of both student and practitioner away from the elementary principles of physical examination on which, in the past, medical diagnosis and care were almost completely dependent. An x-ray or a laboratory test is so easy to order, or a consultation is so readily available, and the results of either or both often appear so definitive that the art of simply "looking at the patient" is in danger of being lost. What is more important, patients will seriously suffer from this tendency since there is no laboratory or other diagnostic test which can be substituted for an old-fashioned detailed appraisal of the physical signs.

This book is designed to focus attention on the methods and importance of eliciting physical signs in surgical conditions. It is not a textbook of surgery, nor is it a short cut to surgical diagnosis. For the student it is intended as a guide to the early acquisition of that astuteness and thoroughness so essential to the diagnosis of surgical disorders. For the practitioner it is hoped it will prove a useful reference to refresh his mind in the appraisal of surgical lesions with which he may not be able to maintain complete familiarity. Both student and practitioner, however, must have a fundamental grasp of the pathology and physiology of disease if they are to use this book intelligently.

All references have been deliberately omitted from the text to facilitate reading. The many publications which have been of aid to the authors are acknowledged by inclusion in the bibliography.

Acknowledgments

The authors assume complete responsibility for any errors or omissions, but are indebted to the following members of the Harvard Medical

School faculty who have read portions of the text and contributed valuable suggestions: Dr. Harrison Black, Dr. Edwin F. Cave, Dr. John A. V. Davies, Dr. Edward Edwards, Dr. Albert Ferguson, Dr. William Green, Dr. Robert Gross, Dr. Dwight Haren, Dr. J. Hartwell Harrison, Dr. David Hume, Dr. Robert Linton, Dr. Joseph Murray, Dr. T. B. Quigley, Dr. Somers Sturgis, Dr. Orvar Swensen, Dr. Grantley Taylor, Dr. Carl Walter, and Dr. Richard Warren.

Material for drawings has been generously furnished by Dr. Edward Edwards, Dr. Robert Gross, Dr. Frank Lahey, Dr. Joseph Murray, Dr. T. B. Quigley, Dr. Mark Ravitch, Dr. Merrill Sosman, Dr. Harry Stone, Dr. Moses Strock, and Dr. Kenneth Warren.

The editors of Surgery, Gynecology and Obstetrics, the Journal of Bone and Joint Surgery, and the Archives of Surgery have kindly allowed reproductions of drawings from papers by Dr. T. B. Quigley, Dr. Edwin F. Cave, and Dr. J. E. Dunphy, respectively. The W. B. Saunders Company and Charles C Thomas, publishers, have permitted reproductions of illustrations from *Peripheral Nerve Injuries: Principles of Diagnosis* by Dr. Webb Haymaker and Dr. Barnes Woodhall, and *A Textbook of Surgery* by Dr. John Homans, respectively. We are grateful to the authors for their courtesy in granting permission for these reproductions.

The artists, James Didusch, Nancy Homans and Mildred Codding, have contributed what we believe is a most important part of the book, namely, clear and precise illustrations of how to do it and what it looks like.

We are indebted to Dolores Dubinsky, Charlotte Lathrop, Julianna Richards, Phylis Belair Smith and Esther Tyson who have typed, retyped and helped in editing the manuscript.

Finally, we must express our deep gratitude to Dr. Carlyle Flake, Dr. Donald Matson, Dr. Benjamin Miller, and Dr. Francis D. Moore who have read large sections of the text and have contributed greatly to its organization and format.

J. E. DUNPHY, M.D.
T. W. BOTSFORD, M.D.

Boston, Massachusetts

Contents

Part One

THE
ELECTIVE
EXAMINATION

chapter 1   # THE LEAVEN OF
THE PHYSICAL
EXAMINATION

The first part of this book is devoted to those features of an elective physical examination which are of primary importance in the recognition of surgical diseases exclusive of those involving the eye, ear, nose, and the heart and lungs. Since the techniques of examining these areas of the body are so well described in other texts, a familiarity with them on the part of the reader is assumed and only passing reference is made to them. The emphasis in this book is placed on the methods of physical examination which are not so well covered in the standard texts, but which should be familiar to every physician as well as every surgeon. Although these techniques may seem cumbersome and lengthy to the novice, once learned they can be quickly and easily executed. Since many of them are required only if an abnormality is detected, the principles of examination described in this book can be incorporated into any elective physical examination without significantly lengthening the time required to perform it.

The material has been garnered from many sources. Acquired by experience, passed on by word of mouth or described only in specialized texts or journals, it is the stuff of which clinicians are made. Some of it is new; most of it is so old that it is in danger of being forgotten. All of it is important. It is important to both surgeons and physicians because, despite all the advances of modern medicine, the patient who seeks medical advice today and is not properly examined might better have lived in the Hippocratic era. He would then at least have lost nothing, and he would have benefited from the great catalyst of the patient-doctor interaction, the sympathetic interest of the physician. In the welter of modern medicine there is a need for this old-fashioned elixir. It is an essential leaven of the physical examination and is never more needed than when an unwilling victim of disease is first presented to the doctor as "the new patient."

3

The first meeting of doctor and patient is a singularly important occasion. It not only calls for a careful evaluation and a complete examination of the patient but it is the golden moment for the establishment of that rapport which is the essence of good medicine. The patient is vulnerable. Regardless of his station in life, he is tense. He is either deeply concerned about the nature of his disease, whether it is real or imagined, or he is irritated and annoyed by its presence and wants to be rid of it at once. Yet, paradoxically, what he wants more than the cure of his disease is the sympathy of his physician. It is this paradox which accounts for the success of the charlatan. It is an insufficiency of this personal interest on the part of our profession as a whole which has created the modern demand for more psychiatrists. What is needed is fewer psychiatrists and more psychiatry, and in the first meeting of doctor and patient the role of the former is a comparatively simple one. He has only to indicate by his manner that he is interested in the patient not as a disease, but as a person with a disease. There are some who can do this by a mere twinkle in their eye, while others must labor to accomplish the same end. However it is done, if it is genuine, the patient will feel it, and from that moment on his care becomes an experience which will enrich the lives of all who have a part in it.

Patients in our teaching hospitals usually identify as their doctor the medical student or junior house officer who first sat down to review their illness with them. What they think of him and the institution he represents depends not so much upon what he knows as on how he conducts the examination. It is stimulating and reassuring to the beginner in medicine to realize that he will be regarded by the patient as a principal figure in his care. It also places a serious responsibility on him. On more than one occasion in the history of teaching hospitals, a medical student has discharged this obligation in so effective a manner that the patient has hesitated to be examined by the Senior Surgeon. While hardly desirable, such an incident has, on the whole, a salutary effect on the Senior Surgeon! It also clearly indicates that the student has those qualities of heart and mind which the laity associates with a good doctor. Such qualities merely reduce their possessor to the level of a charlatan if he cannot back them up with the completeness, thoroughness, and skill of his examination.

SOME POINTS IN HISTORY TAKING

History taking is an art which must be acquired by experience. No detail is unimportant because the correct diagnosis often rests upon a careful balancing of probabilities. The occasion is so propitious for the establishment of the proper doctor-patient relationship that it is essential to have a certain degree of privacy and to create an illusion of leisureliness by allowing the patient to talk and even ramble a bit. Several points which are helpful to the examiner merit a brief emphasis.

The Chief Complaint

The principal complaint of the patient seeking surgical care is usually fairly concrete, such as a swelling in the groin, an ulcer of the toe, or pain after eating. Incredible as it may seem, however, some patients may conceal their real symptoms hoping that if nothing wrong is found during the examination, the symptoms are of no significance. Other patients exaggerate their chief complaint so that it requires considerable experience and skill on the part of the examiner to place it in its proper perspective. On still other occasions the patient's complaint reflects a basic insecurity or fear and has no organic basis. Listening to the patient's story and at the same time scrutinizing him as a person provides one of the best leads as to the significance and reality of the chief complaint.

Once established the chief complaint is the focal point from which the examiner develops the present illness. Here there is no substitute for precision. When did the symptom first appear? What other symptoms were associated with it? Has any treatment been taken? Are there other disturbances of function? Frequently the examiner must have the patience of Job and the astuteness of Sherlock Holmes in order to ascertain and arrange the facts in an intelligible sequence. Sometimes the patient is totally unreliable and the history must be obtained from a friend or relative.

Evaluation of Symptoms

The following are examples of the way in which the details of the history must be elaborated:

Pain.   (1) When did it begin and what was the exact mode of onset? The answer to this question is of vital importance. To obtain it one must ask the patient exactly what he was doing when the pain struck him, then ascertain its severity and rapidity of onset. (2) What is the nature of the pain? Was it colicky, steady, boring, dull, or excruciating? Did it radiate and were there any associated symptoms precipitated by the pain such as a desire to urinate or defecate?

The following are examples of leads which may be obtained by analyzing the precise character of abdominal pain:

A. An excruciating persistent pain not relieved by morphine suggests a vascular lesion such as mesenteric thrombosis, or a dissecting aortic aneurysm.

B. A constant, steady, boring pain, particularly if accentuated by motion or activity, suggests an inflammatory or infectious lesion such as appendicitis or diverticulitis.

C. An intermittent abdominal pain with a rhythmic crescendo pattern suggests small bowel obstruction.

D. An intermittent pain severe to excruciating one moment and then relieved without medication is characteristic of a colic.

The rapidity of the onset of pain gives important leads as to diagnosis particularly in abdominal lesions. An explosive onset associated with collapse is characteristic of a ruptured viscus or a vascular accident. A pain which is rapidly progressive suggests mesenteric thrombosis, acute pancreatitis, or strangulated hernia. Abdominal pain which is slow and gradual in development is more characteristic of inflammatory or infectious lesions such as appendicitis or diverticulitis.

Vomiting.   When did it begin? What was the exact relationship of the onset of vomiting to the onset of pain? What was vomited? How much? How often? Was there nausea? Did the vomiting bring relief of pain? Of nausea? Was there bile in the vomitus? Blood? The answer to each question has a definite significance. If vomiting is without pain or has preceded the onset of pain by a considerable period of time, an acute surgical lesion is unlikely. Early persistent vomiting suggests high intestinal obstruction. Repeated vomiting and persistent nausea are common in pancreatitis. If there is no bile in the vomitus and vomiting is a prominent feature of the illness, there is pyloric obstruction. Repeated regurgitation of undigested food indicates a high gastric or esophageal obstruction. Self-induced vomiting associated with persistent epigastric or right upper quadrant pain is characteristic of biliary colic and acute cholecystitis. Vomiting first of food and gastric contents, then bile, and finally feculent material indicates low intestinal obstruction. If accompanied by distention and constipation, the diagnosis is certain. Only a few careful questions, not an x-ray, are needed to obtain such information. Severe vomiting and retching followed by hematemesis are characteristic of the Mallory-Weiss syndrome.

Bleeding.   The passage of blood from any orifice is apt to be a frightening experience to the patient and the amount lost is often exaggerated in the patient's account of it. The finding of blood is indicative of an erosion or ulcerative process but its diagnostic significance is somewhat limited.

Painless bleeding is a cardinal sign of neoplasia and requires, in many instances, exhaustive studies in order to find the cause. As a rule, simple obvious explanations such as hemorrhoids cannot be accepted as the cause without complete study to eliminate more serious factors.

Tumors.   Evaluation of a tumor or swelling by history may be quite misleading. Often the patient is unaware of its presence until it is detected by the examiner. On other occasions the patient may deliberately conceal the length of time which the lesion has been present or deny that there has been recent increase in size. Here again, gentle probing on the part of the examiner may bring out the facts particularly with reference to tumors of the breast. Has it been noticed in the course of taking a bath or a shower? Although a leading question, this may bring out a detail which the patient had previously withheld. Any change in size, particularly regressions, or related symptoms such as pain must be determined.

Trauma. Trauma is so common that it must be evaluated with considerable judgment. Many times the patient will relate his illness or the development of a lesion to a supposed trauma because he can think of no other cause for its development. At other times a history of mild trauma may be the clue to diagnosis as in traumatic fat necrosis of the breast.

In acute injuries the details of the accident provide many important clues. In penetrating wounds the trajectory of the missile can often be ascertained and will provide leads as to its probable course and potential visceral injury. The position of the patient when struck is most important. Loss of consciousness or retrograde amnesia (that is, loss of memory for events just preceding the accident) are evidence of a head injury which may result in a subdural or extradural hematoma. Unless the patient is specifically questioned on such points, he may not in the excitement of the occasion furnish the information himself. Children are so frequently exposed to trauma that the parents very often date the onset of an illness to some form of accident. Multiple injuries and lacerations in a child may have been inflicted by a parent—the "battered child syndrome." The nature and extent of the injuries are usually out of proportion to the kind of accident which the patient describes, such as a subdural hematoma and long bone fractures from an alleged fall.

These are but a few examples of the details with which each of the patient's symptoms must be analyzed if all of the information is to be obtained from the history. It cannot be emphasized too strongly that there is no substitute for this information and that many times decisive steps in the patient's care are wholly dependent upon the elicitation of a fact or two in the history.

In the performance of the physical examination, there are two important considerations. It must be complete, and it must be well done. If, for some adequate reason, a portion of the physical examination has been necessarily postponed, the examiner must be capable of realizing exactly what has been omitted. The ability to do this is acquired during the doctor's formative years by the regular performance of complete physical examinations according to a set routine. Such a check list is provided in the Appendix. It must be learned by habitual repetition so that eventually without conscious effort the examiner knows he has performed a complete examination or has deliberately omitted a portion of it. Only thus can inexcusable errors of omission be avoided.

Equally important as the completeness of the examination is the quality of its performance. Unless the fullest advantage is taken of all the techniques available, one may look without seeing, listen without hearing, or palpate without feeling. It is with this aspect of the examination of the patient with reference to surgical disorders that we are primarily concerned.

The Problem-Oriented Method of Medical Records

The traditional medical record serves as a somewhat disorganized collection of medical data from which the physician is expected to extract information sufficient to diagnose and treat his patient's ills. For single or relatively few problems it is adequate, but it is inefficient in dealing with patients with multiple chronic and acute problems. The problem-oriented method of medical record keeping (Weed) has been developed to overcome this shortcoming.

The major components of the problem-oriented medical record are (1) the *Data Base,* which includes the chief complaint, complete history, physical examination, and laboratory results (this is essentially the same as the traditional method), and (2) the *Problem List,* which is defined as anything that needs treatment or further diagnostic study and includes social problems. The list is added to or changed if new problems arise or current problems are resolved. A problem may be listed as a diagnosis, a symptom, abnormal laboratory finding, social circumstance, risk factor, and so forth.

A plan is formulated for each active problem listed and should include relevant data as follows:

a. *Subjective data* (usually historical, including information from past medical records).
b. *Objective data* (current pertinent physical and laboratory findings).
c. *Assessment* (diagnosis and significant differential diagnosis).
d. *Plan* (purpose of plan, including diagnostic, therapeutic, and educational maneuvers designed to implement the plan).

In the further care of the patient, the problems are discussed in a similar fashion in the progress notes; separate notes are written for each problem and consultations are on the same basis. The nurse's notes are oriented to individual problems, and the discharge summary is in the same format. Conciseness and relevancy are essential to this method.

The method records medical data in an orderly and concise fashion and provides better communication between health professionals. It assists the physician in identifying his patient's problems and in assessing the results of his diagnostic and therapeutic efforts. It provides an adequate basis for self-assessment and contains data useful for the instruction of other physicians. Many physicians consciously or unconsciously for years have followed a plan of sorting out the problems of their patients and resolving them. However, the problem-oriented record does lend the concept of order and discipline to the multiple problems of many patients.

The problem-oriented record is meaningless, however, if the Data Base is incomplete, and the Data Base is meaningless if the physician has not performed a proper physical examination.

chapter 2 # EXAMINATION OF THE HEAD AND NECK

Ostensibly the physical examination starts with the examination of the head and neck. Actually, however, it should begin the moment the patient and the doctor meet. The patient's gait, his bearing, his habitus, and the manner in which he shakes hands provide the experienced clinician with valuable information before the history is taken.

I. GENERAL APPRAISAL OF THE PATIENT

After the patient has been put at ease and while he is describing his symptoms, the examiner should study his appearance. Much can be learned from the face of a patient. Most systemic diseases are reflected there. Jaundice, the pallor of anemia, the cyanosis of cardiac or pulmonary lesions, the plethora of polycythemia or hypertension, and the cachexia of cancer are often evident at a glance. One should acquire the habit of assaying the patient's endocrine balance. Some classic alterations are depicted in Figures 2–1, 2–2, 2–3, and 2–4. Less obvious changes are frequently detectable or may be suspected if one habitually bears the possibilities in mind. The gravity of an illness is often best weighed by merely looking at the patient's facial expression. Finally, the patient's occupation, the type of life he has led, and the sort of person he is all leave marks which can be detected by the experienced clinician.

The rapport which has been established during the taking of the history will be lost if the physical examination is not conducted with dignity, gentleness, and thoughtfulness. The patient should be completely stripped, but appropriate draping will allay any embarrassment. At the start it is well to continue conversation which has been initiated during the history taking. Light conversation may be distracting and occasionally is in order,

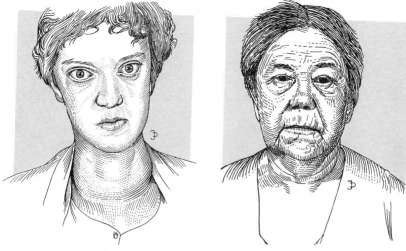

Fig. 2–1   Fig. 2–2

Figure 2–1. Young girl with exophthalmic goiter.
Figure 2–2. Myxedema.

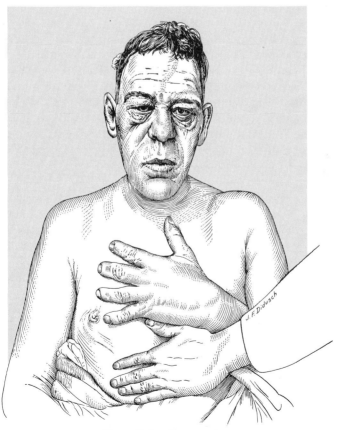

Figure 2–3. Acromegaly.

11

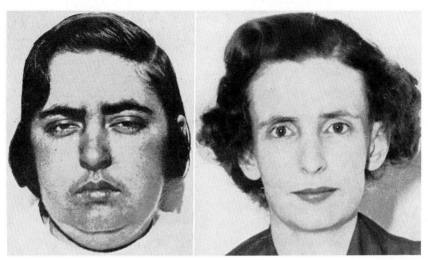

Figure 2–4. "Cushing's Disease" before and after treatment. (Peter Bent Brigham Hospital case.)

but as a rule it is best to pursue some detail of the history. A query about the exact character of the symptoms so worded as to indicate the examiner's keen interest in the problem is a most effective way of getting the patient to lose his anxiety by focusing on some aspect of his story.

While the patient is getting adjusted in this way to his position on the examining table, it is convenient to examine his hands. A good look at the hands constitutes an important feature of the general appraisal of the patient. If done at the beginning a clue is frequently found which leads the examiner to scrutinize with particular care some other part of the body.

Many diseases show themselves in the hands. Warm moist hands suggest *hyperthyroidism*. A cold moist hand reflects increased sympathetic tone, possibly *Raynaud's disease,* but more likely an anxiety state. An intense redness of the thenar and hypothenar eminences, "liver palms," suggests *cirrhosis of the liver.*

The shape of the fingers is important. *Acromegaly* produces large fingers with broad tips (Fig. 2–3). In *pulmonary osteoarthropathy* ("clubbed fingers") there is a bulbous thickening of the tips, and the nails are broad and overhanging (Fig. 2–5). The condition is seen in conjunction with long-standing pulmonary sepsis, especially lung abscess, in the cyanotic forms of congenital heart disease, and rarely in advanced forms of liver disease or malnutrition associated with intestinal diseases such as regional ileitis or ulcerative colitis.

The texture of the skin of the hands and the general hygiene of the hands and fingernails give one an insight into the patient's occupation, habits, and character.

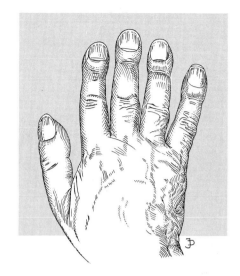

Figure 2–5. Hypertrophic pulmonary osteoarthropathy (clubbed fingers).

Having made a general appraisal of the patient, one may proceed with the examination of the head and neck, bearing in mind that in no other part of the body are the alterations of disease so accessible to the eyes and fingers.

II. THE HEAD

Position

The head and neck may be examined with the patient in the sitting or reclining position; the former is more desirable. Good light is essential, preferably clear daylight, since jaundice is obscured by artificial light. The neck and shoulders must be completely exposed. The examiner shifts his position from in front to behind the patient to facilitate inspection and palpation.

The Skin

Obvious lesions will be overlooked unless the examiner deliberately scrutinizes every inch of the integument over the face, neck, ears, and behind the ears. Look particularly for blemishes of any kind, scars of burns or previous operations, and the telangiectatic skin produced by x-ray therapy. Remember that weather-beaten skin is a fertile soil for the growth of cancer.

Some of the more common and more important lesions of the skin are described on pages 15 to 20.

The Hair and Scalp

The amount, texture, and distribution of hair over the scalp and face should be noted. The skin of the scalp need not be minutely inspected, but may be appraised at the hairline and by separating the hair during palpation. Palpate the scalp and cranium with the flat of the fingers of both hands systematically applied over the entire cranial vault. Ask the patient if he has any small lumps, nodules, or scars on his scalp, since minute wens or tumors will occasionally escape the attention of the examiner although they are well known to the patient.

The Eyes

The following should be noted: the condition of the eyebrows, the shape of the eyes, the size and regularity of the pupils, the position of the eyeball, and the condition of the sclera and conjunctiva.

Test the extraocular movements by moving a finger slowly back and forth and having the patient follow it with his eyes while his head is stationary. Look particularly for jerking movements (nystagmus), failure of convergence, lid lag, and asynchronous or limited motions of one or both eyes. Determine the *reaction of the pupils to light and accommodation.*

Be alert for the irregular or fixed pupils of advanced syphilis, the pinpoint pupils of morphine intoxication, or the slight asymmetry of the eyeball which occurs in maxillary or retro-orbital tumors. Occasionally eye signs provide the first clue to a diagnosis of hyperthyroidism (Fig. 2–1) (see p. 43).

Icterus is detectable in the conjunctiva before it is evident in the skin if the patient is examined in clear daylight. *Inflammation of the sclera* and *conjunctiva* is usually obvious. The conjunctiva of the lower lid is exposed by pulling downward on the loose tissues of the face just beneath the eye.

An ophthalmoscopic examination is now performed. Although the technique will not be described in this text, the importance of this maneuver is emphasized with particular reference to the signs of arterial disease and increased intracranial pressure.

The Ears

The external ear is inspected as part of the general scrutiny of the skin of the head and neck.

Hearing is easily tested by rubbing the tips of the thumb and forefinger together very gently in close proximity to the ear. The force necessary to produce a sound audible to the patient is an excellent guide to impaired hearing, since normal hearing can detect the slightest motion. The canals and ear drums are then inspected with the otoscope.

The Nose

Note the contour and symmetry of the nose. The patient's head is tipped slightly backward and the nostrils are inspected with the aid of a light. The septum is transilluminated by flashing the light in one nostril and looking in the other. Look particularly for deviation or perforation of the septum.

The patency of each nostril is determined by having the patient breathe through his nose while the other nostril is compressed. Further inspection of the nostril may be performed with the aid of a nasal speculum.

Some Lesions of the Skin

Many lesions of the skin commonly occur on the face, scalp, or neck, so that it is appropriate at this point to consider certain of their physical characteristics which are of diagnostic importance.

Pigmented Nevi

There are many varieties with which the surgeon must be familiar although their clinical manifestations may not always be distinctive.

Intradermal nevus. This is the common mole, a few of which will be found on practically every patient. It derives its name from the fact that the cells lie entirely within the dermis. The appearance of the lesion varies considerably from a flat, pale, brown, or pinkish macule to a deep brown papillary warty excrescence. It commonly contains hair, an important diagnostic point because the presence of hair nearly always is indicative of the intradermal nevus and benignity. The intradermal nevus rarely is found on the skin of the palms, soles, tips of the fingers or toes, or on the scrotum.

Junctional nevus. This is an epidermal rather than a dermal lesion and derives its name from the histologic appearance of the cells at the junction of the epidermis with the dermis. The junctional nevus appears as a smooth, hairless, light to dark brown, flat or slightly elevated macule. It may vary in size from a few millimeters to several centimeters in diameter. It occurs anywhere on the body, but "moles" on the scrotum or on the palmar surface of the hands or feet are nearly always of this variety. The junctional nevus may be present from birth but not infrequently appears in later life. Occasionally it appears to come out in "crops."

Compound nevus. This lesion contains both junctional and intradermal components. About 12 per cent of nevi in adults will show some junctional change histologically, whereas 50 per cent of nevi in childhood show this change. For practical purposes, compound nevi cannot be distinguished from junctional or intradermal nevi except as previously noted. If a nevus contains hair, it is probably intradermal and benign. If it occurs on the palm of the hands or feet or on the scrotum, it is almost certainly junctional in type and has a malignant potential.

Blue nevus or mongolian spot. Histologically this is an intradermal lesion and is more likely of neurogenic than epidermogenic origin. It appears as a smooth, hairless, flat or slightly elevated, dark brown to slate or blue gray spot. It commonly appears on the face, the back of the hands and feet, or on the buttocks. Its slate gray to blue color is one of its most distinguishing characteristics. Because of its dark color, it is often mistaken for a nevus undergoing malignant degeneration. The fact that it has shown no change in many years is an important, reassuring, practical point. The location on the face, back of the hands, and buttocks is also of some diagnostic import.

Juvenile melanoma. A flat nevus which increases in size in childhood is apt to be a juvenile melanoma. These are hairless and may be elevated or even verrucous. They rarely ulcerate. The important point clinically is that, upon biopsy of the lesion, mitotic figures and marked junctional change suggestive of a malignant melanoma may be found. It is extremely rare for these lesions to metastasize in childhood and, in general, they should be regarded as benign.

Again, from a practical point of view, nevi on the palms of the hands and feet, tips of the fingers, or on the scrotum should be removed in childhood when they are benign rather than delay until later in life when there is a serious risk of malignant change.

Malignant melanoma. Unfortunately, the appearance of metastases may be the first sign of a malignant melanoma. However, any change in size, ulceration, irritation, bleeding, or deepening of pigmentation should be regarded as a potential sign of malignancy in a nevus and justifies a wide excisional biopsy. Lesions which are particularly subject to trauma and lesions on the soles of the hands, feet, and on the scrotum should be removed prophylactically.

Three clinical and pathologic types of melanoma may be recognized.

1. Superficial spreading—These lesions are raised, almost circular in outline, and have a characteristic color combination of tan, brown, black, and bluish pink. Some areas appear distinctly blue, others white. A dark gray shade is suggestive of invasive growth. The remarkable color pattern relates to areas of growth and regression (Fig. 2–6 *A*).

Superficial spreading melanoma is late to metastasize, may regress spontaneously, and if seen early is curable by wide local excision in a high percentage of cases.

2. Nodular melanoma—This is a sharply localized, raised, blue to black nodule. It may look like a blueberry just under the epidermis or may be exophytic and ulcerated. In most cases, the lesion is deeply invasive, and regional lymph nodes are frequently palpable and nearly always involved (Fig. 2–6 *B*).

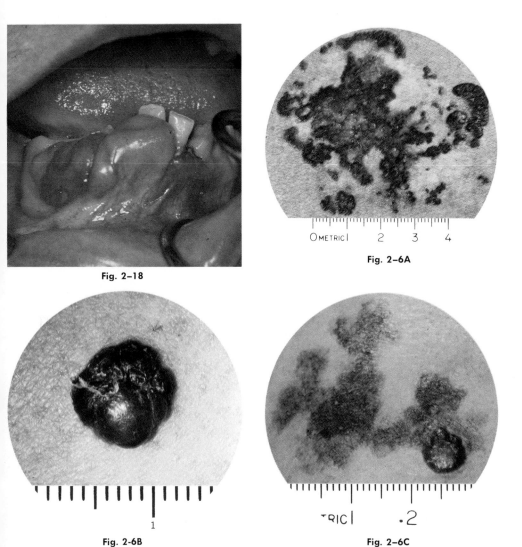

Fig. 2–18

Fig. 2–6A

Fig. 2-6B

Fig. 2–6C

Figure 2–18. Fibrous epulis. (From Pindborg, J. J.: Atlas of Diseases of the Oral Mucosa. 2nd ed. Philadelphia, W. B. Saunders Company, 1973.)

Figure 2–6. *A,* Superficial spreading melanoma, deeply invasive. *B,* Nodular melanoma, deeply invasive. *C,* Lentigo maligna melanoma, deeply invasive. (From Mihm, M. C., Jr. et al.: Early detection of primary cutaneous malignant melanoma. N. Engl. J. Med. *289:*989, 1973.)

3. Lentigo melanoma—This is a superficial spreading lesion usually much larger than superficial spreading melanoma. It is predominantly brown to black in color without the pinkish, blue-white color of superficial spreading. Dark blue nodules indicate a late stage (Fig. 2–6 C).

Prognosis in all forms of melanoma is related to the depth of invasion of the skin.

Pigmented Papilloma (Senile Wart)

These lesions appear usually after the age of 40, as slowly growing, pedunculated, brown nodules with a finely corrugated surface. They may appear singly or in crops over the face, neck, and trunk. They are not related to the pigmented nevus although frequently mistaken for moles. Malignant change is very rare; when it does occur, it takes the form of a slowly growing epidermoid carcinoma.

Sebaceous Cyst

The wen or sebaceous cyst frequently occurs on the scalp, behind the ears, and on the face and neck as a smooth, rounded nodule attached to the overlying skin. Careful inspection may reveal the orifice of an occluded sebaceous duct at the point of fixation to the skin. Infection is common; it may lead to rapid increase in size and is usually accompanied by tenderness, redness, and induration of the surrounding tissues.

Dermoid

Epithelial inclusion cysts simulate wens but are much less common. They occur at points of fusion of the ectoderm in fetal development and so are usually seen in the midline over the forehead or scalp and at the lateral angles of the palpebral fissures. They may be distinguished from wens by their location and by the fact that the overlying skin is not attached to the nodule.

A "wen" or "dermoid" near the angle of the jaw is indistinguishable from a small parotid tumor and should be regarded as such until proved otherwise by operative excision under circumstances which permit complete resection of the parotid gland if indicated.

Metastatic Cancer

Nodules of metastatic cancer frequently appear on the scalp and neck. These may closely simulate epithelial cysts. A "wen" which suddenly appears on the scalp or neck in a patient with recognized cancer should be regarded as a metastatic lesion until proved otherwise.

Metastases involving the skull often appear as smooth, rounded nodules which simulate benign cysts of the scalp. Because of the way the scalp slides deceptively over the nodule, one may gain the impression that the nodule itself is moving unless great care is taken during palpation.

Senile Keratosis

Fair-skinned, blue-eyed individuals tend to develop brownish scaling lesions which may degenerate into epidermoid cancer. At first the lesions resemble ordinary freckles, but later brown warty excrescences appear; these scale off and leave a superficial moist scab which is quickly covered by a new growth of brownish scales.

Seborrheic Keratosis

This is a precancerous lesion which appears in later life as a superficial, brownish, warty nodule covered with a moist, greasy scale. If there is a history of progressive increase in size, the lesion may represent an early stage of carcinoma.

Epidermoid Cancer

Cutaneous cancer commonly occurs on the scalp, face, and neck. At first it appears as a small, freely movable, slightly raised thickening of the skin with superficial scaling. Ulceration soon follows. Later it appears as a firm, indurated, excavated ulceration with a necrotic base from which considerable exudate may discharge (Fig. 2–7). A painless "infected ulcer" of the skin is almost invariably epidermoid carcinoma. Fixation to

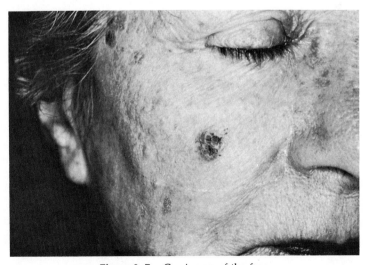

Figure 2–7. Carcinoma of the face.

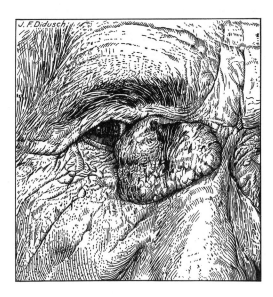

Figure 2–8. Basal cell carcinoma of the eyelid. Note the weather-beaten skin.

the underlying fascial and muscle planes develops with progression of the disease. The regional lymph nodes may be involved.

Basal Cell Carcinoma

This lesion commonly occurs about the eyes, ears, or nose. At first it resembles a small, pearly gray pimple. As it spreads, it has a firm, raised margin which usually extends well beyond the area of ulceration. The surface of the ulcer is similar to that seen in epidermoid cancer, but an advancing raised edge extending well beyond the area of ulceration and a lack of fixation are indicative of a basal cell lesion (Fig. 2–8). The underlying fascia, muscles, and bone may be involved in advanced or neglected cases. Metastases to lymph nodes are very rare.

III. THE ORAL CAVITY

A detailed examination of the oral cavity is essential since it is a common site of asymptomatic neoplasm: One must systematically visualize the *lips*, the *teeth*, the *alveolar ridges*, the *buccal mucosa*, the *hard and soft palate*, the *floor of the mouth*, the *tongue*, the *tonsils*, and the *oropharynx*. The base of the tongue and the tonsillar area should be palpated, as should any visible lesion within the oral cavity.

Usually the examination can be satisfactorily performed with a flashlight, a tongue depressor, and the palpating finger. However, a head light or a reflecting mirror is very advantageous. Moreover, since the base of the tongue, which is a frequent site of cancer, cannot be seen without using a laryngeal mirror, the use of this instrument is an integral part of a complete physical examination. It completes the examination of the oral cavity and permits visualization of another common area of cancer, the hypopharynx and larynx.

Inspection

First inspect the lips, the gums, and the teeth. The patient is asked to grimace and expose the teeth and gums anteriorly. Then the lips may be lifted away from the teeth with the aid of a tongue depressor. The mucosa of the lips may be visualized at the same time. Malocclusion, adentia, or faulty dental hygiene should be noted.

The patient is now asked to open his mouth widely; the examiner should then retract and thoroughly inspect the buccal mucosa. The gentle use of a tongue depressor is essential. Visualize the opening of Stensen's duct on the buccal mucosa. The orifice appears as a minute dimple opposite and, as the cheek is retracted, a little below the second upper molar tooth (Fig. 2–9). The alveolar ridges are inspected at this point.

Have the patient place the tip of his tongue against the roof of the mouth in order to expose the floor of the mouth. Wharton's ducts, the openings from the submaxillary gland, are readily seen on either side of the frenulum of the tongue (Fig. 2–10). Saliva may be seen issuing from them, particularly if the floor of the mouth is dried with a cotton applica-

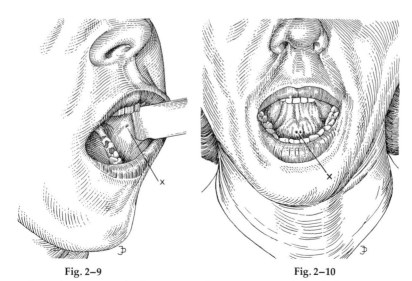

Fig. 2–9   Fig. 2–10

Figure 2–9. Exposure of the orifice of Stensen's (parotid gland) duct.
Figure 2–10. Exposure of the floor of the mouth and the orifices of Wharton's (submaxillary) ducts.

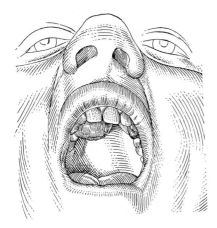

Figure 2–11. Hemangioma of the palate.

tor. The hard and soft palate and the uvula are best seen if the patient tips his head slightly backward. Any abnormality is obvious (Fig. 2–11).

Now ask the patient "to stick out his tongue" and carefully inspect all surfaces. Note the circumvallate papillae on the dorsum and lateral surfaces of the tongue; their hypertrophy is common and may simulate neoplasm. The retromolar triangle, which is the area on the alveolar ridge at the lower pole of the tonsil behind the third molar tooth, is a fairly common site for cancer; it is best seen if the tongue is pushed medially with a tongue depressor.

Next ask the patient to open his mouth widely without protruding his tongue, and gently depress this organ with a tongue depressor to permit visualization of the tonsils, the tonsillar pillars, and the oropharynx.

Palpation

This is as much a part of a complete physical examination as is palpation of the rectum or vagina. It should be performed routinely in patients over 50 years of age, especially males, because of the frequency of oral cancer. It is absolutely essential if there are symptoms referable to the oral cavity, if any lesion is seen, or if there are enlarged cervical lymph nodes.

The palpating finger should be protected by a rubber glove or finger cot. The floor of the mouth is felt bimanually; the submaxillary area can be palpated thoroughly in this same manner (Fig. 2–12 *A*). The buccal mucosa is felt between the thumb and forefinger (Fig. 2–12 *B*); the distal portion of Stensen's duct can also be appraised in this position. The alveolar ridges and tonsillar area can be felt by sliding the fingers along the floor of the mouth, crossing behind the last molar tooth, and coming out along the lateral side of the alveolar ridges. The tongue is felt by holding it in the protruding position with one hand over a bit of gauze

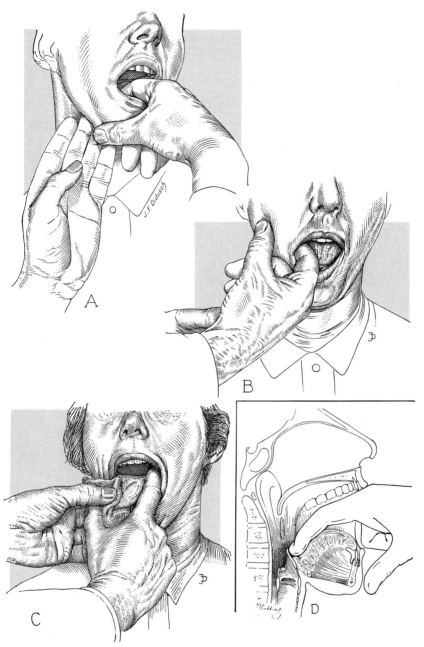

Figure 2–12. Palpation of the oral cavity. *A,* Bimanual palpation of the floor of the mouth and the submaxillary region. *B,* Palpation of the cheek and distal portion of Stensen's duct. *C,* Palpation of the tongue. *D,* Palpation of the base of the tongue and the hypopharynx.

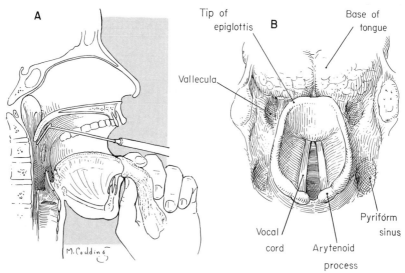

Figure 2–13. *A,* Indirect laryngoscopy. The mirror should be warmed to prevent fogging. Note the examiner has grasped the tongue over a piece of gauze and pulls it forward. *B,* Composite diagram of the important structures to be visualized in the larynx and hypopharynx. All may not be seen in a single view but can be visualized by slight rotation of the mirror. The valleculae and the pyriform sinuses are common sites of cancer.

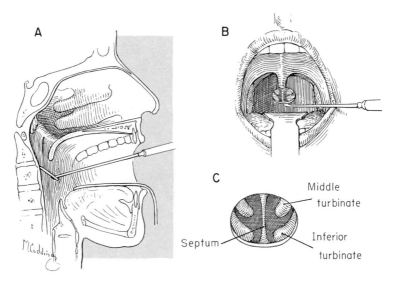

Figure 2–14. *A,* Indirect nasopharyngoscopy; note that the tongue is depressed with a retractor. *B* and *C* show the relationship of the nasal septum and the middle and inferior turbinates.

and palpating it with the thumb and forefinger of the opposite hand (Fig. 2–12 *C*). Since palpation of the base of the tongue, the tonsils, the hypopharynx, and the region of the pyriform sinus stimulates the gag reflex, it may be postponed until the remainder of the physical examination has been completed (Fig. 2–12 *D*).

The examination of the oral cavity is completed by a mirror examination of the base of the tongue, hypopharynx, larynx, and nasopharynx. The technique is depicted in Figures 2–13 and 2–14.

The reg on of the parotid gland and the preauricular lymph nodes are now palpated before proceeding to examine the neck.

Lesions of the Oral Cavity

Cancer

The most important lesion of the oral cavity which must not be overlooked in an elective examination is cancer. It may occur almost anywhere within the oral cavity, but usually spares the dorsum of the tongue anterior to the circumvallate papillae. Its favorite sites are the sides and undersurface of the tongue, the base of the tongue, the floor of the mouth, the alveolar ridges and the buccal mucosa (Fig. 2–15). Any ulceration is suggestive of cancer until proved otherwise by biopsy or a brief period of judicious observation. The importance of palpation in evaluation has already been emphasized.

Cancer of the tongue. This is the most common malignant tumor of the oral cavity. It occurs at the base of the tongue, along the edges or

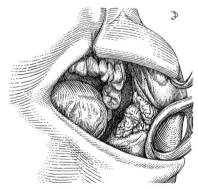

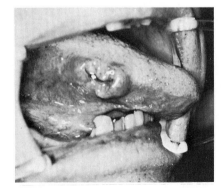

Fig. 2–15   Fig. 2–16

Figure 2–15.   Carcinoma of the buccal mucosa. The corner of the mouth is distorted by retraction. Note the lesion just beyond the ring retractor.

Figure 2–16.   Carcinoma of the tongue. The raised, ulcerated lesion involves the side of the tongue.

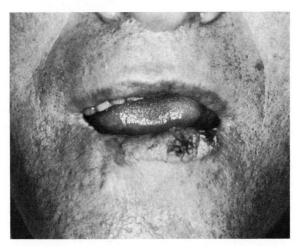

Figure 2-17. Carcinoma of the lip. The lesion appears as an indolent ulcer. To the right of the lesion is an area of leukoplakia.

on the under surface and frequently spreads to the floor of the mouth (Fig. 2-16). Its gross characteristics are those of a hard, indurated necrotic ulcer. Metastases occur frequently and early. The submaxillary and submental nodes are usually involved first in lesions in the anterior two-thirds of the tongue. The deep cervical nodes are involved in cancer of the posterior third and base of the tongue.

Cancer of the lip. This occurs predominantly in the male after the age of 50. It appears either as a superficial break in the mucosa at the mucocutaneous juncture or as a warty excrescence. It may fungate, but it commonly spreads as an indolent indurated ulcer (Fig. 2-17). Metastases occur late. Centrally placed lesions usually involve the submental nodes. Lateral lesions spread first to the submaxillary nodes. The lower rather than the upper lip is almost invariably involved.

Leukoplakia. Leukoplakia first appears as a whitish translucent patch overlying the mucous membranes of the tongue or cheeks; it may, however, cover the entire intra-oral mucosa. In advanced cases it becomes an elevated plaque with irregularly confluent areas. Fissuring and superficial ulceration secondary to infection may also occur. Carcinoma may arise in pre-existing areas of leukoplakia.

Benign Lesions of the Tongue

Much can be learned from a careful inspection of the tongue. Its moistness is a good indication of hydration, provided the patient is not a mouth breather.

Characteristic changes are seen in vitamin deficiency states. In *ariboflavinosis* the papillae become flattened, and the tongue has a finely pebbled appearance and deep reddish brown color. In *pellagra* the epithelium of the tongue ulcerates superficially and leaves a raw painful surface. A sore, painful tongue coated with whitish patches from which candida (monilia) may be smeared and cultured is a common complication of prolonged and vigorous *antibiotic therapy.* It is also seen as a complication in the chronically ill depleted patient with a polyvalent vitamin B deficiency.

Horizontal fissuring of the tongue is a congenital lesion of no clinical significance, but *longitudinal fissuring* is characteristic of *syphilis.* In *geographic tongue* the surface epithelium desquamates in irregular circinate patches with central areas of healing. These irregular areas of desquamation and healing give the tongue the appearance of a geographic map. The considerable itching and burning which is often experienced usually makes the patient suspect that he is suffering from advanced cancer. The lesion is recognized by its characteristic pattern, its changing character, and complete lack of deep ulceration or induration.

Benign ulcers of the tongue occur from trauma, irritation from diseased, jagged teeth, ill-fitting dentures, and inflammation; they are painful and superficial.

Tuberculosis produces a very painful superficial ulceration of the tongue. It is almost invariably associated with active pulmonary tuberculosis. Cancer must always be considered in any ulceration of the tongue, and to be safe, biopsy is frequently necessary.

Benign Lesions of the Lips, Teeth, and Mucous Membrane

Herpes labialis. This acute, short-lived lesion appears as a tender, raised, reddish, round, crusted plaque on the mucosa of the lip. Short duration and absence of ulceration and induration characterize it as the common "cold sore."

Gingivitis. This is characterized by reddening and tenderness of the gums. The surface of the gums bleeds easily and a purulent exudate may discharge from the margin of the gum.

The lead line of plumbism appears as a grayish black row of stippled dots extending horizontally just below the free margin of the gum.

Chancre. Primary syphilis produces a firm, indurated, painless, button-like nodule on the lip. It may simulate cancer if ulceration appears. The submental or superficial cervical lymph nodes are usually involved. Hinton and Wassermann tests are negative at this stage. The diagnosis is established by darkfield examination.

Epulis. A nodular reddish brown tumor appearing on the outer side of the alveolar ridges is characteristic of an epulis (Fig. 2–18, page 17). It is firm and nontender to palpation. Usually inflammatory in origin, it may rarely be a true neoplasm.

Hutchinson's teeth. Hutchinson's teeth, a manifestation of congenital syphilis, are now a rarity. The upper central incisors are affected; the base of each tooth is broad and the biting surface is narrow and notched.

Epithelial cysts. These commonly occur on the floor of the mouth. *Dermoids* may occur in the midline as firm, slightly cystic, round nodules. A *ranula* appears as a superficial, tense, bluish, translucent swelling on one or the other side of the frenulum. On its surface, Wharton's duct may be distinguished. Cysts of the floor of the mouth should be carefully palpated bimanually. *Thyroglossal duct cysts* may bulge into the floor of the mouth and are identified by their midline position and extension downward into the neck.

Melanosis of buccal mucosa and intestinal polyposis (Peutz-Jeghers syndrome). This is a remarkable syndrome characterized by melanin deposits in the skin and buccal mucosa associated with polyposis of the small intestine. There is often an associated anemia. Because the

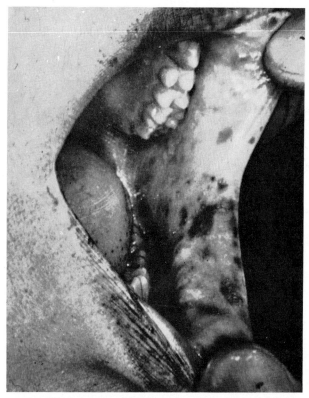

Figure 2–19. Peutz-Jeghers Syndrome: The pigmented lesions on the oral mucosa are readily seen on inspection. (Courtesy of Dr. Harold Jeghers and New England Journal of Medicine.)

patients complain of recurrent abdominal pain and constipation, exploratory laparotomy may be performed without the diagnosis being established.

The majority of patients are dark complexioned. The melanin spots are readily distinguished on physical examination if the face and buccal mucosa are carefully inspected (Fig. 2–19).

Lesions of the Oropharynx

The tonsils. The mere presence of a slightly enlarged tonsil is not abnormal. The tonsillar crypts may contain detritus, but this in itself is of no significance.

Acute tonsillitis. The onset is sudden with fever and a "sore throat"; the tonsils are swollen and reddened. The surface is frequently covered with white spots which represent exudate issuing from the tonsillar crypts. There may be infection and hyperemia of the adjacent mucosa of the oropharynx.

Chronic tonsillitis. This term is loosely applied to indicate chronic disease of the tonsil which may take several different forms. Hypertrophy of the tonsils may occur, which together with hypertrophy of the pharyngeal tonsil (adenoids) leads to partial nasal obstruction and reduced hearing. An unfortunate sequela of such nasal obstruction is the "adenoid facies." The alae nasae are widened, and the patient tends to hold the mouth open, thus creating an impression of stupidity. Recurrent attacks of acute tonsillitis result in scarring and distortion of the tonsils, often with the accumulation of detritus and exudate in the crypt. Pressure against the base of the anterior pillar with a tongue depressor everts the tonsil and expresses such debris. If there is a significant degree of chronic tonsillar infection, the regional cervical nodes will be enlarged and palpable.

Peritonsillar abscess. In acute peritonsillar abscess the patient has difficulty in opening his mouth. The tonsillar area is markedly swollen and edematous. The involved tonsil appears to be pushed toward the opposite side.

Tuberculosis of the tonsil. The tonsils are frequently the primary site of cervical tuberculosis. There may be little change in the appearance of the tonsil or it may be deformed or hypertrophied. *Lymphoma* may invade the tonsil, producing a smooth-surfaced enlargement.

Retropharyngeal abscess. The patient is an infant or child in most instances. The lesion appears as a protrusion of the posterior pharyngeal wall. Palpation of any suspected inflammatory process involving this area should always be performed with the patient prone or in the Trendelenburg position (Fig. 2–20). Suction should be available because the lesion may perforate with immediate aspiration of the contents. Retropharyngeal neoplasms may produce swelling in this area.

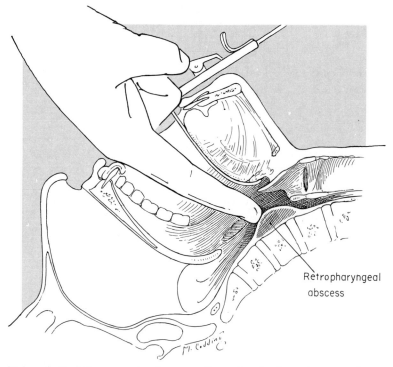

Figure 2–20. Diagrammatic demonstration of palpation of a retropharyngeal abscess. Because of the danger of rupture of the abscess and aspiration of its contents, the patient should be in Trendelenburg position and suction should be available.

The Salivary Glands

Parotid Gland

The position of the parotid gland is shown in Figure 2–21. Normally it cannot be seen or defined by palpation. The opening of the parotid duct (Stensen's duct) may be identified as a minute dimple opposite the second upper molar tooth (Fig. 2–9). It is readily seen if inflamed or pouting.

Parotitis. On inspection, the enlarged gland stands out as a diffuse swelling anterior to the ear and extending downward and backward over the angle of the jaw. The orifice of Stensen's duct will appear swollen and reddened if the buccal mucosa is retracted with a throat stick. In calculous parotitis, tiny flecks of calcareous deposits may lie at the opening of the duct.

The inflamed gland can readily be defined by palpation. The distal portion of Stensen's duct can also be felt by introducing the gloved finger into the mouth and palpating the cheek between the finger and thumb just above the orifice of the duct (Fig. 2–12 *B*). The differential diagnosis

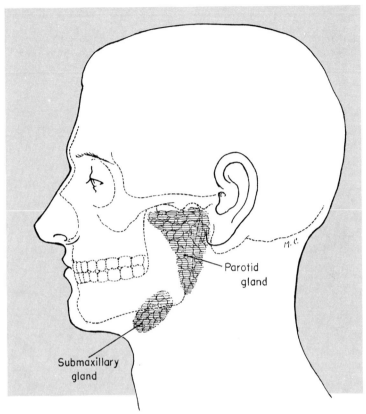

Figure 2–21. Diagrammatic sketch of the positions of the parotid and submaxillary salivary glands.

between preauricular adenitis, cervical adenitis, and parotitis may be difficult. Careful identification of the borders of the parotid gland is particularly helpful. Inflammation of the orifice of Stensen's duct or a purulent exudate discharging from it is excellent diagnostic evidence of inflammation of the parotid.

Pleomorphic ("mixed") tumors of the parotid. The gland is usually diffusely enlarged, firm, nontender, and slightly movable. A pleomorphic tumor of the parotid gland is usually slowly growing but may reach considerable size (Fig. 2–22). Although distant metastases or involvement of the facial nerve are rare, the lesion should be regarded as malignant. Recurrences after inadequate excision are common and become progressively invasive causing great suffering. The tumor should not be "shelled out" surgically, but removed en bloc by total excision of the superficial lobe of the gland.

The lesion may be mistaken for a dermoid cyst if the superficial portion of the gland is involved at an early stage. This is particularly true if

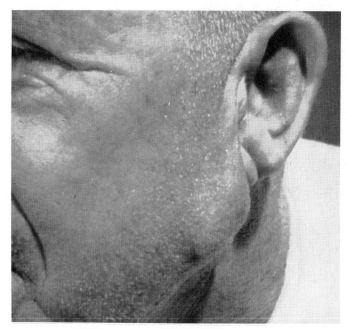

Figure 2–22. "Mixed" tumor of parotid.

the cervical extensions of the gland constitute the only enlargement. A "dermoid cyst" at the angle of the jaw should always be regarded as a potential tumor of the parotid gland until proved otherwise.

Warthin's tumor (papillary cystadenolymphomatosum). Warthin's tumor is a benign lesion of the parotid. It is slowly growing, rarely becomes larger than 1 to 2 cm., and usually is freely movable. Cystic areas may become adherent to the skin. It can be cured by wide local excision and does not require superficial parotidectomy.

Cancer of the parotid. Cancer may be indistinguishable from a pleomorphic tumor, but fixation and stony hardness indicate carcinoma. Paralysis of the seventh nerve is an excellent diagnostic sign since it occurs in cancer and is rare in pleomorphic tumors. As the neoplasm may infiltrate and destroy only portions of the nerve, careful inspection may be required to detect impairment of nerve function (Fig. 2–23).

Submaxillary Gland

This gland lies under and below the anterior ramus of the jaw (Fig. 2–21). It may be felt as a smooth, movable, nontender, flattened ovoid mass. It becomes firmer and easier to palpate in older patients and may be mistaken for a tumor. Wharton's duct opens at the base of the tongue on either side of the frenulum (Fig. 2–10). If the floor of the mouth is dried with a swab and the tongue is stimulated with a bit of lemon juice, saliva

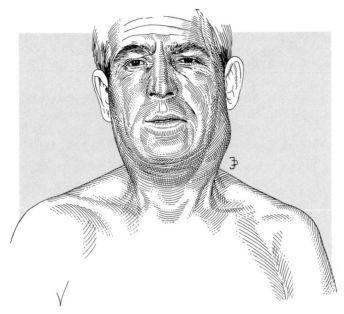

Figure 2–23. Carcinoma of the parotid salivary gland. Note the slight asymmetry of the mouth, indicative of involvement of the facial nerve.

can be seen exuding from the duct. Failure to elicit a discharge of saliva by this means is indicative of obstruction.

The enlarged submaxillary gland is easily outlined by palpation. The examiner may stand behind the patient and pass his fingers beneath the ramus of the jaw, but bimanual palpation with the finger of one hand on the floor of the mouth and the fingers of the other hand under the ramus of the jaw is more efficient and more informative (Fig. 2–12 *A*). Submaxillary glands are frequently the site of calcareous inflammation. They may be involved with tuberculosis; occasionally tuberculous adenitis embraces the submaxillary gland and makes the original site of the inflammation difficult to determine. Tumors of the submaxillary gland are less common than tumors of the parotid. They are much more likely to be carcinomatous.

IV. THE NECK

Examinations of the head and neck should always be integrated because of the frequency with which lesions of the head, face, or oral cavity involve the cervical lymph nodes.

Particular skill is required to examine the neck because the muscles, fascial layers, and the bony and cartilaginous structures mask physical signs and are themselves easily mistaken for pathologic processes.

Inspection

First inspect the neck for asymmetry, swelling, pulsations, sinuses, and limitation of motion. The boundary of the anterior and posterior triangles of the neck may be recognized if the neck is extended, thus placing the sternocleidomastoid muscle under tension.

It is important to identify the following anatomic structures: the sternocleidomastoid muscle, the hyoid bone with its greater cornua, the thyroid cartilage, the trachea, the clavicle, and the pulsations of the carotid bulb and third portion of the subclavian artery (Fig. 2–24).

Palpation

Palpation should be done with the palmar surface of the tips of the fingers; use a delicate rotary motion to detect the smooth, firm surface of an enlarged node. Deep, firm palpation will press nodes into the muscles so that they cannot be felt. Palpate the anterior triangle with one hand behind the occiput to flex the neck in order to produce the proper degree of relaxation (Fig. 2–25). The submental region is palpated with the head flexed in a more neutral position (Fig. 2–26). The patient's head is returned to a neutral position and the trachea is identified. The head is then inclined and rotated toward one side to permit palpation of the posterior triangle (Fig. 2–27). Now palpate the supraclavicular region. The third portion of the subclavian artery can be felt in the angle formed by the

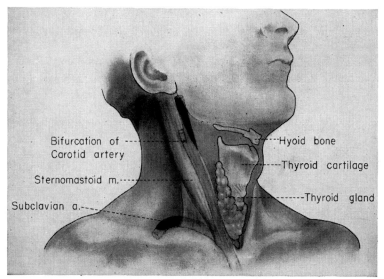

Bifurcation of Carotid artery
Sternomastoid m.
Subclavian a.
Hyoid bone
Thyroid cartilage
Thyroid gland

Figure 2–24. Composite diagram of the structures which must be identified in palpation of the neck.

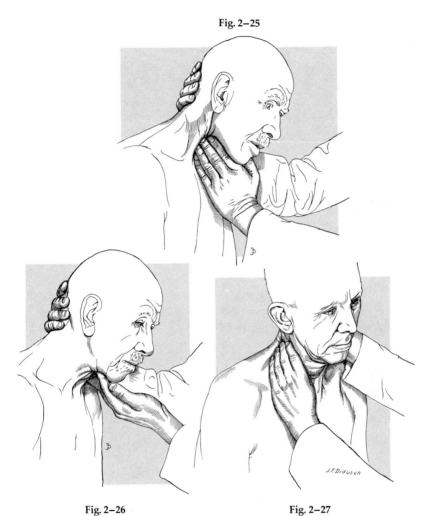

Fig. 2-25

Fig. 2-26   Fig. 2-27

Figure 2-25. Palpation of the anterior triangle of the neck. One hand flexes the patient's head to obtain proper relaxation.

Figure 2-26. Palpation of the submental region.

Figure 2-27. Palpation of the posterior triangle of the neck. A light rotary motion of the fingers is essential to the detection of slightly enlarged lymph nodes.

posterior edge of the sternocleidomastoid and the clavicle. The back of the neck is palpated with the patient's head slightly extended. The examiner now stands behind the patient and again palpates the front and sides of the neck. The supraclavicular region and the pulsations of the subclavian artery can be palpated effectively from this position.

Auscultation

Careful auscultation over the subclavian, common carotid, external, and internal carotid arteries should be performed. A bruit heard over both the subclavian and the common carotid is usually transmitted from a stenotic aortic valve. An isolated bruit over a single artery indicates localized stenosis (See Chap. 10).

The Cervical Lymph Nodes

If the examiner finds an apparently enlarged cervical node or group of nodes, he must seek an answer to the following questions:

1. IS IT AN ENLARGED LYMPH NODE OR IS IT A NORMAL STRUCTURE?

The greater cornua of the hyoid bone and arteriosclerotic plaques at the bifurcation of the common carotid artery are common sources of error; these can readily be excluded with experience and care. The greater cornu of the hyoid may be recognized since it moves when the patient swallows. It can be identified by careful palpation as a bilateral symmetrically placed structure connected with the hyoid bone. Arteriosclerotic plaques at the bifurcation of the carotid are also best identified by their precise location directly in contact with the common carotid artery opposite the upper edge of the thyroid cartilage. These may also be bilateral.

2. WHAT ARE THE PHYSICAL CHARACTERISTICS OF THE NODE OR NODES IN QUESTION?

The size, consistency, and discreteness of enlarged lymph nodes are of considerable diagnostic importance. In *metastatic cancer* the involved nodes are usually discrete, nontender, unilateral, and of a firm or hard consistency. They may vary from the size of a peak to several centimeters in diameter. *Hodgkin's disease* produces large, discrete, nontender nodes of a firm, rubbery consistency (Fig. 2–28). *Tuberculosis,* on the other hand, results in a softening, matting-together, and conglomeration of the nodes, often with fluctuation and occasionally with sinus formation. The

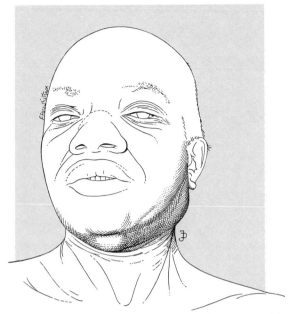

Figure 2–28. Hodgkin's disease of the lymph nodes of the neck.

inflammatory process is usually nontender. *Acute pyogenic infections* produce enlarged, tender, and discrete nodes. These may become confluent if the condition becomes chronic; rarely abscesses develop. In contrast to tuberculosis, these changes are accompanied by classic signs of inflammation, namely, swelling, redness, heat, and tenderness. *Fluctuation* indicates that the central area of the infection has become fluid and that an abscess has formed. Fluctuation is elicited by compressing the swelling with the finger of one hand and palpating the swelling with one or two fingers of the other hand. If an impulse is transmitted from the compressing finger to the palpating finger, fluid is present.

Low grade chronic inflammation of the scalp may lead to lymphatic involvement which closely simulates Hodgkin's disease or lymphoma. *Pediculosis* is especially prone to do this. The hair should be carefully examined for nits in such cases.

3. WHERE IS THE PRIMARY LESION?

A complete survey of the head, neck, and oral cavity is necessary regardless of the location and physical characteristics of the node. The *character and location of the adenopathy* are guides to the probable primary source. The principal lymphatic chains and their sites of drainage are shown in the accompanying diagram and table (Fig. 2–29).

Adenopathy in the posterior auricular or posterior cervical triangle incriminates the scalp. Submental nodes suggest a lesion in the lip or an-

Figure 2–29. Diagram of the principal lymph nodes of the neck.

1. *Submental lymph nodes* drain the central lower lip, floor of mouth and apex of tongue. Their *efferents* drain into the submaxillary and deep cervical nodes.

2. *Submaxillary lymph nodes* drain the medial palpebral commissure, cheek, side of nose, upper lip, lateral lower lip, gums and anterior part of margin of tongue. Their *efferents* drain into the superior deep cervical nodes.

3. *Preauricular lymph nodes* drain the lateral surface of the ear and adjacent temporal region. Their *efferents* pass into the superior deep cervical nodes.

4. *Posterior auricular lymph nodes* drain the posterior part of the temporoparietal region, the upper part of the cranial surface of the ear and the back of the external acoustic meatus. Their *efferents* pass to the superior deep cervical nodes.

5. *Occipital lymph nodes* drain the occipital region of the scalp. Their *efferents* pass to the superior deep cervical nodes.

6. *Superficial cervical lymph nodes* are indicated by the heavily shaded area along the sternomastoid muscle. They drain the lower parts of the ear and parotid region. Their *efferents* pass into the superior deep cervical nodes.

7. *Deep cervical lymph nodes* form a chain along the carotid sheath from the base of the skull to the root of the neck. These nodes are indicated by lightly shaded areas. They are divided into superior and inferior groups. The *superior deep cervical nodes* are those above the posterior edge of the sternomastoid muscle. They drain most of the tongue, larynx, thyroid gland, trachea, nasopharynx, nasal cavities, palate, esophagus and other lymph nodes listed above. The *inferior deep cervical nodes* are those below the posterior margin of the sternomastoid muscle. They drain the back of the scalp and neck, superficial pectoral region and the superior deep cervical nodes.

8. *Supraclavicular lymph nodes* are part of the deep cervical chain. They drain the back of the neck, superficial pectoral region, and may receive efferents from the axillary nodes. They may receive metastases from the abdominal or thoracic viscera.

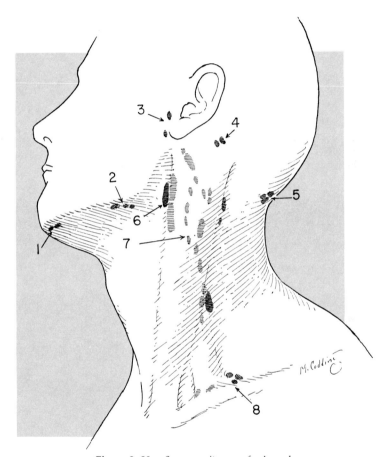

Figure 2–29. *See opposite page for legend.*

terior two-thirds of the tongue. The superficial cervical nodes are usually involved by lesions spreading from the alveolar ridge, tonsils, face, or lateral aspect of the tongue. Upper deep cervical involvement suggests the base of the tongue, the nasopharynx or tonsillar area, the pharynx, or larynx. Midjugular involvement suggests the hypopharynx and larynx. There is considerable overlap, however. Lesions close to the midline may involve the contralateral nodes. Lesions which are well lateralized may rarely produce infection or metastasis in nodes in the opposite side of the neck. Similarly, lesions which ordinarily would be picked up by the superficial nodes may first appear in the deep nodes. Consequently, one must scrutinize the entire "watershed" whenever an obvious lesion is not found in the probable drainage site. Remember that the thyroid gland is an important source of neoplastic metastases to either the superficial or deep cervical nodes.

The supraclavicular nodes are frequently involved by metastases from the thoracic or abdominal viscera. Any neoplastic process which spreads to the retroperitoneal or retropleural lymphatics may produce these so-called "sentinel nodes" (Fig. 2–30). Cancer of the lung, the stomach, the esophagus, the testicle, or the cervix is especially prone to do so. Rarely cancer spreading from the thoracic or abdominal viscera reaches the deep or superficial cervical nodes without producing demonstrable involvement of the supraclavicular chain.

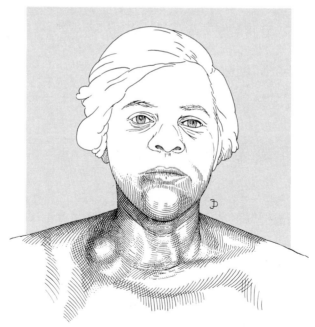

Figure 2–30. Metastatic cancer in a supraclavicular lymph node (sentinel node). The patient had carcinoma of the cervix uteri.

The *physical characteristics of the nodes* are also helpful in identifying a primary site. Inflammatory lesions commonly come from the teeth and tonsils. Always suspect the tonsils in tuberculosis. If the nodes have a particularly discrete, rubbery consistency suggestive of lymphoma, confirmatory evidence may be found in an enlarged liver or spleen or in lymphadenopathy elsewhere in the body. When cancer is suspected, either because of the physical characteristics of the nodes or because no other explanation can be found, one must examine and re-examine all the potential sites.

4. WHAT IF NO PRIMARY SITE IS EVIDENT?

Search the nasopharynx and nasal sinuses by mirror examination, endoscopy, and x-rays. A small asymptomatic neoplasm in these areas may produce extensive cervical metastases. If this search is fruitless, biopsy of the node is necessary. Occasionally the histologic character of the metastasis suggests the primary site. The thyroid gland may be inculpated even though it appears normal to palpation. Frequent re-examination of all the potential primary sites is indicated if the biopsy discloses metastatic cancer but fails to indicate its source. There are many examples on record in which a primary site for obvious cervical metastases was found only after repeated examinations over a period of many weeks.

Primary branchiogenic carcinoma (carcinoma developing in a branchiogenic cyst), if it occurs at all, is so rare that it should be dismissed except as a diagnosis to be established by autopsy. Repeated examinations with particular attention to the base of the tongue, the nasopharynx, and the tonsils will disclose the primary site.

The Thyroid Gland

The normal thyroid gland is frequently palpable in slender individuals on either side of the trachea as a firm, smooth mass which moves upward when the patient swallows. In obese or thick-necked individuals it cannot be felt.

When an enlargement of the thyroid is noticed, its size, extent, consistency, and vascularity must be determined. The examiner should stand behind the patient and endeavor to identify the trachea for possible displacement. He then outlines the thyroid with fingers, and as the patient swallows, the gland is allowed to slip between the fingers for comparison of the two sides (Fig. 2–31 *A*). Nodular areas are easily detected. For more complete evaluation of each lobe, the sternocleidomastoid is retracted with one hand and palpation performed with the other (Fig. 2–31 *B*). One feels specifically for irregularities and for a thrill. The lower pole is probably retrosternal if it cannot be felt. Percussion of the area of retrosternal dullness may confirm this impression.

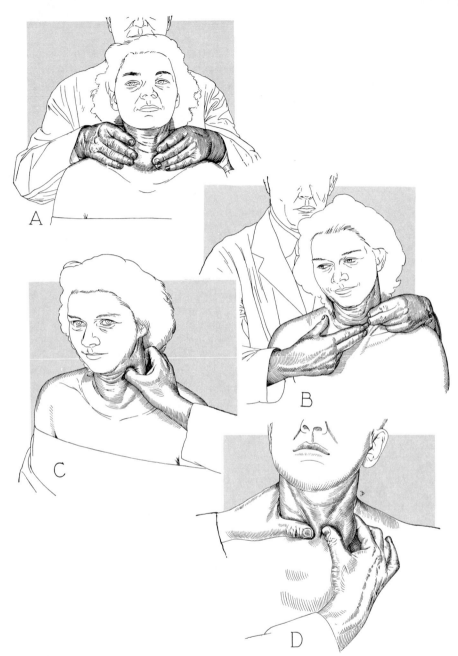

Figure 2–31. Palpation of the thyroid gland. *A,* Palpation of the thyroid gland from behind the patient. The patient is asked to swallow and the gland is allowed to slip between the fingers for comparison of the two lobes. *B,* Palpation of the thyroid gland with retraction of the sternomastoid muscle. *C,* Palpation of the superior pole vessels of the thyroid gland. *D,* Palpation of the left lobe of the thyroid gland which is brought into relief by dislocation of the trachea toward the side being palpated by the examiner's left thumb. The thumb should be placed over the lower edge of the thyroid cartilage. The dislocated lobe is felt between the right thumb in front and the right index finger behind the sternomastoid muscle.

42

The examiner now stands in front of the patient. The vessels of the upper pole can be palpated and the degree of vascularity estimated by placing the thumb under the anterior edge and the finger behind the posterior edge of the sternocleidomastoid muscle (Fig. 2–31 *C*). The lobe can be brought into sharp relief and its entire surface and consistency appraised if the trachea is displaced toward it with the thumb of the opposite hand (Fig. 2–31 *D*).

Lesions of the Thyroid Gland

Goiter. If the examination is performed precisely in the manner described, it is comparatively easy to recognize the diffuse cystic swelling of a *colloid goiter*, the firm discrete nodule of a *solitary adenoma*, the irregular nodular gland of an *adenomatous goiter*, and the soft vascular enlargement of classic *Graves' disease*.

Hyperthyroidism. The signs of hyperthyroidism may be obvious enough to be recognized at a glance (Fig. 2–1), or so masked that they escape the attention of all but the most experienced clinicians.

The evidence of hyperthyroidism within the gland itself rests on the detection of an increased vascularity. A *palpable thrill* and an *audible bruit* are classic, but are present only in the more advanced cases. Palpation of the superior pole vessels (Fig. 2–31 *C*) may give a clue to increased blood flow and is a useful maneuver in following the involution of the gland during preparation for surgery.

Care must be taken both on palpation and auscultation not to mistake the transmitted signs from the carotid vessels, especially in the case of the hypertensive patient.

Signs of hyperthyroidism are not confined to the local examination. Whether the gland is nodular, diffusely enlarged or appears normal, one must be alert for the eye signs, the tremor, the warm, moist hands, the fine-textured skin with its dermographia, and the full pulse associated with a widened pulse pressure.

Exophthalmos may or may not be present. It is usually bilateral, but may be unilateral. The various special signs associated with exophthalmos relate to the abnormal position of the eyeball; these *per se* are not indicative of hyperthyroidism.

Eye Signs Associated with Exophthalmos

Lid lag (Von Graefe's sign). The upper lid lags behind the lower lid as the patient looks down; this exposes the eyeball.

Failure of convergence (Moebius' sign). In attempting to look at an object close to the midline, one or both eyes fail to converge toward it.

Retraction of the upper lid (Stellwag's sign). The upper lid is retracted, and often there are spasmodic contractions of the lid as the patient looks upward. The patient winks less than normally.

Failure to wrinkle the forehead (Joffroy's sign). There is no wrinkling of the forehead when the patient attempts to look over his head.

LATENT HYPERTHYROIDISM. Mild hyperthyroidism may simulate heart disease, neurasthenia, anemia, or tuberculosis. In fact, in all cases of heart disease or tuberculosis, hyperthyroidism must be specifically excluded as a potential concomitant disorder.

The history is often of more diagnostic value than the physical examination, but whenever a patient with fair skin and warm moist hands has a presenting complaint of fatigue, lassitude, or loss of weight, the examiner should suspect hyperthyroidism. In many instances response to therapy is required to establish the diagnosis, since the basal metabolism, radioiodine uptake, and other diagnostic measures may all be within the normal range.

Thyroiditis. Four distinct types may be recognized on physical examination:

ACUTE THYROIDITIS (BACTERIAL). Rarely, the thyroid gland is involved by a specific bacterial infection. This may be secondary to an inflammation of the mouth, tonsils, or cervical lymph nodes. Fever, tenderness over the gland, and rarely suppuration, are the manifestations. Tuberculosis or a fungal infection may involve the thyroid. Specific antibacterial therapy is usually curative, but surgical drainage may be necessary.

SUBACUTE NONSPECIFIC THYROIDITIS. This condition occurs much more frequently in women than in men. The onset is usually abrupt, with symptoms of pain in the throat, neck, and thyroid gland. The temperature may rise to 104 or 105° F. The gland is enlarged, firm, and exquisitely tender, especially in the early stages. The process is usually diffuse, but may involve one side more than the other. The tenderness and the sudden onset, often following an upper respiratory infection, are the significant diagnostic points. Spontaneous resolution is the rule, but in protracted cases cortisone may provide relief of symptoms.

RIEDEL'S STRUMA. The onset is insidious, the first symptoms being those of gradual tracheal compression. The gland is replaced by firm, dense, fibrous tissue which generally results in an irregular enlargement. The consistency of the gland is so hard that the process is usually indistinguishable from cancer. Operation may be required to relieve tracheal compression or exclude cancer.

HASHIMOTO'S STRUMA. The first symptom is usually the presence of a lump in the neck. The gland is diffusely, but not uniformly, enlarged and is of a firm, rubbery consistency. It may suggest an ordinary adenomatous goiter, but tends to be less nodular. Symptoms of mild hypothyroidism are common. The condition may occur at any age but is more common in females of middle age. Circulating antibodies against thyroglobulin or antigens of thyroid cells have been demonstrated in some patients. Sometimes it may be difficult to distinguish Hashimoto's struma from cancer. The condition often responds to administration of thyroid hormone but may require operation to relieve pressure symptoms or exclude cancer. Radical surgery is to be avoided.

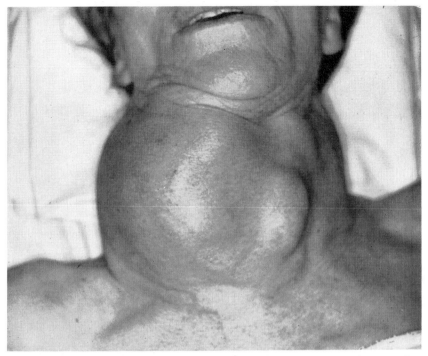

Figure 2–32. Adenomatous goiter. Such massive enlargement is rarely seen today. (Boston City Hospital case.)

Carcinoma of the thyroid. A *solitary nodule* in the thyroid well may be the only manifestation of early malignancy. Since the differential diagnosis between a benign cyst or benign adenoma and malignancy is impossible, such lesions must be regarded as cancer until proved otherwise by operation.

Occasionally a solitary nodule in the thyroid gland is associated with obvious metastatic involvement of the cervical nodes; this makes a diagnosis of malignancy fairly obvious.

Papillary and follicular cancer present as a firm to hard solitary nodule. This type of nodule may be indistinguishable from a benign cyst or adenoma. A history of previous x-ray exposure in a young female provides suggestive contributory evidence of cancer.

Papillary carcinoma is slow growing. It may involve regional nodes, but distant metastases are rare.

Follicular carcinoma may resemble papillary carcinoma on physical examination but tends to metastasize by way of the blood stream.

Medullary carcinoma is characterized histologically by sheets of pleomorphic tumor cells in a stroma that stains like amyloid. Although histologically medullary carcinoma resembles undifferentiated cancer, biologically it behaves more like papillary cancer. Lymph node metastases are frequent and often extensive. However, long-term survival following radical thyroidectomy and neck dissection is common. There may be an associated pheochromocytoma and hyperparathyroidism (Sipple's syndrome).

LATERAL ABERRANT THYROID TUMORS. Small, relatively slow-growing carcinomas of the thyroid, especially of the papillary type, may produce metastases to the cervical glands before there is any detectable abnormality in the thyroid. The deep cervical glands above the level of the thyroid cartilage are usually involved. The involved glands resemble normal thyroid histologically and from this the term "lateral aberrant thyroid tumors" is derived.

Undifferentiated cancer is characterized by a stony hard, irregularly nodular gland which is fixed to the underlying tissues. Esophageal or tracheal compression with difficulty in swallowing or breathing may occur. Hoarseness indicative of paralysis of the recurrent laryngeal nerve is particularly suggestive of cancer.

Congenital Lesions of the Neck—Carotid Body Tumors

Congenital Lesions

A knowledge of the embryologic derivation of cysts and sinuses of the neck is of considerable help in their identification. The lines of closure of the first and second branchial clefts are shown in Figure 2–33.

The sites at which remnants of the thyroglossal duct and the first and second branchial clefts are usually found are outlined in Figure 2–34.

Thyroglossal duct cysts. These congenital cysts occur anywhere between the base of the tongue and the isthmus of the thyroid. They are characteristically located in the midline, but approximately one out of five is sufficiently lateral in location to cause confusion with a branchial cleft cyst. The diagnosis is established by the fact that the cyst moves upward when the patient protrudes his tongue. Occasionally infection may occur with the establishment of a draining sinus in or near the midline.

Branchiogenic cysts and sinuses. Branchiogenic cysts are always located anterior to the sternocleidomastoid muscle at about the level of the carotid bifurcation. Their position is approximated by the junction of the upper and middle third of the anterior edge of the sternocleidomastoid muscle. Secondary infection is common and the usual signs of inflammation may appear with a sudden increase in the size of the swelling. Occasionally a small sinus is the only evidence of this congenital abnormality (Fig. 2–35). In such instances, slight traction on the sinus may make it stand out sufficiently to be felt directly under the skin extending upward under the edge of the anterior belly of the digastric muscle.

Cystic hygroma. This congenital anomaly of the lymphatics is

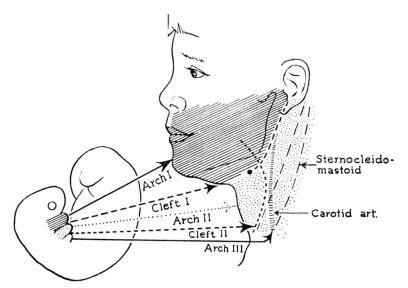

Figure 2–33. Embryological derivation of lower face, ear and upper neck from the first and second branchial arches. The theoretical lines of closure of the first and second branchial clefts are shown in dotted lines. (Reprinted from Annals of Surgery, by permission.)

most commonly located in the neck. It appears as a large cystic swelling which is translucent. It usually extends over a large area and may involve the entire neck and supraclavicular area. It may be bilateral (Fig. 2–36).

Torticollis. This abnormal rigidity of the sternocleidomastoid muscle may be congenital or acquired. It produces a characteristic twist to the neck (Fig. 2–37). It is often associated with facial asymmetry of long standing; the features on the affected side are smaller. In infants a small mass is sometimes palpable within the substance of the muscle.

Figure 2–34. Areas in which we expect to find remnants of the thyroglossal duct, the second branchial cleft, and the first branchial cleft. (From Bill, A. H., Jr.: Surg. Clin. North Am. December 1956.)

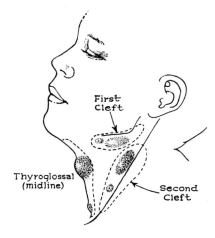

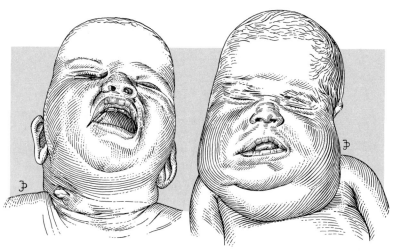

Fig. 2–35   **Fig. 2–36**

Figure 2–35.   Branchial cleft sinus in an infant. Note the nipple of skin at the sinus opening.

Figure 2–36.   Cystic hygroma involving the entire neck in an infant.

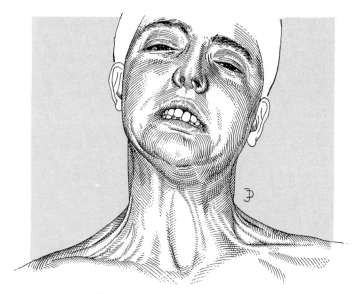

Figure 2–37.   Torticollis (wryneck).

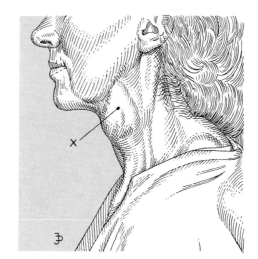

Figure 2–38. Carotid body tumor. Note that the lesion extends upward beyond the level of the carotid bifurcation, an important distinguishing point from branchial cleft cyst.

Carotid Body Tumors

Tumors of the carotid body are frequently mistaken for congenital cysts of the neck. They arise at the bifurcation of the common carotid artery; this point lies just beneath the anterior edge of the sternocleidomastoid muscle opposite the upper border of the thyroid cartilage. In contradistinction to branchial cleft cysts, they lie more deeply in the neck and more anteriorly; they enlarge upward so that the largest portion of the tumor is above the carotid bifurcation (Fig. 2–38). They may bulge into the pharynx. As the tumor is fixed to the carotid bifurcation, it can often be rotated medially and laterally but not up and down.

The Appraisal of Obscure Cervical Pain

Pain in the neck radiating into the shoulder or down the arm is a fairly common complaint. It is often ascribed to "cervical neuritis" or "neuralgia." It may be due to arthritis of the cervical spine. In such cases one should exclude the thoracic outlet syndrome and cervical disk.

Thoracic Outlet Syndrome (Scalenus Anticus, Cervical Rib, or Costoclavicular Syndrome)

The thoracic outlet syndrome is the preferred term for this symptom complex of both neural and vascular components. A supernumerary rib attached to the seventh cervical vertebra may be unilateral or bilateral. Usually it is an incidental physical finding detected on careful palpation of the neck or it may be seen on an x-ray film taken for some other reason. Ordinarily it is of no clinical significance. Occasionally, however, cervical ribs produce symptoms from pressure against the brachial plexus. The usual complaints include pain in the neck or shoulder radiating down the arm, numbness and tingling in the arm or hand, and coldness and numbness of the hand or forearm. In some instances the symptoms are predominantly neurologic, suggesting a peripheral neuritis; in others they are largely circulatory, simulating Raynaud's disease. Thromboses may occur in the compressed or poststenotic dilated portion of the subclavian artery with peripheral embolization.

Similar symptoms may occur if the brachial plexus is post-fixed, which means it comes off the spinal cord so low that it may impinge against the first rib. One should suspect the syndrome in patients who have obscure pain in the neck, shoulder, or arm with bizarre vascular or neurologic changes in the hand or forearm.

The patient is often a female who has undertaken unaccustomed manual labor, but the syndrome occurs in males. It is fairly common among military personnel. Any activity which produces a downward pull or drag on the arm or shoulder may bring on the syndrome.

The physical findings are fairly characteristic. Circulatory changes in the arm, such as ischemia or cyanosis, may be present. Neurologic signs are usually in the distribution of the ulnar nerve with atrophy of the hand. There may be absent, or weakened, brachial or radial pulses. A bruit may be heard over the artery in the supraclavicular or axillary distribution. The cervical rib is rarely palpable in patients in whom there are symptoms. Usually there is some tenderness over the inner portion of the supraclavicular fossa associated with spasm in the scalene muscle.

Special tests. Any motion which tenses the scalenus anticus muscle will aggravate the pain. It can usually be produced by passive depression of the shoulder and forced turning of the head to the affected side. Conversely, relaxing the muscle by passive elevation of the shoulder usually alleviates the pain. A bruit may be heard if the subclavian artery is compressed. The vascular compression test of Adson is significant. It is performed as follows: Seated upright with arms on knees, the patient takes a deep breath and holds it and turns his elevated chin to the affected side. An alteration or obliteration of the radial pulse or a change in blood pressure indicates that the subclavian artery is being compressed.

Dislocation of Cervical Nucleus Pulposus

A herniated disk in the lower cervical regions produces two distinct syndromes.

First, if the herniated disk is in the *midline,* the signs of *spinal cord compression* are produced. The physical findings include weakness of the lower extremities, spasticity, hyperactive reflexes, subsequent sensory changes, and involvement of the sphincters. Involvement of the upper extremities is usually secondary in this type of herniated cervical disk.

Second, lateral herniation of the disk produces the signs of *nerve root compression;* late in the course of the disease there may be long-tract signs. The lateral herniation may be of two types. In one the history is of short duration and is usually associated with a frank herniation of the nucleus pulposus. In the other type there is a more chronic history, and the condition is associated with narrowing of the intervertebral foramen and involved space by hypertrophic spurs. The cervical herniated disk usually occurs between the fifth and sixth vertebrae with involvement of the sixth cervical nerve root, or between the sixth and seventh vertebrae with involvement of the seventh cervical root.

The patient tends to carry his head in slight forward flexion, since extension of the neck increases the pain. The physical signs can be explained on a mechanical basis. Anything which increases the compression of the nerve root increases the pain. Coughing, sneezing, or straining at stool all increase the compression; carrying heavy objects with the involved arm increases the pain because of traction on the nerve root. Lateral bending of the head toward the side of the lesion increases the pain, and lateral bending away from the side of the lesion decreases it.

Disk Involved	$C_5 - C_6$	$C_6 - C_7$
Pain	Top of shoulder Lateral aspect of arm Dorsal aspect of forearm and wrist	Posterior aspect of arm Lateral aspect of forearm Sometimes medial to and beneath scapula Sometimes anterior chest wall
Paresthesias	Dorsal aspect of forearm and hand into base of thumb and index fingers	Lateral aspect of forearm and dorsal aspect of hand into index and middle fingers
Local Tenderness	Over spine and lamina of C_5 and C_6	Over spine and lamina of C_6 and C_7
Motor Weakness	Biceps Sometimes deltoid and spinati	Triceps Sometimes extensors of hand and fingers
Atrophy	Maximal of biceps	Maximal of triceps
Reflexes	Diminished to absent biceps reflex	Diminished to absent triceps reflex
Sensation	Hypalgesia over C_6 dermatome	Hypalgesia over C_7 dermatome

Figure 2-39.   Localization of lateral herniated cervical intervertebral disks.

Pressure on the top of the slightly extended head produces exquisite pain. Bilateral jugular compression increases the pain, and there may be tenderness to percussion over the lesion lateral to the lower cervical spines.

It is usually possible to localize the site of a lateral herniated disk on the basis of the symptoms and physical findings (Fig. 2–39).

Infections of the Head and Neck

Acute alveolar abscess.   Infection arising in the root of a tooth may spread to the cheek or floor of the mouth. Massive swelling with redness, edema, and tenderness of the upper or lower jaw occur (Fig. 2–40). The patient can barely open his mouth. The infection may break through the floor of the mouth, producing a deep cervical infection. Failure to recognize the true nature of the disorder has led to ill-advised incision of the face or neck. The abscess should be drained through an incision along the gum margin. The diseased tooth should be removed.

Vincent's angina (trench mouth).   Vincent's angina is an exudative and ulcerative stomatitis associated with the presence of a spirochete and a spindle-shaped bacillus. It occurs in early adult life, being very rare after the age of 40. The lesions are characterized by irregularly distributed ulcerations, particularly over the hard and soft palate, tonsils, and oropharynx. The ulcerations have a grayish white center and are surrounded by an area of hyperemia and redness. The intervening mucosa

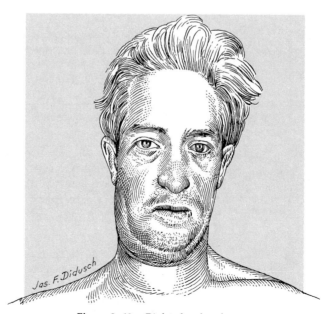

Figure 2–40.   Right alveolar abscess.

appears quite normal. In advanced cases the buccal mucosa may be involved. There is usually a fetid odor to the breath. The cervical lymph nodes may be enlarged, but rarely suppurate.

Infections of the upper lip. The loose tissue of the upper lip is a dangerous site for infection. Squeezing or trauma to a furuncle in this area may lead to a fulminating cellulitis. Cavernous sinus thrombosis may complicate a carbuncle of the upper lip from infection spreading through the angular veins. Edema of the upper face and eyelids, ptosis of the eye, high fever, and coma characterize this highly fatal complication. Fortunately, since the introduction of antibiotics, this entity is rarely seen.

Carbuncle. The back of the neck is a common site for carbuncles. A downward and lateral spread of the lesion is favored by the thick skin, the numerous hair follicles, and the presence of fat columns extending downward to the fascia. The lesion appears as a many-headed boil with a central area of necrosis surrounded by a rim of purple cyanotic edematous skin which, in turn, is surrounded by a lateral rim of redness and cellulitis.

Deep cervical abscess and cellulitis. Infections from the oral cavity, including those from infected teeth, may enter the neck deep to the cervical fascia. The lesion is usually confined to one side of the neck and is characterized by a superficial brawny edema and redness. Because of the depth of the lesion, fluctuation cannot be elicited. As the infection spreads within the visceral compartment, edema of both pharynx and larynx may occur, with difficulty in breathing and swallowing. Frequently the original site of this lesion cannot be found. However, there is no difficulty in recognizing the nature of the process by its deep character, its diffuse extent, the brawny induration and redness, and the lack of fluctuation.

Ludwig's angina. Ludwig's angina is a particular form of deep infection which involves the floor of the mouth, the submaxillary regions, and the deep tissues of the neck down to about the level of the hyoid bone. In contrast to the usual deep cervical abscess, this lesion often becomes bilateral, spreads rapidly, and produces extensive induration and swelling of the floor of the mouth. The tongue may be pushed upward and backward, thus forcing the patient to hold the mouth open and interfering with swallowing and breathing. Edema of the glottis with respiratory obstruction frequently ensues. The condition may prove to be fatal before redness or fluctuation of the neck appear. Here again the liberal use of the antibiotics have made this an extraordinarily rare condition.

chapter 3

EXAMINATION OF THE BREAST

The examination of the breast is a critically important part of the physical examination because of the opportunity it provides to detect early asymptomatic cancer. Cancer of the breast is the commonest cancer in women in the Western world; therefore, periodic examinations at one

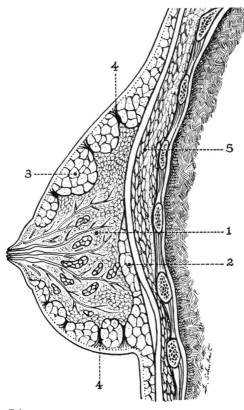

Figure 3–1. Sagittal section of the normal breast showing its relation to the chest wall and rib cage. 1. The mammary gland tissue. 2. Retromammary fat separating the breast from the pectoral fascia. 3. The investing envelope of subcutaneous fat separating the breast from the overlying skin. 4. The fibrous septa (Cooper's Ligaments) which fix the breast to the overlying skin. 5. Fat and pectoral muscle layer beneath the deep fascia. The ductal system begins in the periphery of the breast and the ducts enlarge as they approach the nipple. There is an ampullary dilation before the duct enters the nipple proper. (From Ackerman, L. V. and del Regato, J. A.; Cancer Diagnosis, Treatment and Prognosis. 4th ed. St. Louis, C. V. Mosby Company, 1970).

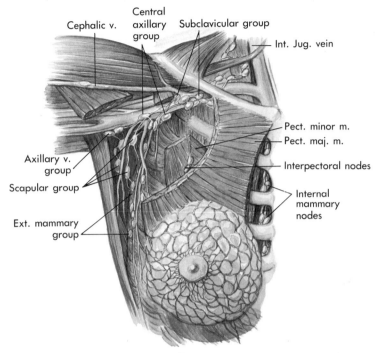

Central
Cephalic v.   axillary   Subclavicular group
              group

Int. Jug. vein

Pect. minor m.
Pect. maj. m.

Axillary v.
group

Interpectoral nodes

Scapular group

Internal
mammary
nodes

Ext. mammary
group

Figure 3–2. The distribution of lymph node drainage from the breast. The sub-areolar lymphatics progress radially to the draining lymph nodes. The major drainage is laterally through the external mammary group and then upward to the central axillary group of nodes before reaching the apex of the axilla. Direct drainage through the pectoral musculature to the subclavicular nodes can occur. The central and medial portions of the breast communicate directly with the internal mammary nodes. (From Spratt, J. S., Jr. and Donegan, W. L.: Cancer of the Breast. Philadelphia, W. B. Saunders Company, 1967.)

year intervals are advisable for all women over the age of 30. In certain high-risk groups, examinations at intervals of four to six months are recommended. High-risk indices include the following: (1) a previously removed cancer of the opposite breast; (2) a family history of cancer; (3) recurrent breast nodules which on biopsy show marked adenosis microscopically; (4) young women on oral contraceptives with recurring breast nodules.

The normal female breast varies considerably in size, shape, and consistency (Figs. 3–1 and 3–2). The virgin breast is smooth, cone-shaped, and of a firm, elastic consistency. It is often sensitive to palpation, especially in the premenstrual period. The borders of the breast are sharply defined and the entire structure may be moved freely over the chest wall. Later in life, and particularly following gestation and lactation, the breast undergoes involutional changes, develops an irregular consistency, and loses it sharply defined borders and shape. The proportion of fat in the breast varies with the habitus. In the obese individual, the breast usually becomes large and pendulous. In the thin individual, it becomes small and atrophic.

In addition to the changes in the breast which occur with age, there are varying degrees of fullness and thickness in normal breasts. The cyclic changes which accompany menstruation result in epithelial hyperplasia and involution associated with fibrosis. These can be detected on physical examination as areas of ill-defined granular consistency. Marked changes of this sort result in the clinical picture of fibroadenosis or chronic cystic mastitis.

If the normal female breast is felt between the finger and thumb, one nearly always obtains a sensation of distinct nodosity. However, if the breast is flattened against the chest wall with the palm of the hand, the patient being in the supine position, this sensation of nodosity disappears. A distinct nodule which can be clearly recognized when the breast is compressed in this manner must be regarded as a tumor until its nature has been determined by histologic examination.

Whether or not there are complaints referable to the breast, it is always necessary to carry out a detailed and systematic examination.

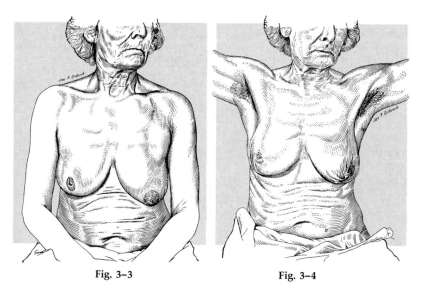

Fig. 3-3   Fig. 3-4

Figure 3–3. Inspection of the breasts with the patient in sitting position, arms at sides. Notice retraction of the right nipple and elevation of the right breast. Case of carcinoma of right breast.

Figure 3–4. Inspection of the breasts with the patient in sitting position during elevation of the arms. Note the shift in position of right nipple and dimpling of the skin as compared to Figure 3–3.

Inspection

The patient sits in an erect position stripped to the waist (Fig. 3–3). The size and symmetry of the breasts are observed. Note the presence or absence of skin discoloration, ulceration, dimpling, edema, deformity, or retraction of the nipples. Ask the patient to raise and lower her arms. During this maneuver the examiner looks for fixation of the skin or nipples, a shift in the relative position of the nipples, or distortion of the breast due to fixed masses (Fig. 3–4). The axillae are inspected for evidence of swelling due to enlarged lymph nodes or superficial infection.

The pectoral contraction maneuver. The breasts are inspected with the patient sitting, arms resting on hips. The patient then presses her

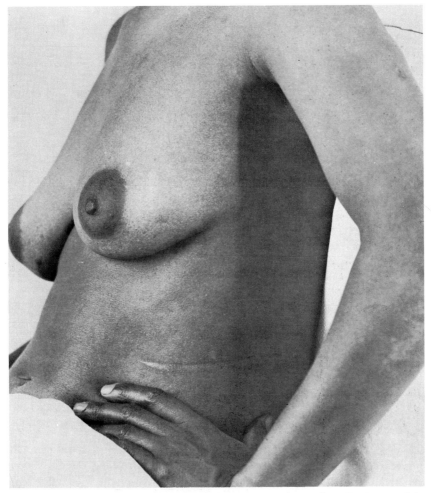

Figure 3–5. Pectoral contraction maneuver, arm *resting* on hip. Carcinoma of the middle outer section of the breast. (From Haagensen, C. D.: Diseases of the Breast. 2nd ed. Philadelphia, W. B. Saunders Company, 1974.)

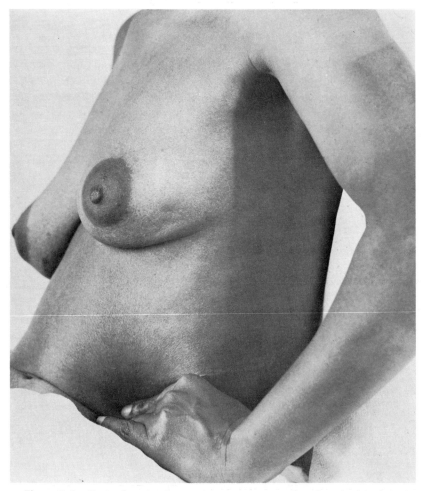

Figure 3–6. Pectoral contraction maneuver, arm *pressed* against the hip, bringing out small dimples in the skin over the carcinoma. (From Haagensen, C. D.: Diseases of the Breast. 2nd ed. Philadelphia, W. B. Saunders Company, 1974.)

hands against her hips, contracting the pectoral muscles. The breast involved with cancer rises more than the normal breast, and areas of dimpling or fixation may become obvious (Figs. 3–5 and 3–6).

Palpation

Palpation of the supraclavicular and axillary regions is best carried out with the patient in a sitting position. Palpate the supraclavicular region gently with the tips of the fingers while the patient keeps her arms at her sides (Fig. 3–7). It is advisable to repeat this part of the examination from behind the patient as in the examination of the neck (Fig. 3–8).

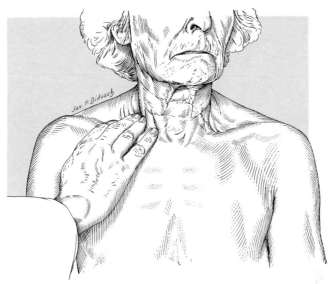

Figure 3–7. Palpation of the supraclavicular region from in front of the patient.

The patient's pectoral muscles must be relaxed in order to palpate the axilla properly. This is accomplished by supporting the arm with one hand while the axilla is gently explored with the tips of the fingers of the other hand (Fig. 3–9). The anterior and posterior axillary folds are also palpated in this position.

The patient then assumes the supine position; the shoulders should

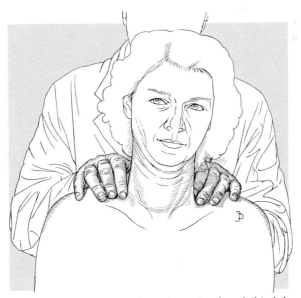

Figure 3–8. Palpation of the supraclavicular region from behind the patient.

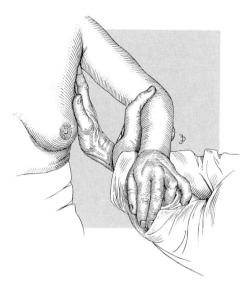

Figure 3–9. Palpation of the axilla. Note that the patient's arm is supported to relax the pectoral muscles. (Modified from Haagensen, C. D.: Carcinoma of the breast. J.A.M.A. *138*:195, 1948.)

be elevated by a small pillow. Palpation is performed gently and precisely with the flat of the fingers and the palm of the hand parallel to the contour of the breast. First palpate the breast with the patient's arm in a relaxed position at her side (Fig. 3–10), and then with her arm raised above her head (Fig. 3–11). Kneading the breast between the fingers gives an impression of the general consistency, but it is absolutely worthless as a means of detecting small masses. It may be necessary for the examiner to use both hands in palpation if the breasts are large and thick.

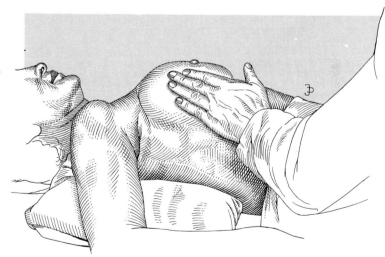

Figure 3–10. Palpation of the breast: arm at side. (Modified from Haagensen, C. D.: Diseases of the Breast. 2nd ed. Philadelphia, W. B. Saunders Company, 1974.)

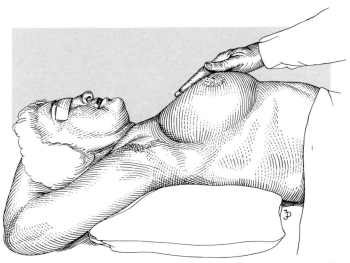

Figure 3–11. Palpation of the breast: arm above head. (Modified from Haagensen, C. D.: Diseases of the Breast. 2nd ed. Philadelphia, W. B. Saunders Company, 1974.)

I. THE APPRAISAL OF A MASS OR NODULE IN THE BREAST

Detection of a lesion during the examination requires definition or elucidation of the following points:

1. LOCATION?

It is customary to designate the location of a lesion according to the quadrant of the breast in which it lies (Fig. 3–12).

2. IS THE LESION SINGLE OR MULTIPLE?

Multiple nodules suggest benign cystic disease or fibroadenosis; a single nodule may be a neoplasm no matter how benign it appears on palpation.

3. WHAT IS THE SENSITIVITY AND CONSISTENCY OF THE MASS?

Tenderness suggests an inflammatory or cystic lesion. A hard, painless, irregular nodule is characteristic of cancer.

4. IS THE LESION FIXED TO THE CHEST WALL?

Fixation of a lesion to the chest wall usually indicates advanced carcinoma. The mobility of a lesion is demonstrated by taking the breast between the hands and gently moving it over the chest wall (Fig. 3–13).

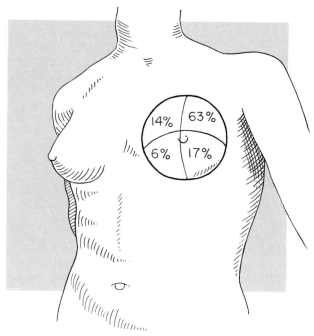

Figure 3–12. Diagram showing the frequency of cancer in each quadrant of the breast (Peter Bent Brigham Hospital series).

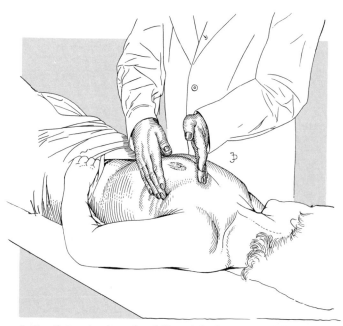

Figure 3–13. Determination of mobility of the breast. (Modified from Haagensen, C. D.: Carcinoma of the breast. J.A.M.A. *138*:195, 1948.)

5. IS THERE DIMPLING OF THE SKIN?

Cancer as it infiltrates the breast tissue produces a shortening of the fascial bands which attach the skin to the breast; this results in retraction of the skin over the tumor. At times this may be obvious or it may require demonstration by gentle compression of the breast tissue between the thumb and fingers of both hands (Fig. 3–14), or by pectoral contraction (Fig. 3–6).

6. IS THERE RETRACTION OR DISPLACEMENT OF THE NIPPLE?

Fat necrosis and carcinoma are likely to produce distortion or retraction of the nipple. An inverted position of the nipple is normal in some patients.

7. ARE THE AXILLARY OR SUPRACLAVICULAR NODES ENLARGED?

Particular care should be exercised in palpation, especially under the border of the pectoralis major and in the apex of the axilla. Neoplastic nodes are characteristically firm or stony hard in consistency, but any enlargement of the nodes may represent carcinoma.

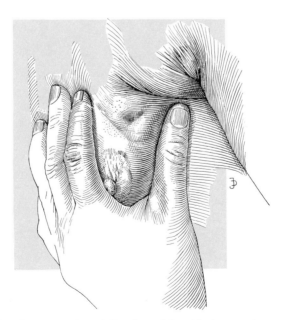

Figure 3–14. Demonstration of dimpling of the skin in a carcinoma of the breast. (Modified from Haagensen, C. D.: Carcinoma of the breast. J.A.M.A. *138*:195, 1948.)

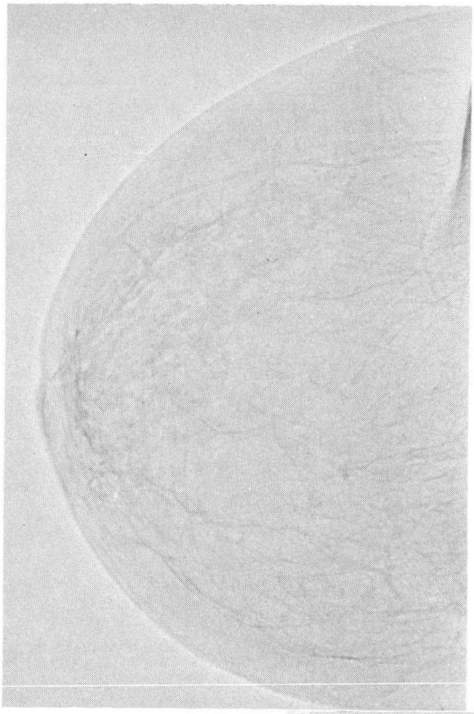

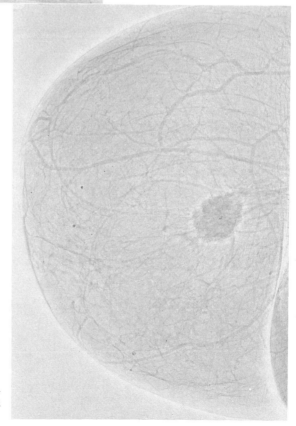

Figure 3–15. Normal xeroradiogram.

Figure 3–16. Carcinoma of breast seen in xeroradiogram.

Figure 3–17. Xeroradiogram showing a fibroadenoma in upper half of breast. Fibrocystic disease is also present.

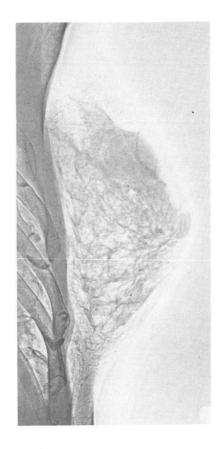

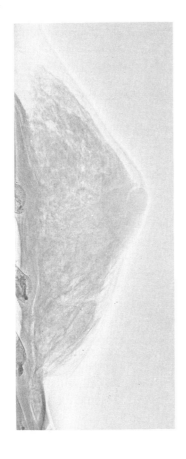

Figure 3–18. Xeroradiogram showing multiple breast cysts typical of fibrocystic disease.

8. WHAT IS THE APPEARANCE OF THE LESION ON XERORADIOGRAPHY OR MAMMOGRAPHY?

Mammography and xeroradiography have become established aids in the appraisal of lesions of the breast. Minute lesions, so small as to be impalpable, may be detected. A smooth contour usually indicates a benign lesion, whereas irregular, stellate, or infiltrating lesions suggest malignancy. Microcalcification that produces a fine stippling are common in cancer (Figs. 3–15 to 3–18).

The findings on soft tissue roentgenography complement and supplement the physical examination but do not exclude cancer nor eliminate the need for biopsy. A negative mammogram combined with a normal physical examination is very reassuring—for example, in a patient with recurrent breast nodules, or after mastectomy for cancer of the opposite breast.

II. THE APPRAISAL OF BLEEDING FROM THE NIPPLE

Although bleeding from the nipple is an uncommon complaint, it is always an alarming one because of the common association of blood with cancer. Actually it is caused by benign lesions more often than it is caused by cancer. The most common lesions found in association with a sanguineous discharge from the nipple are ductile papillomas, chronic cystic mastitis, and cancer.

The examination of the breast may immediately clarify the problem. The finding of a single mass in the breast in association with bleeding is strongly suggestive of carcinoma. The diagnosis of chronic cystic disease is likely if there is an irregular nodosity scattered throughout the breast. Biopsy is required in either event.

If there is no mass in the breast, careful scrutiny of the nipple may reveal a dilated duct which thus indicates the quadrant of the breast from which the blood is issuing. If a dilated duct cannot be visualized, milking the breast tissue with gentle pressure toward the nipple may cause a discharge and thus localize the involved duct. Occasionally the patient may be able to describe the precise point on the nipple from which the blood has issued. Once the site of bleeding is localized, careful and gentle palpation of that area may reveal a firm cord extending radially from the nipple, indicative of a ductile papilloma.

Occasionally it will be found that the bleeding is coming from more than one duct. Under such circumstances, if no palpable lesion can be found in the breast or visualized by transillumination, it is extremely unlikely that carcinoma is responsible for the discharge. Cytologic study of the discharge should be performed. The secretion is collected on a glass slide and immediately placed in fixative. Nipple discharge in the absence of a palpable lesion is more suggestive of cancer in women over 60 years of age. Mammography may demonstrate a lesion.

III. SOME IMPORTANT LESIONS OF THE BREAST

Carcinoma of the breast. Any palpable nodule in the breast may represent carcinoma. The early diagnosis of carcinoma must be made by the detection of small, often freely movable nodules; their precise histologic character must be determined by biopsy. In general, cancerous nodules tend to be firmer and harder than cysts or inflammatory lesions and are usually insensitive.

The characteristic and classic physical signs of carcinoma of the breast appear only after the lesion has progressed for some time (Fig. 3–19). Carcinoma tightens and shortens the fibrous septa of the breast as it grows and produces dimpling of the overlying skin. Later it may interfere with lymphatic drainage and produce a leathery thickening of the skin, the so-called "peau d'orange" (Fig. 3–20 *A*). Retraction of the nipple (Fig. 3–20 *B*) may occur. Bloody or purulent discharge from the nipples may be seen if the neoplasm invades the ductile system; this is particularly characteristic of ductile carcinoma. Tenderness is not usual, but may occur in inflammatory cancers. Stony hard, discrete, axillary, or supraclavicular nodes are features of advanced or rapidly growing carcinoma of the breast.

There is considerable controversy regarding the surgical treatment of breast cancer but all authorities agree that in early causes control of local and regional disease is a primary objective. At the present time in favorable cases this is best provided with limited deformity by modified radical mastectomy. In advanced cases remarkable palliation is often obtained by irradiation and hormonal manipulation.

Inflammatory cancer. Certain cancers of the breast simulate inflammatory lesions. There may be pain, fever, and tenderness suggesting an abscess. Sometimes the advancing border of the infiltrating tumor may be so fiery red, raised, and tender that it looks like an acute cellulitis. This variety of neoplasm is more common in premenopausal women. It may develop during pregnancy. The prognosis is grave. Surgical treatment is contraindicated and the response to irradiation, hormonal manipulation, and chemotherapy is poor.

Intraductile papilloma. This lesion is characteristically associated with bloody discharge from the nipple. Careful inspection of the nipple may reveal the dilated duct from which the discharge is issuing. Occasionally this may be demonstrated by gentle pressure. Once the involved duct is identified, gentle palpation adjacent to the areola in this area will usually reveal either a small tumor or a fine cord extending radically into the breast tissue.

Fig. 3–19

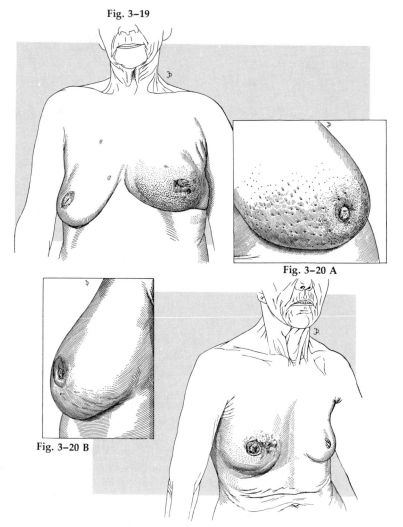

Fig. 3–20 A

Fig. 3–20 B

Fig. 3–21

Figure 3–19. Advanced carcinoma of left breast.
Figure 3–20 A. Peau d'orange in carcinoma of the breast.
Figure 3–20 B. Retraction of the nipple in carcinoma of the breast.
Figure 3–21. Paget's disease of the right breast.

Paget's disease of the breast. Paget's disease is manifested by a red granular excoriation on the nipple or by a dry, scaly lesion which bleeds easily when touched (Fig. 3–21). It may occasionally involve the entire areola. A cordlike strand may be felt extending deeply from the nipple into the breast tissue. Paget's disease of the breast is always associated with underlying carcinoma which may or may not be detectable on palpation. Mammography may disclose the lesion which cannot be palpated.

Carcinoma of the breast in pregnancy. The breast of the pregnant woman is engorged and thickened owing to proliferation of the lobulo-alveolar system prior to delivery. With the onset of lactation, a maturation process occurs in which milk is produced by apocrine shedding of the surface of the alveolar cells. These physiologic and anatomic changes make it difficult to detect a mass in the breast by physical examination. If, however, a mass is detected, it has the same significance as one in the breast of a nongravid woman, and should be managed in the same way.

Fibroadenoma of the breast. A firm, often lobulated, freely movable nontender mass in the breast of a young woman is likely to be a fibroadenoma. Unfortunately, carcinoma may masquerade in this guise even in the young.

Juvenile Type Fibroadenoma of the Breast. Juvenile fibroadenomas are usually solitary and larger than the adult type. The lesion is slightly firm, freely mobile, encapsulated, and not attached to the skin. Rapid painless enlargement of the breast over a period of 10 or 12 days is the usual complaint.

Chronic cystic mastitis. This very common pathologic process produces single or multiple nodules scattered throughout both breasts. Occasionally a single quadrant is involved, making a differential diagnosis from cancer impossible. There is usually considerable thickening of adjacent breast tissue. There is no fixation of the lesion but there may be increased sensitivity of the breast to palpation. There may be some variation in size and in the degree of tenderness associated with the menses. Discrete nodules require a biopsy.

Adenosis or fibronadenosis of the breast. This variant of chronic cystic disease is characterized by many small, pea-sized shotty nodules scattered throughout both breasts. It is usually associated with considerable breast discomfort and tenderness to palpation. There is often a disk-like margin to the breast tissue. This is especially noticeable along the lateral borders of the breasts.

Cystosarcoma phyllodes (giant adenofibroma). This rapidly enlarging and irregularly nodular tumor presents a frightening clinical picture, but in fact is usually a rare manifestation of fibrocystic disease (Fig. 3–22). It should always be regarded as benign, although in very rare instances malignant degeneration may be found histologically. The lesion may occur in younger or older women. The rapid growth often gives an inflammatory appearance to the tumor and there may be apparent fixation to the skin. If possible, the lesion should be locally excised, but simple mastectomy may occasionally be required because of the extent of the growth.

Sarcoma. Lymphosarcoma, fibrosarcoma, and rhabdomyosarcoma may involve the breast, the latter usually by direct extension from the pectoral muscles or by blood stream metastasis. The diagnosis is usually established by biopsy. Simple mastectomy and irradiation is the usual treatment, but the prognosis is poor because of the high incidence of distant metastases.

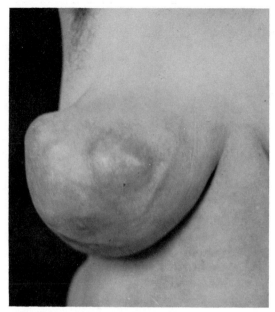

Figure 3–22. Cystosarcoma of breast in a 48 year old woman. (From Haagensen, C. D.: Diseases of the Breast. 2nd ed. Philadelphia, W. B. Saunders Company, 1974.)

Fat necrosis. Fat necrosis may occur at any age and usually is encountered in large, pendulous, fatty breasts. There may or may not be a history of trauma preceding the appearance of the nodule. The physical characteristics of fat necrosis simulate those of carcinoma. There may be dimpling of the skin and retraction of the nipple; the consistency of the mass is such that it is easily confused with neoplasm. Enlarged axillary nodes secondary to the inflammatory process frequently add to the confusion. The diagnosis can only be established by biopsy.

Trauma to the breast. Although patients frequently relate the appearance of a lump in the breast to some type of mild trauma, the history usually indicates that it has been inconsequential. There is little evidence that trauma is a significant factor in the development of carcinoma of the breast.

When trauma to the breast has been sufficiently severe to produce injury, there is little doubt about it. A hemorrhage and hematoma in the breast produce very striking physical findings. There is often a large mass with marked tenderness. Edema and swelling and ecchymosis of the breast may be massive. In the course of a few days, the characteristic signs of an absorbing hemorrhage with discoloration and pigmentation of the skin appear. Not infrequently following such injuries there is a residual lump which persists in the breast and often marks the first sign of fat necrosis. If a lump persists, it may require biopsy.

Mastitis. An inflammatory reaction in the breast tissue commonly occurs during lactation. A systemic reaction with chills, fever and sweats occurs if the lesion is associated with pyogenic organisms. The affected breast is swollen, red and tender. Fluctuation may develop and axillary lymphadenitis is usually present. The possibility of inflammatory carcinoma must always be kept in mind. A mastitis may be associated with puberty or mumps. *Mastitis neonatorum* occurs in the newborn. It is associated with the escape from the nipple of a whitish discharge, the so-called "witch's milk."

Tuberculosis of the breast. Early tuberculosis of the breast may simulate cystic mastitis or carcinoma. As a rule, the axillary lymph nodes are not involved in the early stages. Unless tuberculous lesions are detected elsewhere, the diagnosis may be made only on biopsy. Advanced tuberculosis is associated with discoloration of the skin, breakdown of tissue, and the formation of sinuses. The process tends to be diffuse and poorly demarcated. The inflammatory reaction, as in tuberculosis elsewhere, is "cold" and nontender.

Mastodynia. Occasionally a patient complains of severe pain in a breast in which no nodules can be demonstrated. A little induration may be felt and the pain characteristically is worse during the premenstrual period. The diagnosis is usually made by exclusion; occasionally the pain is an early symptom of cystic disease.

Polymastia or supernumerary breast. This may occur above or below the normal breast. Sometimes the supernumerary breast is present while the nipple is absent.

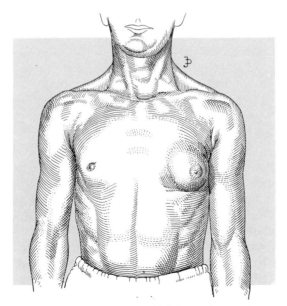

Figure 3–23. Gynecomastia of left breast in a young man.

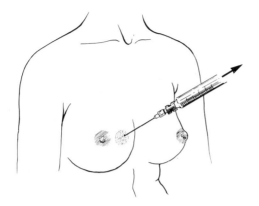

Figure 3–24. Needle aspiration of breast cyst. (From Dunphy, J. E. and Way, L. W.: Current Surgical Diagnosis and Treatment, Los Altos, Lange Medical Publications, 1973.)

Gynecomastia. Gynecomastia, or female type of breast in the male, is usually unilateral. Its appearance is quite characteristic (Fig. 3–23). It should be distinguished from the mere overdevelopment of fat in the normal male breast. In the young adult, gynecomastia assumes a symmetrical appearance identical with that seen in the female breast. In elderly males, hyperplasia of the breast produces an irregularly nodular lesion which may be quite suggestive of neoplasm. Biopsy is often required to clarify its nature.

If gynecomastia is bilateral, a systemic cause should be sought. The testicles should be carefully examined for tumor. An excess of estrogens associated with some cases of liver insufficiency may lead to bilateral gynecomastia.

Cancer of the male breast. Cancer in the male breast produces an irregular hard nodule beneath the areola. Fixation to the chest wall is common. Because of the paucity of breast tissue the more classic signs of breast cancer may not develop. Metastases to the axilla occur early.

IV. ASPIRATION OF BREAST CYSTS

Aspiration of breast cysts can easily be performed under local anesthesia without significant discomfort to the patient (Fig. 3–24). The fluid may be submitted for cytologic examination but the yield of positive findings is so low that most authorities do not do it. Residual nodular palpable tissue after aspiration requires biopsy. Needle aspiration is best suited for the younger patient with recurrent painful cysts which have been shown to be typical of cystic disease on previous biopsy. Mammography or xeroradiography may provide additional evidence of benignity.

chapter 4

EXAMINATION OF THE CHEST

The examination of the chest will be considered under two headings: (1) The Elective Examination, and (2) The Examination of the Post–operative Chest.

The chest is examined best with the patient sitting upright. If circumstances make this impossible, the anterior chest wall may be thoroughly examined while the patient remains supine. The patient may then be rolled first to one side and then to the other to permit examination of the posterior chest wall. This shift in the position of the patient renders comparison and interpretation of the physical findings on auscultation and percussion difficult. Consequently, unless the patient is in shock or collapse, it is wisest to support him in the upright position long enough to permit percussion and auscultation of the base of the lungs posteriorly.

I. THE ELECTIVE EXAMINATION

Inspection

The examiner first notes the general contour. The so–called *barrel chest,* in which the thoracic cage is nearly as thick as it is wide, is a result of a marked increase in the anterior–posterior diameter of the chest. Although the possessor of such a chest is often pleased with his large chest measurement, the condition is associated with varying degrees of chronic emphysema. The expansile movements of the chest are often restricted and there is a lowering of pulmonary reserve. Such patients take general anesthesia poorly and are prone to postoperative pulmonary complications. The *flat-chested individual* in whom the thoracic wall lies in the same plane as the clavicle may be suspected of having pulmonary disease, but in most cases such patients have excellent expansile movements of

73

the chest and, in contrast to more robust appearing patients, have adequate pulmonary reserve and undergo general anesthesia quite easily.

Large deformities of the chest wall are usually obvious, but a careful scrutiny is necessary to avoid overlooking asymptomatic lesions.

Observation of the Respiratory Movements

Normal respiratory movements will be hardly noticed by the examiner unless he focuses attention on them. A moment's observation will reveal that on inspiration the clavicles rise, the rib cage expands laterally and there is an upward and expansile movement of the abdominal wall due to a descent of the diaphragm. The abdominal movement is more pronounced in men than in women. If not evident, these changes can be brought out by asking the patient to breathe deeply. The normal rate of respiration varies from 16 to 20 per minute. Variations in the rate and character of respirations provide many important clues in diagnosis.

A quickening of the rate and a shortening of the depth of respiration occur in many conditions, particularly infections. The extent of the change in respirations is significant in that the patient is not aware of shortness of breath.

Deep, smooth, obvious respirations, predominantly thoracic in type, occur in certain anxiety states, particularly during the course of the physical examination. If the patient is not aware that he is being observed, respirations subside to normal or may be followed by a brief period of apnea. Rarely, the neurotic or hysterical patient will continue to hyperventilate until tetany is produced from the washing out of carbon dioxide from the blood.

Deep, sighing respirations (Kussmaul breathing) occur in acidosis, particularly diabetic acidosis. Similar respirations occur from "air hunger" in acute blood loss.

Slow, stertorous breathing is characteristic of the coma of cerebral injuries. It may become irregular or assume an intermittent character, periods of apnea alternating with periods of respiration. The respiratory phase is usually introduced by a slow rate, gradually increasing and then quieting down to the apneic phase (Cheyne–Stokes breathing). Various toxic states, particularly if there is nitrogen retention, are accompanied by this type of breathing.

Extremely slow respirations, regular in type, should immediately arouse a suspicion of morphine intoxication. The presence of pin–point pupils confirms the diagnosis.

Dyspnea (shortness of breath) with or without cyanosis occurs in a variety of cardiac or pulmonary lesions.

Gasping inspiration and forced expiration occur in chest injuries with open sucking wounds.

Forced respirations accompanied by contraction of the accessory muscles of respiration occur in obstruction of the upper respiratory tract. The jaw retracts with each attempted respiration. This type of respiration is a terminal sign in various septic and toxic states.

Respiratory insufficiency. It is now established that serious pulmonary insufficiency may be present without cyanosis or obvious respiratory distress so that analysis of blood gases is essential in all cases of potential respiratory impairment.

Auscultation and Percussion

Since the technique of the examination of the heart and lungs and the variations produced by various medical and surgical conditions is so thoroughly presented in standard texts of physical diagnosis, it would serve no useful purpose to repeat them here. A familiarity with the technique will be assumed.

Although the details of examining the heart and lungs are not included in this text, the importance of the examination to the surgeon requires emphasis. There is a growing tendency to rely upon the impressions of medical colleagues and the interpretation of the roentgenologist in appraising the state of the patient's circulatory and respiratory system. While such deference is understandable, it is a mistake. Such information must be integrated by the surgeon himself and in doing so he must use the stethoscope himself. A careful preoperative auscultation and percussion of the heart and lungs by the surgeon provide a basis for comparison during the postoperative period which is of the greatest importance. Slight changes in respiration, a few rales or diminished breath sounds, a little quickening of the pulse or change in the intensity of the heart sounds when fitted into the total picture provide the surgeon with data that he alone can interpret correctly.

Lesions of the Chest Wall

Deformities

Gross deformities of the chest are obvious. Many of these are associated with lesions of the vertebral column, such as kyphosis or scoliosis (see Chap. 10). Advanced degrees of such deformities produce a serious impairment of pulmonary reserve. If there has been recurrent pulmonary infection, there may be clubbing of the fingers.

Funnel chest, or péctus excavatum (Fig. 4–1), is a congenital anomaly in which the body of the sternum is depressed. In severe cases it may reach the vertebral column or extend into the paravertebral gutter. The heart may be rotated and displaced, with considerable interference with cardiac and respiratory function.

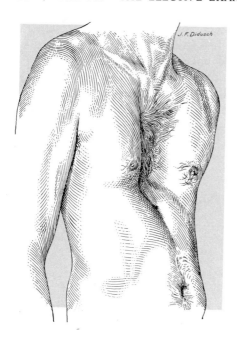

J. F. Didusch

Figure 4–1. Pectus excavatum (funnel chest).

Infections

Tuberculosis of the costal cartilages may produce a low grade inflammatory swelling of the anterior chest wall. Until the lesion breaks down with sinus formation, its true nature may not be suspected.

Pyogenic infections of the chest wall usually take the form of furuncles or abscesses. Typical carbuncles are less common although they may occur over the lower back, particularly in hirsute patients.

Tumors

Wens, moles, senile warts and hemangiomas are especially common on the skin of the chest wall because of its great extent. The *angiomas* of liver insufficiency are found over the anterior chest wall as delicate vascular patterns radiating from a central red spot. They are distinguished from congenital nevi or angiomas by their branching spidery appearance. *Occasionally comedones or wens acquire sufficient size and density to cast a shadow on a roentgenogram of the chest. Such a shadow may be mistaken for an intrathoracic tumor.*

Lipomas of the chest wall are very common. Their characteristics are such that they can usually be recognized by means of the physical examination. A soft, compressible, sharply demarcated, lobulated mass not attached directly to the skin or underlying tissues is characteristic of a lipoma. A definite sense of fluctuation can often be elicited, leading the novice to suspect that there is fluid in the lesion. Bimanual compression of the mass may produce wrinkling of the skin because of delicate fibrous septa which extend from the skin to the capsule overlying the lipoma. At times these lesions lie beneath fascial planes or grow into fascial planes, acquiring sufficient fixation to suggest the possibility of a sarcoma. The diagnosis of a lipoma may be confirmed by the fact that the soft consistency of their growth is rendered hard by the application of cold. If doubt exists, an x-ray taken in the plane of the subcutaneous tissue will reveal the lipoma as an area of decreased density.

Neurofibroma. Neurofibromas are firm, well circumscribed, non-compressible, movable nodules. They occur along the course of the parietal nerves. They may be associated with brownish areas of pigmentation of the skin, the "cafe au lait" spots of von Recklinghausen's disease.

Sarcomas are the most common malignant tumors of the thoracic wall. All varieties occur. Fibrosarcoma and chondrosarcoma are encountered most often. These tumors vary in their appearance. In their early stages they may be firm, well circumscribed and freely movable and their infiltration and malignant characteristics are not appreciated. In advanced cases they become irregularly nodular with areas of softening, hemorrhages and palpable infiltration of the surrounding tissue well beyond the main tumor mass. Recurrence of sarcoma in the scar of a previous excision is especially common (Fig. 4–2). Any tumor of the chest wall which

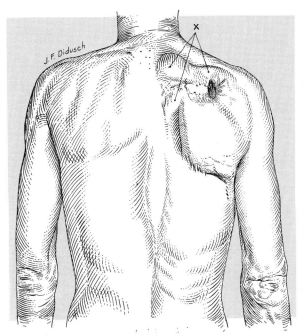

Figure 4–2. Recurrence of a fibrosarcoma in the scar of a previous excision. The scapula was partially excised and the defect covered with a skin graft. The cross indicates the recurrent nodules of tumor.

is not clearly a lipoma should be regarded as potentially malignant. Removal should be performed under conditions which permit a radical excision.

Chondromas. Tumors arising in the costal cartilages or ribs may appear grossly benign, but are frequently malignant (Fig. 4–3).

Tender costochondral junction. Patients frequently present themselves complaining of a tender prominence of a costochondral junction. Careful palpation is usually sufficient to exclude the presence of a tumor, but if there is any doubt, an x-ray should be taken.

Eosinophilic granuloma. This benign lesion occurs as a solitary tumor of the ribs; it may easily be mistaken for a malignant lesion because of its rapid onset and the frequency with which it produces severe pain and tenderness. An exquisitely tender, very painful tumor of the rib in a young adult patient should arouse a suspicion of this lesion. It is important to suspect it clinically since the x-ray appearance may be mistaken for that of an osteolytic malignant growth.

Superior pulmonary sulcus syndrome. Any neoplasm which invades the thoracic inlet may involve the ribs, the sympathetic chain and the brachial plexus; this produces the so–called superior pulmonary sulcus syndrome. The essential clinical features include fullness in the supraclavicular fossa, pain in the distribution of the ulnar nerve with wasting of the intrinsic muscles of the hand supplied by this nerve, and a Horner's syndrome on the affected side. Horner's syndrome is a con-

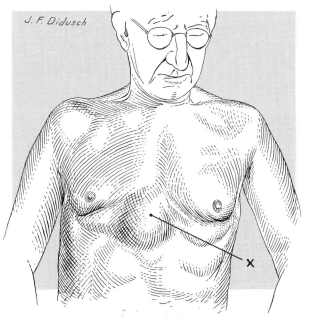

Figure 4–3. Chondrosarcoma of the anterior chest wall.

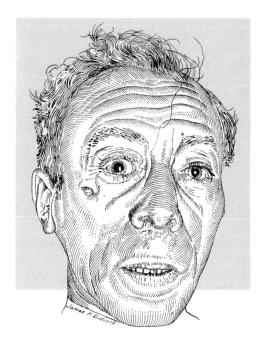

Figure 4-4. Horner's syndrome in a patient with carcinoma of apex of the left lung (superior pulmonary sulcus syndrome).

sequence of paralysis of the cervical sympathetic chain and is characterized by drooping of the upper eyelid and constriction of the pupil. The narrowing of the aperture between the lids creates an appearance of enophthalmos (Fig. 4-4).

The most common cause of the superior pulmonary sulcus syndrome is bronchiogenic carcinoma involving the apex of the lung.

II. THE POSTOPERATIVE CHEST

Pulmonary complications are the commonest cause of fever in the post-operative period. Usually mild and of little significance, they may be the deciding factor in a fatal issue in the seriously ill patient. Aspiration pneumonia, massive collapse and pulmonary embolism are potentially lethal complications. The prompt recognition of all pulmonary complications is an essential feature of good postoperative care.

The Time Factor

The time of onset of a pulmonary complication is a useful diagnostic guide. Respiratory distress and cyanosis within a few hours of recovery from anesthesia suggest an unrecognized aspiration of vomitus. The atelectatic complications associated with mucous plugs in the bronchi usually appear within the first to the third postoperative day. Pulmonary embolism may occur at any time. It is known to have happened during an operation and may develop as late as the third or fourth week. Usually, however, pulmonary embolism appears between the fifth and sixteenth day after operation. The septic complications of lung abscess or subphrenic abscess have always been late in onset. Now the frequent use of antibiotics may delay them for many weeks.

Postoperative Pulmonary Atelectasis

This very common pulmonary complication occurs within the first few hours after operation. It usually is detectable not later than the evening of the first day. If one regularly examines the lung bases of the postoperative patient on the morning of the first postoperative day, one will frequently find physical signs of atelectasis before the full–blown clinical picture is evident. The right lung is affected much more often than the left. Elevation of the diaphragm, limited motion of the diaphragm, diminished breath sounds, and sometimes a few rales on the affected side are the significant signs. Frequently, one can correlate these with an unusually painful incision or a patient who is particularly sensitive to pain, a tight abdominal binder, and, perhaps, a history of respiratory infection or chronic sinusitis. Simple measures designed to bring up the mucous plug and expand the lungs are usually effective if instituted at this stage. Expectorants, loosening of the binder, adequate medication to control pain, and encouraging the patient to move and cough are in order. If preventive measures are not taken early, a classic picture develops later in the day.

Inspection

In the early stages a slight increase in the respiratory rate may be the only sign. Established pulmonary atelectasis is usually obvious on inspection. Temperature, pulse, and respiration are all elevated. The patient is flushed and uncomfortable, but does not appear seriously ill. He is aware of mucus in his throat which he cannot bring up easily because of pain when he coughs. Bits of sanitary tissue with flecks of thick, tenacious sputum are scattered over the bedside table.

Percussion and Auscultation

Percussion and auscultation of the chest will disclose dullness, diminished breath sounds, restricted movements of the diaphragm and sometimes, but not always, fine to coarse rales at the lung base on the affected side. It is best to sit the patient up for the examination. Indeed, the mere act of moving and examining the patient may bring about a cough which loosens the principal bronchial plugs and improves the patient's condition. Thumping the affected side is frequently beneficial. If these and other measures fail, suction of the trachea by a catheter or bronchoscopy may be necessary.

X-ray

An x-ray of the chest is usually not necessary. It will show elevation of the diaphragm, increased pulmonary markings, and sometimes a slight shift of the trachea to the affected side.

Massive Pulmonary Collapse

In massive pulmonary collapse of the lung a major bronchus is occluded and air is completely absorbed from the involved lung. The lung is more or less completely compressed and there is a shift in the mediastinum toward the involved side (Fig. 4–5).

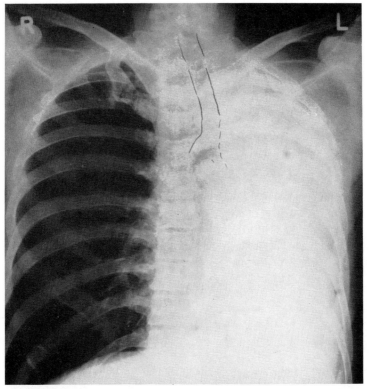

Figure 4–5. Massive collapse of the left lung. The mediastinum is shifted toward the side of the lesion. Note the marked tracheal displacement.

Inspection

The appearance of the patient is characteristic and dramatic. There are marked dyspnea, cyanosis, considerable respiratory distress, and moderate to severe pain.

Palpation

The trachea is shifted toward the affected side. There are absence of tactile fremitus and little or no expansion of the thorax on the involved side.

Percussion

The percussion note is dull and the cardiac and mediastinal dullness is shifted toward the involved side.

Auscultation

Breath and voice sounds are absent; occasionally, loud bronchial rales may be heard.

The diagnosis is definitely confirmed if the physical signs clear as the patient is forced to cough violently or after tracheal aspiration. Bronchoscopy may be necessary.

Aspiration Pneumonia

Aspiration pneumonia is a highly fatal, but fortunately preventable, complication. If the stomach is emptied prior to surgery and adequate supervision is provided during recovery from anesthesia, it should not occur. However, despite all precautions, aspiration may take place and because of the human factor in medical care, may not be recognized when it happens. Dyspnea, cyanosis, and fever within a few hours of recovery from anesthesia should arouse a suspicion of aspiration. Examination of the chest will reveal coarse rales throughout both lung fields. Emergency bronchoscopy must be done as a diagnostic as well as a therapeutic measure. High dose corticoid therapy is indicated.

Respiratory Distress Syndrome (Shock Lung, Hemorrhagic Lung, Post Traumatic Pulmonary Insufficiency)

In recent years, a new form of respiratory failure has been recognized. The respiratory distress syndrome is a frequent and often fatal condition following extensive surgery, severe trauma, shock, cardiopulmonary bypass, and profound sepsis.

There are unique features which, if recognized early, can lead to successful corrective measures. The onset is usually insidious. Anxiety and a slight elevation of pulse and respiration may be the only initial signs. Cyanosis and dyspnea are notably absent. Examination of the lungs reveals good breath sounds without rales; yet, at this point, measurement of PaO_2 (partial pressure of arterial oxygen) and $PaCO_2$ (partial pressure of arterial carbon dioxide) will disclose hypoxemia and hypercapnia.

Steady progression to a state of severe hypoxia, hypercapnia, acidosis, and cardiac arrest follows. The usual signs of pulmonary insufficiency, such as dyspnea, cyanosis, and labored respiration, are late in appearing. Terminally, pulmonary consolidation due to massive congestive and interalveolar hemorrhage is present.

The important point is the lack of early symptoms and physical signs. A high index of suspicion and prompt monitoring of respiratory function are the keys to early recognition. Pulmonary microembolism is a major underlying etiological factor but sepsis, fluid overload, and oxygen toxicity may all play a role.

Treatment requires assisted ventilation, the careful administration of oxygen, and precise monitoring of all parameters of respiratory and circulatory function.

Pulmonary Embolism

The recognition of pulmonary embolism by physical signs requires a high index of suspicion on the part of the examiner. Quite large emboli may produce remarkably little change in the physical findings on examination of the lungs, and a careful search for evidence of phlebitis in the extremities may be the only means of finding a clue to the diagnosis (see Chap. 11). Generally there are two types of pulmonary embolism: that due to peripheral infarction of the lung with pleural involvement and that occasioned by occlusion of major branches of the pulmonary artery.

PULMONARY INFARCTION (DUE TO SMALL EMBOLI INVOLVING PERIPHERAL PORTIONS OF THE LUNG WITH PLEURAL INVOLVEMENT)

Inspection

The signs are essentially those of an acute, sharply localized, dry pleurisy. The patient is in obvious pain which is aggravated when he tries to breathe deeply. He may have a sense of suffocation, but respirations are only slightly elevated and there is no cyanosis. He may bring up a little bloodstained sputum.

Palpation

At an early stage a friction rub may occasionally be felt over the area of involved pleura.

Auscultation

Respirations are diminished on the involved side and a transient friction rub may be heard. Occasionally, a few rales are the only evidence of pulmonary injury.

Sometimes no striking variation from the normal can be detected, but pleuritic pain in the postoperative period is due to pulmonary infarction until proved otherwise. A minute search of the extremities for minimal thrombophlebitis should be made in all patients, even though well and ambulatory, in whom there is a diagnosis of "dry pleurisy."

PULMONARY EMBOLISM (WITH OCCLUSION OF MAJOR BRANCHES OF THE PULMONARY ARTERY)

When the embolus is large and lodges in the major branches of the pulmonary artery, the physical signs are those of acute circulatory collapse. Sometimes this takes the classic form of acute cor pulmonale, but frequently the evidence of right-sided heart failure is minimal. Occasionally, the signs of peripheral failure may render a differential diagnosis between pulmonary embolism and acute massive hemorrhage exceedingly difficult. The patient is pale, respirations are rapid and of the "air hunger" type and the blood pressure is low.

Inspection

Pain is not a prominent sign, but the patient almost invariably has a sense of extreme anxiety and impending diaster which may be quite out of proportion to any of the physical findings. A pallid cyanosis with distention of the neck veins is characteristic and, if present, is almost diagnostic. The pulse is usually rapid, with a low pulse pressure and marked hypotension. Unless there is clear-cut evidence of cyanosis and venous stasis, an immediate inspection of the wound and other possible sites of bleeding in the postoperative patient should be made.

Auscultation

Remarkably little change may be found on auscultation of the heart and lungs. The heart rate may be rapid or comparatively slow. The lungs are usually clear on auscultation in the major forms of embolism and in the most severe cases death ensues without the development of significant pulmonary signs. The differential diagnosis between pulmonary embolism and coronary artery occlusion may be impossible unless signs of an associated phlebitis are found. In the postoperative patient the condition often develops after slight effort, such as straining at stool.

Special Tests

An electrocardiogram may be helpful in distinguishing between pulmonary embolus with acute cor pulmonale and coronary occlusion.

Pulmonary scanning with radioactive technetium has become a very valuable diagnostic technique in early or doubtful cases.

All gradations occur between small pulmonary infarctions and massive occlusions of the pulmonary artery with immediate death. Generally the presence of pain and bloody sputum indicates that the infarction is more peripheral, smaller and less serious. A small embolus may be followed by a massive embolus; therefore, in all cases anticoagulation is required.

Lung Abscess

Improved methods of anesthesia, greater care to prevent aspiration in operations on the mouth and throat and the use of antibiotics have made this a comparatively rare postoperative complication. Aspiration of foreign material, infected emboli, or necrosis in an area of prolonged atelectasis or pneumonia are the principal etiologic factors.

The onset of the disease is usually delayed for many days or weeks after operation. Fever, cough, and chest pain are presenting symptoms. The physical signs, except in large or peripheral abscesses, are usually so slight that they cannot be relied upon. X-rays of the chest, both anterior-posterior and lateral views, are essential if the diagnosis is to be made early. In advanced and neglected cases the abscess ruptures into a bronchus, producing singularly foul sputum. The putrid character of this sputum indicates the diagnosis.

Subdiaphragmatic Abscess

A subdiaphragmatic abscess is a complication of abdominal sepsis. Appendicitis, perforated ulcer, cholecystitis, and pancreatitis are the chief primary sources of infection, but any peritoneal infection may lead to a subdiaphragmatic abscess.

The control of peritoneal infections by antibiotics reduced the incidence of subphrenic abscess for a time, but more recently, with the increased magnitude of operations, the frequency of severe abdominal trauma, and the appearance of antibiotic-resistant, gram-negative organisms, this serious complication is being seen with increasing frequency. Moreover, its naturally insidious course continues to be rendered more so by the use of antibiotics. Indeed, the symptoms of subdiaphragmatic abscess in patients who have been and are still under antibiotic therapy are so minimal that, as a general rule, the diagnosis must be considered whenever a patient who has had abdominal infection is not progressing satisfactorily. Fever may or may not be present. Anorexia is sometimes the only symptom. Failure to gain in weight and strength after all the obvious signs of peritoneal, pelvic, or wound infections have subsided is sufficient to arouse suspicion.

The physical signs of subphrenic abscess depend considerably upon its location, the rapidity with which it forms, and the presence or absence of air in the abscess cavity. The examiner must understand the anatomy of the subphrenic area, which is illustrated diagrammatically in Figures 4–6 and 4–7. A simple clue for remembering the distribution is shown in Figure 4–8.

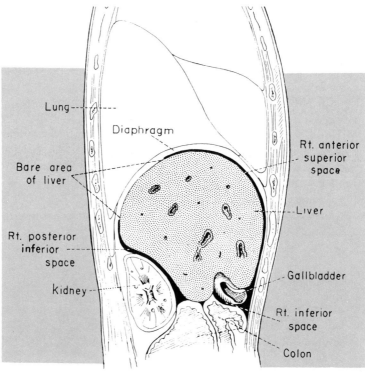

Figure 4–6. Sagittal section of the right subphrenic spaces. The spaces are shown in solid black. The right anterior superior space lies between the liver and the diaphragm. It is separated from the right posterior inferior space by the bare area of the liver. The right posterior superior space lies behind the bare area of the liver and extends into the renal fossa. The right inferior space lies in a subhepatic position.

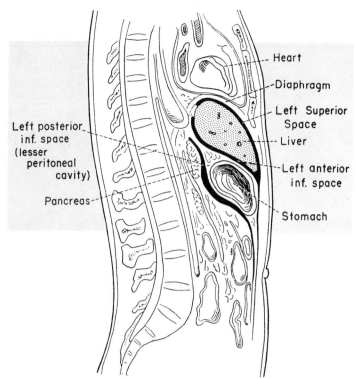

Figure 4–7. Sagittal section of the left subphrenic spaces. The left superior space lies between the left lobe of the liver and the diaphragm. The left anterior inferior space lies beneath the liver between it and the stomach. The left posterior inferior space is the lesser peritoneal cavity.

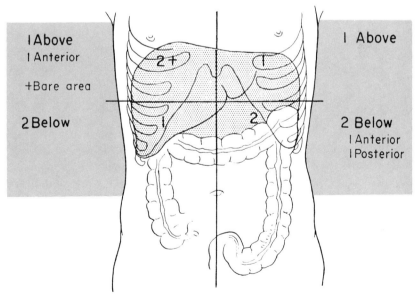

Figure 4–8. Diagram of a simple formula to remember the number and location of the subphrenic spaces. The positions of the spaces are shown in sagittal section in Figures 4–6 and 4–7.

87

It is helpful to know the probability of infection in a given area from a particular type of primary disease in attempting to localize an infection in any of these spaces. The posterior inferior space infection commonly occurs from the appendix, the right superior space infection from the gallbladder or duodenum, and left posterior inferior space infection from the pancreas.

The localization of physical findings in subphrenic abscess will be governed by the space involved.

Inspection

The early stages of a subphrenic abscess may produce remarkably little alteration in the patient's appearance or well–being. There may be slight fever, but with antibiotics this may not appear for some time. Pain is not a prominent feature, nor is it produced when the patient breathes deeply. There is no cyanosis or dyspnea. In more advanced cases an appearance of cachexia may occur without obvious localizing cause. Pain in the shoulder is so rarely encountered in the presence of a subphrenic abscess that it is of little value. In neglected cases perforation of the abscess into uninvolved areas such as the pleura, the lung, or the peritoneal cavity may produce severe pain, shock, and collapse. There are cases in which the abscess has been evacuated through the bronchial tree.

Careful inspection of the chest may reveal diminished expansion on the affected side. This may be quite striking in more advanced cases. Edema or fullness may be detected in the flanks in posterior space infections or under the costal margin in anterior superior space infections.

Percussion

The diaphragm on the affected side is limited or fixed in its motion and is elevated regardless of which space is involved. In superior space infections a pleural effusion is often present above the diaphragm. A very high diaphragm, without evidence of shift of the heart or mediastinum, is suggestive of subphrenic abscess. Percussion may demonstrate that the area of liver dullness is abnormally high, particularly in right superior space infections. When gas is present in the abscess, one may find an area of hyperresonance above the area of hepatic dullness, with another area of dullness above this due to a pleural effusion and compression of the lung. This can best be detected by upright roentgenograms (Fig. 4–9).

Palpation

Careful palpation (searching for areas of tenderness or edema over each of the suspected locations) is one of the most reliable means of detecting a subphrenic abscess. The following areas should be checked in

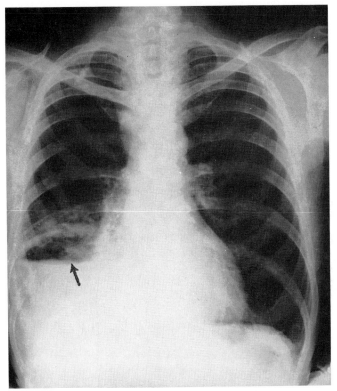

Figure 4–9. Classic x-ray appearance of a large right anterior superior subphrenic abscess. Note that although the diaphragm is elevated there is no shift of the mediastinum. It is rare to find air in the abscess cavity. More often the only roentgen signs are elevation and fixation of the diaphragm.

relation to the specific space infection:

Right anterior superior space. Under the costal margin anteriorly; between the ribs, especially in the sixth to the tenth intercostal spaces.

Right posterior inferior space. Over the tenth, eleventh, and twelfth intercostal spaces posteriorly; in the flank posterolaterally.

Right anterior inferior spaces. Below the costal margin anteriorly, much as in palpation of the liver or gallbladder.

Left superior space. Under the ribs anteriorly; in the epigastrium; in the sixth to the tenth intercostal spaces anterolaterally.

Left inferior anterior space. The left hypochondrium beneath the costal cage.

Left inferior posterior space. Over the twelfth rib posteriorly and in the left flank.

All available evidence must be scrutinized in doubtful cases. Repeated examinations of the suspected area are advisable. If the patient has had acute appendicitis, the right posterior inferior space is particularly suspected and should be repeatedly examined. A lesion of the left inferior space should be sought following an acute pancreatitis with necrosis and secondary infection following splenectomy for a penetrating abdominal wound with associated colonic injury.

The x-ray is of great value in recognizing subdiaphragmatic abscess; it is particularly helpful in the lateral view in localizing infections to an anterior or posterior space. Fluoroscopic evidence of an immobile diaphragm is additional evidence of a subphrenic abscess, but frequently the x-ray is indecisive and carefully repeated daily examinations of the suspected areas are necessary to corroborate the diagnosis.

In doubtful cases exploration of the suspected space is indicated. Needling of suspected subdiaphragmatic abscess should not be done, since the needle may traverse the pleural space or enter the liver, carrying infection with it. Direct exposure of the indicated space or spaces by special extraplural and extraperitoneal surgical operations is safer than an attempted aspiration of a suspected subdiaphragmatic abscess. Unless localization and adequate drainage are readily established, transperitoneal exploration should be performed.

chapter 5

THE EXAMINATION OF THE SURGICAL CARDIAC PATIENT

INTRODUCTION

The recent appearance of the surgeon on the cardiologic scene has placed a new emphasis and importance upon physical examination of the heart. In conjunction with chest x-ray and electrocardiogram, the physical examination is of crucial importance for a proper evaluation of the cardiac patient. An understanding of the physical signs outlined below presupposes a knowledge of the basic anatomy of the more common cardiac abnormalities. This chapter is concerned only with those findings that are significant in defining practical problems involved in the selection of patients for surgery or their postoperative management. The reader is referred to the many excellent textbooks on cardiology for more exhaustive treatment of cardiac diagnosis.

SOME POINTS IN HISTORY TAKING

The examiner must direct the history to yield information concerning: (1) cause, (2) morbid anatomy, and (3) functional capacity. Because the patient's functional capacity is his main concern, attention should be directed to this area first. A functional standard is based upon the severity of the patient's symptoms with regard to exertion. Helpful in this regard is the New York Heart Functional Classification: Class I, no symptoms; Class II, symptoms with moderate or severe activity; Class III, symptoms with mild sedentary living; and Class IV, symptoms at rest.

The examiner should take time to acquaint himself with the daily way of life of the patient. Some patients are so cleverly adjusted to their disease that they appear to be leading normal active lives. Close questioning of the wage earner still able to work full time may reveal that weekends and early evening hours are spent in bed so that work can go on. Analysis of the daily life of a housewife who seems able to get on despite her heart disease may reveal that she has the ideal husband who does all of the family chores. Teen-age daughters may be so skilled at homemaking that their mothers may lead the life of a cardiac invalid unnoticed.

Specific symptoms such as dyspnea, fatigue, orthopnea, palpations, paroxysmal nocturnal dyspnea, and angina should be elicited in terms of duration, frequency, and predisposing activities. Great care must be taken in eliciting important symptoms upon which surgical indications may be based. Thus syncope is an important symptom of aortic stenosis as a result of diminished cerebral blood flow. It may also occur with complete heartblock. Should the patient deny the presence of true fainting episodes care should be taken to inquire concerning the presence of light-headedness which may have the same significance.

A history of cerebral embolus, a feature of great importance in the evaluation of mitral valve disease, will not be easily missed. However, care should be taken to avoid overlooking the small stroke that results only in transient dizziness, aphasia, or short periods of mental confusion that may be easily forgotten by the patient unless prodded in the proper direction.

The history of paroxysmal rhythm disturbances is of the utmost surgical significance because these are apt to recur during or following operation. The knowledge of the exact mechanism may be of help in their diagnosis in the complicated postoperative period when the electrocardiogram may contain surgically induced bizarre patterns that make such diagnosis difficult.

The duration of atrial fibrillation in patients with mitral valve disease is of practical importance because this will determine the ease with which this rhythm disturbance may be terminated following corrective surgery. In isolated aortic valve disease the onset of this arrhythmia is a grave prognostic sign and indicates an urgent need for surgical correction.

Details of previous treatment, both medical and surgical, should be recorded. For example, if a subclavian pulmonary anastomosis was performed in the past was it end-to-end or end-to-side? Was a previously closed mitral commissurotomy followed by a clear-cut history of prolonged symptomatic benefit? If so, then a second closed commissurotomy may be indicated. The surgeon's report of previous operations must be obtained as a part of the medical history.

A careful history may be of great importance in establishing an etiologic diagnosis. The history of acute rheumatic fever or the presence of a murmur from the time of birth may lead at once to the proper classification of a cardiac illness. The family history may be of some help because rheumatic fever, coronary artery disease, and more rarely, congenital heart disease may be familial. A prenatal history may be important in revealing teratogenic factors. Rubella, for example, is associated with patent ductus arteriosus more often than with any other cardiac lesion.

SPECIAL PROBLEMS IN INFANTS AND CHILDREN

Because cardiac disease may seriously retard growth and development, questions concerning such matters are very much in order. In infancy fatigue or dyspnea may be evaluated quantitatively by the number of ounces of formula tolerated before such symptoms are noted. Dyspnea may not be apparent during the day but the parents may notice this symptom during the night, and will frequently describe the infant as sleeping fussily and noisily.

The age of onset of symptoms may be of importance in the differential diagnosis of many congenital defects. Simple atrial septal defects, for example, are rarely symptomatic in early infancy. In transposition of the great vessel, cyanosis is frequently noted at birth, while in tetralogy of Fallot it usually appears later in life, sometimes not until the second or third year. The earlier the cyanosis appears in tetralogy the more severe the stenosis. Squatting is not uncommon in such patients. Symptoms such as apnea or convulsions, when present in a cyanotic child, help to establish the urgency of corrective surgery because they are indicative of brain damage.

In general, surgical heart disease can be so widespread in its manifestations that there is no substitute for a *careful and orderly history* in providing perspective with which to pursue further evaluation by physical examination.

PHYSICAL EXAMINATION

Inspection

A sound general principle of surgery is never to feel what can be seen. The hand can never be as gentle as the eye. By means of inspection much can be learned before there is any physical contact with the patient. This is especially important in dealing with infants who tolerate handling poorly. Note is taken of the following:

Growth and development, facies, and physique. Congenital heart disease of clinical significance is frequently associated with retardation of growth and motor development. Such signs are of surgical importance and may determine the timing of corrective surgery. The facies and physique may reveal the typical features of congenital malformations associated

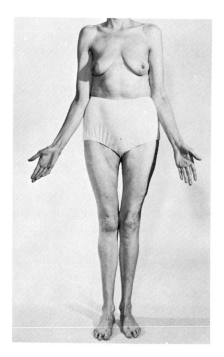

Figure 5–1. Marfan's syndrome. This patient has severe aortic regurgitation related to cystic medial necrosis of the aorta. Note the typical body habitus of Marfan's syndrome with arachnodactyly, increased carrying angle of the forearms. The patient is also unusually tall, has hyperextensible joints, a high palate, and congenital cataracts.

with cardiac involvement. These include Marfan's syndrome, mongolism, and the curious facies associated with supravalvular aortic stenosis. Good muscle development to the upper part of the body associated with underdeveloped lower extremities may be found in some instances of coarctation of the aorta.

Nutritional status. In infants, nutritional status may indicate feeding performance and hence provide a functional evaluation of cardiac disability. In adults, cachexia similar in severity to that seen in terminal carcinoma may occur with severe valvular heart disease.

Color. Arterial oxygen unsaturation may give the skin a ruddy, almost abnormally healthy appearance. When more severe, clear-cut cyanosis is evident. A very low venous oxygen saturation as a result of low cardiac output imparts to the skin a pearly gray color that is unmistakable to family members. Jaundice may be present and, when associated with severe congestive failure, may result from long-standing systemic venous hypertension.

Unusual pulsations. Unusual pulsations may be present in the neck and precordium. Accentuated arterial pulsations in the neck may be associated with aortic regurgitation, idiopathic hypertrophic subaortic stenosis (IHSAS), or coarctation of the aorta. Prominent venous pulsations may indicate tricuspid regurgitation. Occasionally, such venous pulsations result from a nodal rhythm. Uner such circumstances atrial contractions occur simultaneously with the ventricular contraction. Since the atrioventricular valves are closed at this time the atrial contraction is reflected in prominent venous pulsations known as cannon waves.

Abnormal precordial pulsations provide visible evidence of ventricular overactivity. A visible sternal systolic lift indicates right ventricular dilatation and hypertrophy. An overactive apical beat indicates left ventricular hypertrophy or dilatation. In severe regurgitant valvular lesions the entire precordium, including the patient, may shake with each heartbeat.

Skeletal abnormalities. Skeletal deformities of the precordium are not uncommon. The overdevelopment of the right ventricle seen in patients with atrial septal defect produces a characteristic bulging of the precordium. Mitral valve disease occurring in early childhood may also produce this change.

Respiration. Note is taken of the rate and character of respiration. If the patient has walked to the examining table or bed a quick glance will reveal the presence of dyspnea with this mild degree of exertion. Is the patient comfortable lying flat during the examinaion?

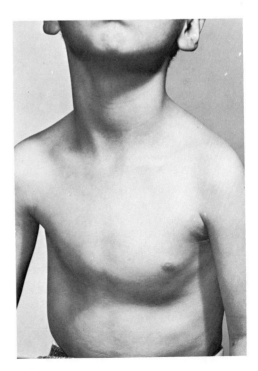

Figure 5–2. Protuberant precordium in patient suffering from atrial septal defect.

Palpation

Extremities and pulses. The initial physical contact with the patient should be palpation of all the peripheral pulses and examination of the hands and feet for clubbing, cyanosis, and edema. Palpation of the pulses early in the examination will give an indication of heart rate before the patient is disturbed, a point of some consequence with infants and children.

The amplitude and shape of the arterial pulse curve may be determined by palpation. In coarctation the femoral pulses when palpable are reduced in volume and are delayed by as much as one-half cardiac cycle because of the longer route taken by blood perfusing the collateral circulation. Frequently, the femoral pulses are impalpable, and blood pressure determinations in the arm and leg are necessary to confirm the diagnosis. A striking differential in pulse amplitude between upper and lower extremities is diagnostic in coarctation of the aorta.

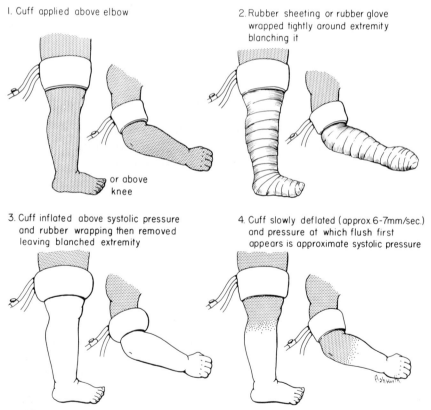

1. Cuff applied above elbow

or above knee

2. Rubber sheeting or rubber glove wrapped tightly around extremity blanching it

3. Cuff inflated above systolic pressure and rubber wrapping then removed leaving blanched extremity

4. Cuff slowly deflated (approx. 6-7mm/sec.) and pressure at which flush first appears is approximate systolic pressure

Figure 5–3. Demonstration of the use of flush pressure technique in diagnosis of coarctation of the aorta in infancy.

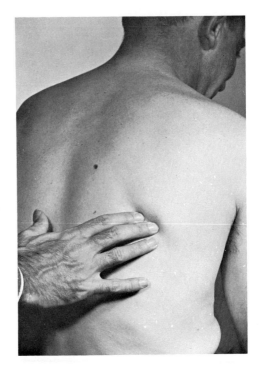

Figure 5–4. Palpation for collateral circulation in coarctation of the thoracic aorta. Light pressure over the latissimus dorsi muscle reveals pulsating collaterals as definite evidence of intrathoracic coarctation.

In infants, auscultation of the blood pressure in the legs is rarely possible. The flush technique (Fig. 5–3) allows a valid comparison between arm and leg systolic pressures: the "flush" pressure underestimates systolic pressure by 10 to 20 mm. Hg, but if the leg pressure is 20 mm. Hg or more below arm pressure, coarctation is almost certainly present.

Use of the "Doppler" technique allows more accurate determination of arm and leg systolic pressures. The blood pressure cuff may be conveniently placed around the upper arm and thigh while the Doppler ultrasound probe is held over brachial and popliteal arteries. At times the signal is better heard if the cuff is placed around the forearm and calf and the probe over the radial and dorsalis pedis artery.

When coarctation of the aorta is present in older children or adults, it is possible to confirm the presence of this lesion in the thoracic aortic segment by palpation of pulsating collateral circulation in the latissimus dorsi muscle as shown in Figure 5–4.

In infancy, markedly diminished pulses in all extremities usually indicate severe cardiac failure. Following proper medical therapy all pulses may improve or only the upper extremity pulses may improve, thereby establishing a pulse discrepancy and hence coarctation as the cause of the failure.

The shape of the pulse curve as established by palpation is of consequence. A collapsing pulse may be indicative of an aortic diastolic run-off as in patent ductus arteriosus, aorticopulmonary window, aortic regurgitation, or truncus arteriosus or it may indicate the premature functional closure of the left ventricular outflow tract characteristic of IHAS (idiopathic hypertrophic aortic stenosis). A slow-rising pulse with decreased amplitude and a small pulse pressure may be present in aortic stenosis. In combined aortic stenosis and aortic regurgitation the carotid pulse may have a double peaked quality and is termed a bisferious pulse.

The abdomen. The abdomen is examined for the presence of free fluid and for the size and location of the liver and spleen. The elevated systemic venous pressure associated with congestive failure frequently results in hepatosplenomegaly. In acute congestion there may be marked tenderness to palpation over the liver. This may be sufficiently severe to suggest an acute surgical abdomen. A common error in abdominal palpation is to miss hepatomegaly in infants by examining too close to the costal margin. Palpation is best begun in the right lower quadrant. If the abdomen is tense in the crying infant, advantage may be taken of the short periods of relaxation during inspiration.

Situs inversus may be detected by a left-sided liver. In azygous extension of the inferior vena cava, a rare venous abnormality, the liver is a midline structure filling the epigastrium.

Precordium. The precordium is next palpated for evidence of ventricular activity and thrills. Many a complex surgical problem can be clearly defined by an "educated" hand on the chest. The importance of this maneuver cannot be overestimated. A right parasternal lift suggests an overactive right ventricle, while a hyperactive apical impulse suggests left ventricular overactivity. A thrill may be palpable over the precordium and is an index of the intensity and the low frequency content of its associated murmur. Certain thrills are extremely helpful diagnostic findings; thus a systolic thrill is felt in the suprasternal notch or second right interspace in 90 per cent of patients with congenital valvular aortic stenosis. A thrill is felt at the second and third left interspace in about 50 per cent of those with pulmonic valvular stenosis and there is a thrill at the lower left sternal border in approximately 70 per cent of cases of ventricular septal defects.

Percussion of the cardiac borders adds little to the physical examination because cardiac enlargement and contour are best determined by the routine chest film.

Auscultation

THE LUNGS

The lungs are examined for evidence of failure, infection, and degenerative disease. In infancy, rales are present only in severe heart failure.

Rales heard in infancy are usually related to pulmonary infection or infection superimposed upon pulmonary edema, rather than to edema alone.

Adults, especially male smokers, are evaluated for evidence of chronic lung disease. This is a point of considerable significance with regard to the selection of patients for surgery or for their postoperative management with tracheotomy or artificial ventilation. Pulmonary emphysema may seriously hamper operability. The loudness of the breath sounds at rest and the ability to increase the intensity of breath sounds by overbreathing provide an excellent functional assessment of the severity of emphysema.

THE HEART

Auscultation of the heart is best carried out by seeking specific information one item at a time.

Rate and rhythm. While auscultation is important in this regard a more accurate determination of rate and rhythm is made with the electrocardiogram. This study should be a routine part of every cardiac examination.

Intensity of heart sounds. The heart sounds in general are evaluated for intensity. Distant heart sounds may suggest pericardial effusion or constrictive pericarditis. The influence of thickness of the chest wall in determining the intensity, however, should not be forgotten. Auscultation is routinely carried out over the apex (mitral area), the left parasternal area in the fifth intercostal space (the tricuspid area), the second and third intercostal space to the left of the sternum (the pulmonic area), and the right parasternal area in the second intercostal space (aortic area). Murmurs heard in these areas are followed either into the axilla, up into the neck, or into the left subclavicular area depending upon their source.

Normal heart sounds. The first heart sound corresponds in time to the onset of systole and closure of the atrioventricular valve. The second sound corresponds to the end of systole and is produced by closure of the semilunar valve. In diastole there may be a third heart sound following the second by about one-tenth of a second. This is related to rapid filling of the ventricles early in diastole. A fourth sound may be present just prior to systole and this is related to atrial contraction with increased rate of filling of the ventricles. The first sound is heard best at the apex while the semilunar closure sounds are best heard in the pulmonic area. The character of the sounds themselves are of clinical importance.

ACCENTUATED FIRST SOUNDS. In mitral stenosis the first sound is markedly accentuated and may even be palpable at the apex. This physical finding is of importance in differentiating pure or predominant mitral stenosis from a mixed stenosis and regurgitation.

EJECTION CLICK. The opening of a stenotic but flexible semilunar valve may be audible immediately after the first sound. The mechanism is probably caused by ballooning of the cusps into the aorta or pulmonary artery due to fusion of the commissures shortly after the onset of systole. With pulmonary valvular stenosis this is more easily heard over the pulmonic area, while with aortic valvular stenosis of a congenital type with flexible leaflets this is heard best over the aortic area and at the cardiac apex. The aortic click is constant throughout the respiratory cycle, while the pulmonic click is loudest in expiration and may disappear in inspiration. In each case the click is followed by the systolic murmur associated with the obstructing lesion.

OPENING SNAP. In instances of mitral or tricuspid stenosis associated with a flexible valve an opening snap is audible immediately after the closure of the pulmonic valve. This finding is of great significance in the selection of patients for reparative rather than replacement operations because an opening snap implies a flexible valve.

THE NORMAL SECOND SOUND. The second sound is normally split since the aortic and pulmonic valve closures are not simultaneous. The aortic valve closes first and is followed by the less intense pulmonic valve closure. The interval between the aortic valve closure and the pulmonic valve closure varies normally with respiration. During inspiration right heart filling is increased and right ventricular ejection time is hence increased. The interval between aortic and pulmonic closure sounds is therefore increased. During expiration the right ventricular ejection time is shortened while the left ventricular ejection time is increased owing to increased left ventricular filling. The interval therefore narrows between these two sounds.

LOUDNESS OF THE SECOND SOUND The very loud second, or pulmonic, sound is usually due to increased pulmonary artery pressure, although on occasion the normal closure sound may be quite loud when the chest wall is thin.

PURITY OF SECOND SOUND. When only one closure sound is heard there may be only one semilunar valve as in true or pseudotruncus arteriosus, or the pulmonic component may not be audible because of pulmonic stenosis.

PARADOXICAL SPLITTING OF THE SECOND SOUND. In severe aortic stenosis there may be paradoxical splitting of the second sound. The reason is that the obstructing lesion results in a prolonged aortic ejection time. As a consequence the closure of the aortic valve follows the closure of the pulmonic valve. With inspiration, right ventricular ejection is prolonged and the pulmonic closure more closely approximates the time of aortic closure. This results in a narrowing of the split with inspiration. With expiration the right ventricular ejection time is shortened so that the pulmonic closure occurs well before the aortic closure, thereby widening the split. This paradoxical splitting of the second sound is of clinical importance because it implies a clinically significant degree of aortic obstruction.

FIXED SPLITTING OF SECOND SOUND. Large atrial septal defects are associated with fixed splitting of the second sound. Since both atria communicate freely, they act like a single filling chamber. The increased venous inflow on inspiration influences left and right ventricles in a similar fashion so that there is no change in the degree of splitting between inspiration and expiration (fixed split). Although the venous inflow increases on inspiration, the left-to-right shunt decreases and left ventricular stroke volume increases as well. Therefore, in "fixed" splitting, both A_2 and P_2 are delayed to about the same extent during inspiration.

The split is normally of the order of .05 to .06 second and though some variation can be detected phonocardiographically this is not apparent to the ear and is a physical finding of prime importance in the diagnosis of isolated atrial septal defect.

Murmurs

Auscultation for murmur is perhaps the most important part of the physical examination of the heart. It should never be done halfheartedly. The room should be quiet and both the patient and examiner comfortable. The proper choice of stethoscope pays big dividends at this point. The habit of picking up any stethoscope that may be on the ward is soon discarded by the experienced examiner. Low intensity sounds that are easily missed may have crucial surgical significance. Murmurs are perhaps best understood when consideration is given to the mechanism of their production. They result from vibrations of the blood transmitted through the heart wall to surrounding structures as the result of turbulent blood flow. Since turbulence is related to the velocity of blood flow the murmurs will increase in intensity with increases in flow, such as may be caused by exercise, excitement, or fever. Changes in body position will affect the intensity of a murmur by altering the ease with which vibrations are conducted to the outside of the chest wall. Leaning forward during a forced exhalation may bring out a basilar diastolic murmur or aortic regurgitation or pulmonic regurgitation. Lying on the left side aids in the transmission of a mitral diastolic murmur to the chest wall.

For proper diagnosis a murmur must be analyzed in terms of *timing*: systolic (pansystolic, ejection), diastolic (immediate, mid, late, presystolic); *location of maximal intensity and transmission; quality; intensity; influence of respiration.*

Timing of murmurs. SYSTOLIC. Clinically significant systolic murmurs are usually either pansystolic or ejection. The pansystolic ejection murmur starts with the first heart sound and persists until ventricular systole is ended as evidenced by closure of the semilunar valves. It maintains a rather constant loudness throughout systole. Murmurs produced by turbulent flow from a contracting ventricle to a low pressure area are of this type. They include the murmurs of mitral regurgitation, tricuspid regurgitation, and most ventricular septal defects without severe pulmonary hypertension.

Ejection murmurs do not begin until after the first sound. They reach peak intensity later in systole and then decrease in intensity just prior to the second sound. The flow producing these murmurs is not sufficiently turbulent to make a noise except during the active ejection phase of the cardiac cycle. Such murmurs are usually produced by turbulent flow across obstructing lesions of the right or left ventricular outflow tract. In atrial septal defect there is a systolic ejection murmur in the pulmonic area that is caused by greatly increased pulmonary blood flow. It is, therefore, an ejection type murmur due to "relative infundibular stenosis" and not related to organic obstruction.

DIASTOLIC MURMURS. Diastolic murmurs occur between the closure sounds of the semilunar valves and the next systole. Between these two events the atrioventricular valves open to allow ventricular filling. Diastolic murmurs are therefore, in most cases, related to incompetence of the aortic or pulmonary valves or to turbulent flow across the atrioventricular valve during the ventricular filling. The various types of diastolic murmurs are best discussed with the associated pathologic anatomy. Indeed, the timing of the diastolic murmur may be predicted from a knowledge of the mechanism of production.

CONTINUOUS MURMURS. A continuous murmur extends throughout the entire cardiac cycle and usually reaches peak intensity in mid or late systole. It is always caused by run-off from a systemic or pulmonary vessel rather than from a cardiac chamber because ventricular diastolic pressure is not sufficiently high to sustain blood flow. It may be caused by aortic run-off into the pulmonary artery as in congenital or artificial patent ductus arteriosus, aorticopulmonary window, truncus arteriosus; or by collateral circulation in conjunction with coarctation of the aorta, or by severe pulmonary stenosis. It may be related to coronary artery run-off as in coronary AV fistula, or to pulmonary run-off as in pulmonary AV fistula. Continuous murmurs should be distinguished from a to and fro murmur. In the latter the systolic component diminishes in intensity and there is usually an interval before the diastolic component starts. An example of a to and fro murmur is that type seen with combined aortic stenosis and regurgitation. A more difficult to and fro murmur to distinguish from a continuous murmur is that caused by aortic regurgitation combined with ventricular septal defect. In this instance both murmurs may be sufficiently long so that it sounds like a continuous murmur.

Location of maximal intensity and transmission. Both the location of maximal intensity and transmission of a murmur are aids in the differential diagnosis of valvular disease. These may be predicted from a consideration of the anatomic placement of the cardiac chambers and great vessels and of the events taking place in the cardiac cycle that produce the murmur. Thus, mitral, tricuspid, and pulmonary murmurs are best heard in their respective areas. Aortic ejection murmurs are best heard in the aortic area. Aortic diastolic and pulmonic diastolic murmurs are best heard in the pulmonic area. Systolic murmurs due to right ventricular outflow tract turbulence are best heard directly over the outflow tract to the left of the sternum.

The murmur is transmitted in the direction of blood flow. Thus, aortic murmurs are transmitted into the neck. Pulmonary murmurs are transmitted into the left subclavicular area. Mitral systolic murmurs are transmitted into the axilla. Aortic and pulmonary diastolic murmurs are transmitted downward toward the apex.

There are some exceptions to these general principles, however. On occasion vibration of the septal leaflet of the mitral valve may be so severe that the adjacent aortic wall picks up the vibration and this murmur of mitral regurgitation is transmitted along the same pathways as an intrinsic aortic murmur.

Quality of murmurs. The experienced examiner may be greatly aided by the peculiar qualities of murmurs that almost defy description and are best appreciated by actual auscultation. The blowing quality diastolic murmur of aortic and pulmonary regurgitation, for example, is not easily confused with the rumbling, low-pitched diastolic murmur of mitral stenosis. The harsh systolic murmur of aortic stenosis lacks the musical quality found in many functional systolic murmurs.

Murmurs may be distinguished from a pericardial friction rub not only by the to and fro character of the friction rub, but also by the curious quality of a rub. Friction rubs seem to be close to the ear on auscultation. They are almost always present after cardiac surgery, may persist for many days, and are of no consequence.

Intensity. While it may seem initially cumbersome, it is of value to grade murmurs in intensity. Although a subjective finding, the grade of a murmur varies little from experienced examiner to examiner. Murmurs are best graded from I to VI in order of increasing loudness. A Grade I murmur is just barely audible in a quiet room. A Grade VI murmur is extremely loud and audible before the stethoscope actually reaches the chest wall. The most common murmurs lie between. The Grade II murmur is quite easily heard but low in intensity. A Grade III murmur is associated with a barely palpable thrill. A Grade IV murmur is associated with a more easily palpable thrill, and a Grade V murmur is extremely loud with an obvious and prominent thrill.

Grading is of some diagnostic and surgical importance. For example, simple atrial septal defects are almost never associated with a thrill while the more complex forms of atrial septal defect, such as those with valvular abnormalities, are often associated with a thrill. A ventricular septal defect of surgical significance is almost always associated with a thrill. The absence of a thrill suggests that very little shunting across the defect is taking place. This may be due to an extremely small sized ventricular

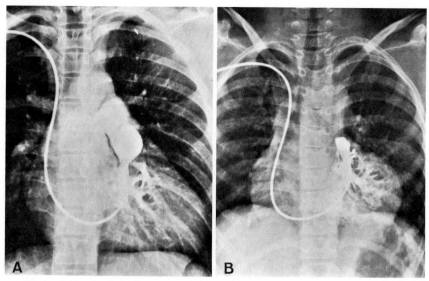

Figure 5–5. Angiocardiograms in tetralogy of Fallot. *A,* There is partial obstruction to the right ventricular outflow tract but enough flow of blood to visualize the pulmonary artery with contrast injection in the right ventricle. This patient has a loud systolic ejection murmur caused by flow in this area. *B,* Complete obstruction at the outlet of the right ventricle. This patient has no systolic ejection murmur since there is no flow through the right ventricular outflow tract.

septal defect with very small shunt, or to severe pulmonary hypertension that results in a markedly diminished shunt. The intensity of the murmur in tetralogy of Fallot is an indication of the magnitude of pulmonary blood flow. The more severe the stenosis, the less intense is the murmur. In pulmonary atresia there is a complete absence of murmur due to turbulent flow in the right ventricular outflow tract.

The influence of respiration. The relationship between the intensity of the cardiac murmur to the phase of the respiratory cycle will give an indication of whether the murmur arises from the right side or the left side of the heart. With inspiration there is increased filling of the right ventricle and hence increased flow through the right heart. With expiration, however, left ventricular filling is augmented and left ventricular flow is increased. Thus a right-sided systolic ejection murmur, as for example, that due to pulmonic stenosis, will increase with inspiration and decrease with expiration. On the other hand, a systolic ejection murmur due to aortic valve disease decreases with inspiration and increases with expiration.

Diastolic Flow Murmur

It has been noted that in some instances systolic murmurs, such as those found in atrial septal defect, may be due to turbulent flow through portions of the heart in which there is no organic stenosis. A similar mechanism holds for certain diastolic murmurs that are of the utmost surgical importance in dealing with congenital heart disease. These are the so-called diastolic flow murmurs that are due to turbulent flow through the normal mitral or tricuspid valve. The murmur appears in early diastole during the period of maximal ventricular filling. It is, therefore, synchronous in onset with the third heart sound since the mechanism of production of both is similar. The murmur can be differentiated, however, from the third heart sound by its duration. It also has an unmistakable low rumbling quality. The tricuspid flow murmur is best heard in the tricuspid area and the mitral flow murmur is best heard at the apex in the mitral area. At times the diastolic flow murmur may be extremely faint at rest but may be brought out by a little exercise. It is also influenced by the phase of respiration. Thus a tricuspid flow murmur being right-sided will increase with inspiration, while a mitral diastolic flow murmur being left-sided will increase with expiration. When inaudible at rest with quiet breathing, these murmurs may sometimes be brought out by deep breathing with accentuation of the particular phase of respiration required to bring out either a right-sided or a left-sided murmur.

The importance of the diastolic flow murmur is two-fold. First, it is indicative of a rather sizable increase in blood flow through the atrioventricular valve, and indicates a left to right shunt of sufficient magnitude to warrant surgery. Second, by its location, whether right-sided or left-sided, it helps to distinguish between the various types of left to right shunts. In atrial septal defect, for example, the increased pulmonary blood flow occurs via the tricuspid valve but not the mitral. The patient therefore has a tricuspid diastolic flow murmur. However, in ventricular septal defects and left to right shunts farther downstream from the left ventricle, the increased pulmonary blood flow must go through the mitral valve. Such patients have mitral diastolic flow murmurs.

CONGESTIVE FAILURE AND ANATOMIC DIAGNOSIS IN INFANCY

The infant in congestive failure presents a surgical challenge similar to that of the acute abdomen. The problem is urgent. Cardiac catheterization and angiocardiography are now possible even in the sickest infants and since the range of heart failure–producing lesions is so great, these studies should invariably be carried out prior to surgical intervention.

Ninety per cent of all children with congestive failure due to congenital heart disease present themselves for medical care during the critical first year of life. Not all are candidates for surgery but all require medical evaluation usually combined with hemodynamic and angiographic studies. Surgical consultation is indicated in the great majority of instances since with the available palliative and corrective procedures, most infants can be helped.

The age of onset of symptoms may have diagnostic significance. During the first week, hypoplastic left heart syndrome, transposition of the great arteries, double outlet right ventricle, and preductal coarctation predominate. Between one week and two months truncus arteriosus, simple postductal coarctation, and a large patent ductus anteriosus are frequently seen. From two months to four months, ventricular septal defects, common atrioventricular canal, and total anomalous pulmonary venous return are common. Other less common heart failure–producing lesions include aortic stenosis, tricuspid atresia with transposed great arteries, and atrial septal defects of the ostium primum type. It is also not generally appreciated that atrial septal defects of the secundum type can be associated with severe failure in infancy.

Signs of Congestive Failure

The infant is usually pale, sweaty, and appears desperately ill. Note should be made of the following signs of failure:

Cardiac dilatation. This may be the earliest sign of cardiac failure. It is best defined by x-ray and is related to an increase in both the volume of blood within the heart and fluid within the pericardial sac. Infants with obstruction to pulmonary venous return (for example, anomalous pulmonary venous drainage below the diaphragm into the liver) may have heart failure with cardiac dilatation.

Tachycardia. A normal pulse rate during the first year of life may be as high as 120 to 130 at normal body temperature. Consistent elevation of the pulse to 150 or more is usually an early sign of congestive failure.

Tachypnea. A respiratory rate consistently above 40 per minute in an infant may be an early and frequently is the earliest sign of failure.

Cyanosis. Mild cyanosis in infancy may be related to cardiac failure alone without intracardiac shunting. This finding is explained by alveolar hypoventilation associated with bronchiolar transudate and also by right to left shunt.

Edema. This is uncommon in infancy except in severe failure. Some experience is required to distinguish it from the normal puffiness and consistency of extremity fat.

Rales. This is a late sign of cardiac failure in infancy and lends urgency to the proper management — both medical and surgical.

Gallop rhythm. This may be present but is difficult to hear because of the rapid heart rate and the noise of breathing. It is not a valuable physical sign to attempt to elicit in dealing with infants.

Liver enlargement. The liver enlarges consistently with right heart failure. The infant liver is more compliant than its adult counterpart; thus, gross liver enlargement is seen even with venous pressures of 6 to 8 mm. Hg.

EMERGENCY SURGERY IN INFANCY

While anatomic variations among infants are numerous there are, nevertheless, clear-cut groups of anomalies requiring emergency surgery. Physical examination aided by chest x-ray and electrocardiogram may provide the exact diagnosis in some instances. However, in most cases, angiocardiography or cardiac catheterization is necessary.

Group I: Massive left to right shunt. Findings associated with overwhelming left to right shunt as a cause of congestive failure in infants are easily detected by examination. The common factor in this group is that surgery is directed at reducing pulmonary blood flow. In order of decreasing frequency, this group includes ventricular septal defect, patent ductus arteriosus, truncus arteriosus, aorticopulmonary window and double outlet right ventricle. In some instances transposition of the great vessels and tricuspid atresia are associated with such massive pulmonary overcirculation that treatment must be directed at diminishing pulmonary blood flow.

The essential features of examination include, in addition to the signs of congestive failure, the following findings: abrupt pulses, heaving precordium with overactivity in both ventricles, and a loud pansystolic murmur. There is frequently an apical diastolic flow murmur. The murmur of ductus or window may extend into diastole and help to distinguish these lesions from the rest of the group, but this is not always possible. The transposition cases or tricuspid atresias that fall into this group are not severely cyanotic. The purity of the second sound in truncus arteriosus may be helpful in distinguishing this entity from the remainder of the group.

The operative approach with lesions in this group depends upon the anatomic diagnosis. Patent ductus as an isolated lesion is treated by left thoracotomy and division. The recent demonstration of the safety of cardiac surgery in infancy has placed a high premium on exact anatomic diagnosis since ventricular septal defects, aorticopulmonary window, atrial ventricular canal, and atrial septal defects are now correctable in this age group. Banding of the pulmonary artery to reduce the left to right shunt is performed with decreasing frequency and primarily for lesions that are not easily correctable, such as tricuspid atresia with pulmonary overcirculation, transposition of the great arteries with large ventricular septal defects, truncus arteriosus, and single ventricle.

Total anomalous pulmonary venous drainage must be considered as a unique abnormality apart from this group. While pulmonary overcirculation is present the treatment is not banding of the pulmonary artery but the establishment of an adequate opening between the pulmonary veins and the left atrium. The anatomic diagnosis in such cases is best aided by angiocardiogram. On occasion the limiting factor is the small size of the foramen ovale allowing for insufficient egress of blood from the right to the left atrium. Under these circumstances useful palliation may be obtained by balloon atrial septostomy performed at cardiac catheterization. Total correction, however, is performed with increasing frequency and provides excellent results with the supracardiac and intracardiac type.

Group II: The obstructive group. The distinguishing feature of this group is the presence of an obstruction to pulmonic or systemic outflow.

On the right side this is most often pulmonic valvular stenosis, a condition amenable to surgical correction. The rapidly fatal course of this anomaly that appears very early in life and the ease with which it is approached surgically make diagnosis imperative. The patient has physical findings of severe congestive failure with evidence of right ventricular heave, a pure second sound at the base, a systolic ejection murmur over the outflow tract, normal or decreased pulmonary vascularity on chest x-ray, and evidence of right atrial hypertrophy and dilatation on electrocardiogram.

On the left side the obstructing lesion of importance is coarctation of the aorta. Reference has already been made to the diagnostic features of this condition (p. 96). When all pulses are diminished due to severe low cardiac output, coarctation may be confused with left-sided hypoplasias. Since the latter are invariably fatal, cardiac catheterization is in order for accurate delineation of the lesion.

Group III: The cyanotic group. The distinguishing feature of this group is the presence of severe cyanosis despite oxygen administration. These anomalies consist of transposition of the great vessels with pulmonary overcirculation, transposition with pulmonic stenosis, tetralogy of Fallot, and tricuspid atresia with pulmonary undercirculation. Differential diagnosis must be more accurate than in the left to right shunt group since many different operative procedures are available. Transposition without pulmonic stenosis may be palliated by balloon atrial septostomy or by creation of an atrial septal defect by right thoracotomy. Definitive correction of transposition is best accomplished by the Mustard intra-atrial baffle procedure whereby caval blood is rerouted through the mitral valve and pulmonary venous blood through the tricuspid valve.

Surgical treatment of tetralogy of Fallot is accomplished by one stage total correction or by a palliative shunt procedure (usually ascending aorta to right pulmonary artery) followed several years later by total correction. Our preference has been for one stage total correction in any infant in whom the pulmonary annulus is at least one-third the diameter of the aortic annulus. Surgical treatment of the other anomalies in this group is aimed at shunting blood into the lungs. This is accomplished most often by a systemic artery to pulmonary artery shunt and rarely by means of a vena cava to pulmonary artery shunt.

Transposition of the great vessels with pulmonary overcirculation is the number one cause of heart failure in infancy and is second only to ventricular septal defect and patent ductus arteriosus as the most common congenital abnormality. The diagnostic key is severe cyanosis associated with some of the physical findings of pulmonary overcirculation, i.e., abrupt pulses, active precordium, systolic murmur, accentuated pulmonic second sound, and apical flow murmur. Total anomalous pulmonary venous drainage may present with mild cyanosis and pulmonary overcirculation and may be confused clinically with transposition. For this reason, angiocardiographic studies are helpful in confirming the diagnosis prior to operation. The remaining members of this group are similar in that there are severe cyanosis and diminished pulmonary circulation. Thus on physical examination the heart is relatively small and quiet. The pulmonic second sound is diminished or absent. Angiocardiography is important in distinguishing among tetralogy of Fallot, transposition of the great vessels with pulmonic stenosis, tricuspid atresia, and pulmonic stenosis with atrial septal defect.

CORRECTIVE SURGERY IN CHILDHOOD

Evaluation of the older child with congenital heart disease lacks the sense of urgency associated with the acutely ill infant. Surgery in this age group over two is directed at total correction whenever possible and therefore an accurate preoperative diagnosis is of crucial importance. Cardiac catheterization and angiocardiogram are almost always employed, but such studies must be selected and interpreted in the light of physical examination.

Ventricular Septal Defect

Closure of a ventricular septal defect is indicated only in the presence of significant shunting. In general a significant shunt is one in which the pulmonary flow to systemic flow ratio is 1.5 to 1 or greater. Since many defects close spontaneously, shunts larger than this may be safely followed if there is clinical evidence to suggest diminishing size or if there is no increase in pulmonary vascular resistance. Tiny muscular defects associated with normal-sized hearts, little or no thrill, and a musical systolic murmur are best left alone. Such patients lack the abrupt pulse, systolic thrill, precordial overactivity, and apical diastolic flow murmur of a large left to right shunt across the ventricular septum. Large ventricular septal defects may be associated with little or no shunt in the presence of extremely high pulmonary vascular resistance. Such cases have a right ventricular heave, very loud or palpable pulmonic second sound, and little or no murmur. They have none of the physical findings of significant left to right shunts. Such patients should not be operated upon except under unusual circumstances when it can be demonstrated at catheterization that the pulmonary vascular resistance can be lowered by oxygen administration or by pulmonary vasodilating drugs. Established right to left shunting with fixed pulmonary vascular resistance (Eisenmenger syndrome) is an absolute contraindication to surgery.

Atrial Septal Defects

In a surgical evaluation of atrial septal defect important physical signs are related to the type of atrial septal defect, the magnitude of the shunt, and the level of pulmonary hypertension. Simple or secundum types of atrial septal defects are associated with a normal pulse, right ventricular heave, no thrill, soft right-sided systolic ejection murmur, and fixed splitting of the second sound. More complicated types of atrial septal defect–associated atrioventricular valve abnormalities (cushion defects) frequently are associated with a precordial thrill, a pansystolic murmur of mitral regurgitation, or a ventricular septal defect or both. The magnitude of shunting is determined by the degree of cardiomegaly and the presence of a tricuspid flow murmur. Severe pulmonary hypertension is rare and an assessment of this feature is related to the severity of the pulmonic second sound. Surgical closure is indicated in the great majority of cases of atrial septal defect since spontaneous closure is rare and pulmonary hypertension may develop in adult life.

Patent Ductus Arteriosus

The physical diagnosis of this lesion is not always simple. The typical machinery murmur is not found in some cases associated with very high pulmonary artery pressure. In addition, when the typical murmur is present it may be due to aorticopulmonary window, coronary AV fistula, or a ventricular septal defect with aortic regurgitation. When the left to right shunt is large a mitral diastolic flow murmur is usually present, along with evidence of left ventricular overactivity. Division or ligation of a patent ductus arteriosus is almost always indicated since the vessel rarely closes spontaneously and the threat of pulmonary hypertension or of bacterial endocarditis is a continuing risk.

Pulmonic Stenosis

This lesion is associated with the findings of right ventricular hypertension (sternal heave), and a long systolic ejection murmur transmitted to the left subclavicular area and right-sided in its behavior with respiration.

It is impossible by physical examination alone to distinguish valvular from subvalvular or infundibular stenosis. It is also impossible to detect, in all cases, associated atrial or ventricular septal defects. These require special studies prior to operation. Surgery is indicated when the right ventricular pressure exceeds 60 mm. Hg; in doubtful cases, right ventricular pressure may be remeasured when the child is fully grown.

Aortic Stenosis

Here again fibrous subvalvular, valvular, and supravalvular stenosis are indistinguishable on physical examination. Equally difficult is an assessment of the degree of obstruction from clinical findings alone. Few children show the diminished pulse pressure and slow rise time that characterize the late stages of this disease. Even the electrocardiogram may be normal in the presence of severe obstruction. Patients suspected of aortic stenosis because of the presence of a left-sided systolic ejection murmur over the aortic area transmitted to the neck should have a gradient that is measured across the outflow tract and a contrast visualization of this area. Absolute indications for surgery are a peak systolic gradient of over 75 mm. Hg, an aortic valve area of less than 0.5 cm.^{2} per m.^{2}, and changes of left ventricular ischemia on the ECG in the presence of angina or multiple syncopal spells.

Tetralogy of Fallot

Certain features of the physical examination aid greatly in the selection of patients for total correction of this anomaly. The intensity of the murmur is related to the degree of obstruction. Patients with a loud murmur and thrill have only mild stenosis and are excellent candidates for total correction. Patients with little or no murmur have severe pulmonary outflow tract obstruction or pulmonary atresia. Preoperative angiographic and hemodynamic assessment is mandatory. As in the case of infants, the size of the pulmonary annulus is of critical importance, although appropriate patching of the outflow tract, pulmonary annulus, and main pulmonary arteries allows total correction in almost every instance in which right ventricle-to-pulmonary artery continuity can be angiographically demonstrated. For those cases in which no continuity exists the Rastelli procedure is indicated.

Truncus Arteriosus

The Rastelli procedure, whereby a valve-containing conduit is constructed from the free wall of the right ventricle to the pulmonary artery bifurcation, now makes total functional correction of this anomaly possible.

Unfortunately, the success rate is low in infancy but rises to acceptable levels in children two to three years of age. For the infant with severe pulmonary hypertension, palliative banding of the pulmonary artery is probably indicated.

Tricuspid Atresia

Correction of tricuspid atresia, most often associated with hypoplasia of the right ventricle and decrease in pulmonary blood flow, has recently been attempted in older children by constructing a valve conduit from the right atrium to the pulmonary artery. The atrium then becomes the functioning right ventricle. Regurgitation down the inferior vena cava is prevented by placing a second valve at the caval atrial junction.

CORRECTIVE SURGERY FOR ACQUIRED VALVE DISEASE

The selection of patients for surgery in this group depends heavily upon physical examination. Indeed, cardiac catherization and hemodynamic studies may be extremely misleading if not correlated with the clinical findings. Since multiple valve involvement is not uncommon the examiner must be alert to this possibility.

Mitral Stenosis

Physical examination will yield information concerning the amount of associated mitral regurgitation, the flexibility of the mitral valve, and the degree of pulmonary hypertension. These features have been previously discussed but cannot be overemphasized. A loud, snapping first heart sound with absent systolic murmur is much more reliable in determining the presence of pure stenosis without regurgitation than the left atrial pressure tracing. The opening snap by denoting a flexible valve suggests that repair rather than replacement will be possible. A loud pulmonic second sound is excellent evidence that the stenosis is clinically significant and is operable. A diastolic decrescendo basal murmur may be present due to pulmonary artery dilatation with resulting pulmonic regurgitation. This so-called Graham Steell murmur is indistinguishable from aortic regurgitation. The only way this can be further elucidated is by supravalvular aortogram. Since integrity of the aortic valve is important during cardiopulmonary bypass this special study should be done on all patients who are candidates for open mitral surgery.

Mitral Regurgitation

Signs of left ventricular overactivity associated with a pansystolic apical murmur transmitted to the axilla and posterior lung fields strongly suggest the presence of mitral regurgitation. Care must be taken, as in dealing with mitral stenosis, to determine the competence of the aortic valve.

The absence of a loud, rumbling apical diastolic murmur in such cases suggests annular dilatation as the predominant lesion in the production of mitral regurgitation. When the annulus is of normal size and the regurgitation is severe there is almost always a diastolic murmur of significant proportion. An opening snap suggests the presence of a large septal mitral leaflet and implies that repair may be possible. This is also the case with ruptured chordae tendinae, easily diagnosed by the characteristic rasping, musical murmur widely transmitted along the aortic system.

Aortic Stenosis

The typical plateau pulse is frequently present in adults with this condition. Signs of left ventricular hypertrophy are associated with a coarse, left-sided ejection murmur transmitted into the neck. The second aortic sound is usually absent when valvular calcification is extreme. In far advanced cases the murmur may actually be lower in intensity than in early cases because of the greatly reduced cardiac output.

Left ventricular dilatation does not occur until the final stages of this disease. Such a finding in pure stenosis implies a poor prognosis and a need for urgent surgery. With ventricular dilatation, a rumbling mitral diastolic murmur (Austin Flint) may be heard due to turbulent flow through a normal mitral valve. This murmur may be indistinguishable from organic mitral disease. Thus, with advanced aortic valve disease the most crucial hemodynamic preoperative study is a pressure tracing across the mitral valve.

Aortic Regurgitation

The typical findings of severe aortic regurgitation with widened pulse pressure, heaving precordium, and loud decrescendo basilar diastolic murmur are difficult to miss. In such cases also the presence of a rumbling apical diastolic murmur may have no significance, or may imply the presence of organic mitral disease. It is only by pressure tracings across the mitral valve that an accurate assessment may be made of mitral valve function associated with severe aortic valve disease.

In far advanced cases the pulse pressure may diminish as cardiac dilatation and failure occur. Thus, significant aortic regurgitation can occur in the presence of a relatively normal pulse pressure.

In evaluating aortic regurgitation care should be taken to check for the typical findings of Marfan's syndrome as previously described (p. 94). However, cystic medical necrosis of the aorta can occur without any of the other findings of this syndrome. Occasionally, careful ophthalmologic examination in such cases will reveal lens deformities and liquid vitreous.

Tricuspid Valve Disease

Organic tricuspid stenosis or regurgitation is easily amenable to surgical correction. The diastolic rumble of stenosis is best heard slightly left of the xyphoid since the tricuspid valve is frequently displaced to the left by a large right atrium. Tricuspid regurgitation produces a soft pansystolic murmur in the same area. If the leaflets are flexible and stenosis is present, an opening snap may be audible. In many cases of chronic mitral valve disease, tricuspid regurgitation may be associated with chronic right heart dilatation due to congestive failure rather than primary valve disease. In such cases of functional tricuspid stenosis, a history of repeated episodes of ascites and hepatomegaly is important in establishing the diagnosis. Intensive preoperative medical management by sharply reducing blood volume may render the valve temporarily more competent at surgery. It is possible that in patients with this condition prophylactic fixation of a tricuspid annulus to prevent subsequent dilatation may be indicated.

Coronary Artery Disease

Surgery for coronary artery disease currently surpasses all other major operations in frequency of application. The complications of myocardial infarction, such as congestive failure, ventricular aneurysm, ventricular septal defect, and ruptured papillary muscle of the mitral valve, provide useful physical signs. However, the vast majority of patients with ischemic heart disease have no pertinent physical findings. In many instances, the electrocardiogram may be normal both at rest and with exercise. Thus coronary arteriography is the crucial study and is employed with increasing frequency when there is a suspicion of significant disease. Its application hinges very much on a careful history eliciting the symptoms of angina in all of its ramifications. Many patients with angina have no "chest pain" but complain of pain in the jaw, back, left arm, and epigastrium. Some have only a feeling of tightness and will deny pain. The critical feature in the diagnosis of angina is the prompt response of the pain to rest and nitroglycerin. Since mild chronic angina is not at present an indication for coronary arteriography, it is important to define in the history the progressive severity of the symptoms and the functional classification. Patients with crescendo or rapidly progressing angina require urgent hospitalization and evaluation and those with chronic severe angina (Class III or IV) require elective hospitalization and studies.

Myocardial Infarction

Persistent cardiac pain unresponsive to rest and nitroglycerin is an indication for emergency hospitalization with a presumptive diagnosis of acute myocardial infarction or acute coronary insufficiency. This condition must be distinguished from acute dissection of the aorta and acute pericarditis. The pain of dissection is most severe and frequently referred to the back of the chest and lumbar region. The presence of acute aortic regurgitation or the sudden loss of a peripheral pulse is diagnostic of dissection. This should be confirmed by aortography since the early treatment of acute dissection with antihypertensive and negative ionotropic agents is important to the survival of the patient. A pericardial friction rub may be present in both infarction and pericarditis. Serial electrocardiogram and serum enzyme levels usually resolve the question.

The patient with an established infarct, even in a coronary care unit, must be carefully observed for problems readily discerned by physical examination. Thus, the earliest sign of left ventricular failure may be a gallop rhythm and a few rales at the lung bases. The sudden appearance of a systolic murmur suggests either ruptured ventricular septum or rupture of the papillary muscle of the mitral valve. Both produce pansystolic murmurs. Ruptured septum produces a loud murmur usually with a thrill with maximum intensity along the left sternal border. Rupture of the papillary muscle of the mitral valve produces a murmur heard maximally at the apex and transmitted into the axilla. In rare cases complete rupture of a papillary muscle occurs with no associated murmur and may be confused with massive pulmonary embolus. The mitral leaflets turn completely inside out and retrograde flow through the valve is laminar. Since urgent surgery is required for ventricular septal defect and ruptured papillary muscle, diagnosis should be confirmed by left ventriculography done on an emergency basis. The development of a ventricular aneurysm usually at the anterolateral portion of the left ventricle may provide the physical finding of an increased and paradoxical apical thrust. Here again, chest x-ray and left ventriculography is required to confirm the diagnosis and aid in the time of surgical excision.

A Note of Warning

The precision and safety of cardiac surgery requires an exact preoperative diagnosis. Exploration is not as safe as in many other areas of surgery. In addition, the cardiovascular system lends itself well to special diagnostic studies since it is so accessible to contrast agents and catheters. However, the very precision of such studies may seduce the young surgeon to rely heavily on these laboratory findings to the exclusion of an adequate history and physical examination. Nothing could be more dangerous. The indications and timing of special procedures hinge rather completely on the clinical evaluation of the patient. The best surgery is an amalgam of history, physical examination, and laboratory studies, with surgical exploration and a proper technique skillfully applied.

chapter 6

EXAMINATION OF THE INGUINAL AND FEMORAL REGIONS AND THE MALE EXTERNAL GENITALIA – THE DIFFERENTIAL DIAGNOSIS OF HERNIA

It is a good habit to examine the inguinal and femoral canals and the male external genitalia before examining the abdomen. If this examination is performed first, many a clue to abdominal signs and symptoms will be found. Moreover, there is no danger of becoming so intrigued by abdominal signs that the groin is overlooked.

Since the examination of this region in male and female patients differs in detail, each will be described separately. The examination of this region in infants and children is described in Chapter 8.

I. THE ADULT MALE EXTERNAL GENITALIA

An examination of the external male genitalia is performed at the same time as that of the inguinal and femoral regions. The patient should be examined in a good light and in both the standing and supine positions if possible. The precise anatomic location of an abnormality is the best

117

clue to its identification, so a good working knowledge of the anatomy is essential.

Technique of Examination

Inspection

The examiner notes the development of the genitalia, the distribution of the pubic hair, and the presence and contour of any visible mass. The skin is inspected for scars, excoriations, fungal infections, and sinuses.

The patient is then instructed to cough while the examiner scrutinizes the region of the femoral canal, the external inguinal ring, and the internal abdominal ring for the telltale bulge of a hernial defect. Any change in the size or contour of an existing mass is also noted. Occasionally a small hernia can be seen more readily than it can be felt.

The patient is asked to retract the foreskin, and the prepuce and glans are inspected for scars, balanitis, chancre, or erosion. *Acute urethritis* is recognized by having the patient strip his urethra with his thumb and forefinger to express the purulent urethral discharge. Congenital malformations of the penis are readily detected. In *hypospadias* the urethral opening lies somewhere on the underside of the shaft. In *epispadias* it lies on the dorsum. *Phimosis* is the presence of a long prepuce with a narrow ori-

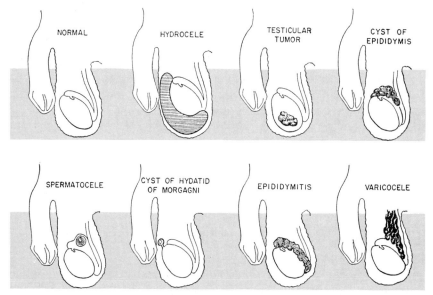

Figure 6–1. Lesions of the scrotum and its contents. The nature of a swelling or nodule in the scrotum can be readily established if the normal relationships of the testicle, epididymis, and tunica vaginalis are kept in mind.

fice which prevents normal retraction and replacement of the foreskin. *Paraphimosis* occurs when a narrow phimotic foreskin is retracted and cannot be replaced. An alarming amount of swelling of the retracted prepuce rapidly appears. If manual reduction fails, surgical division of the restricting band (a dorsal slit) is indicated.

Palpation of the Scrotum and Its Contents

The examiner must pick up the scrotum and testicle, supporting it with one hand while palpating with the other. Note the presence of both testicles, the characteristic shape of the epididymis, and the consistency of the spermatic cord. Bear in mind that the testis is embraced by the tunica vaginalis on its anterior and lateral aspect and by the crescent-shaped epididymis on its posterior aspect. The cord passes down the scrotum on the posterior aspect of the testicle and reaches it at its base, where it develops into the epididymis (Fig. 6–1). If the normal shape and consistency of the testis, epididymis, and cord are familiar to the examiner, abnormalities are readily distinguishable.

Some Lesions of the Scrotum

Hydrocele. A diffuse, tense, slightly fluctuant, nonreducible mass which transilluminates readily is usually a hydrocele. The testis and epididymis can be identified posteriorly with careful palpation (Fig. 6–1). Transillumination is best accomplished by tensing the mass between the fingers and pressing a small flashlight well into its lateral side away from the direct vision of the examiner. If transillumination is successfully demonstrated, the diagnosis is conclusively established.

Cyst of the epididymis. A small cyst of the epididymis appears upon transillumination as a tense, well circumscribed, nonreducible nodule lying posteriorly. It may be lobulated, and it may lie in any portion of the epididymis from the upper to the lower pole (Fig. 6–1).

Spermatocele. This is a nontender, well localized swelling lying posteriorly along the course of the epididymis. It does not transilluminate as clearly as a hydrocele or a cyst of the epididymis (Fig. 6–1).

Cyst of the hydatid of Morgagni. A translucent cystic nodule on the anterior superior aspect of the testicle is a cystic hydatid; it is recognizable by its distinct anterior position (Fig. 6–1).

Epididymitis (tuberculous). The epididymis is enlarged and of a firm, usually nontender, rubbery consistency. The vas is also thickened or "beaded."

Epididymo-orchitis. Tenderness and uniform swelling are present if the inflammation is confined largely to the epididymis (Fig. 6–1). The vas may also be tender and swollen. In advanced cases, the testicle is also involved, and the distinction between testis and epididymis lost; it may be difficult to distinguish from torsion of the testis except by the history.

Varicocele. This is a soft, wormlike mass which extends upward along the cord. It is separable from the testis and epididymis (Fig. 6–1) and is nonfluctuant, transmits no impulse, and does not transilluminate. It collapses in the supine position.

Testicular tumor. The body of the testis is enlarged and may be irregular. The tumor may be of any size and involve the entire body, or may merely be a nodule protruding from the surface of the testis (Fig. 6–1). Normally there is a characteristic tenderness associated with palpation of the testis; in the presence of neoplasia this may disappear. There may be an associated hydrocele which makes identification of the tumor extremely difficult.

Syphilis will produce a smooth, painless enlargement of the testis.

Torsion of the testical and scrotal hernia may be confused with primary lesions of the testicle or epididymis. Very sudden onset of testicular pain in otherwise healthy individuals suggests torsion. The testicle is enlarged and exquisitely tender. Palpation of the cord will show thickening, and sometimes a definite twist can be identified within the cord. The differential diagnosis between an acute epididymo-orchitis and torsion of a fully descended testicle is sometimes quite difficult. If there is a history of recent surgery or infection involving the genitourinary tract, the diagnosis of epididymo-orchitis is likely. Elevation and immobilization of the scrotum will relieve the pain in an inflammatory lesion while it will not relieve the pain in torsion.

Torsion of the testicle is a critical emergency. Prompt operation will avoid infarction and loss of the testicle.

An irreducible scrotal hernia may be mistaken for a lesion arising within the scrotum. A scrotal hernia will not usually transilluminate, but occasionally a gas-filled loop of bowel may be translucent. Palpation of the structures of the cord above the mass is the best evidence that the lesion is not a hydrocele. Marked thickening of the cord extending upward through the external ring is conclusive evidence that the lesion is not confined to the scrotum. Peristalsis may be audible within the mass.

Palpation of the Urethra and Penis

Palpation is indicated if there are complaints of pain or urethral discharge or if swellings or sinuses are noted. A *periurethral abscess* may be felt as a tender, fluctuant nodule usually in the middle of the shaft. An area of scarring or induration, especially at the base of the penis, is seen in *urethral stricture.*

Rarely the dorsal vein of the penis becomes thrombosed, producing a tender cord running down the upper surface of the organ just beneath the skin. This is usually idiopathic, but may occur in leukemia.

II. THE LYMPHATICS OF THE GROIN

The lymph nodes of the groin consist of an inguinal and a subinguinal group (Fig. 6–2). The subinguinal group may be divided into a superficial and a deep group. The superficial subinguinal nodes lie along the course of the saphenous vein and are especially numerous around the saphenous opening. *The gland of Cloquet*, which lies directly above the saphenous opening, belongs in this group; when enlarged, it stimulates an incarcerated or strangulated femoral hernia. Drainage to these nodes is from the skin and subcutaneous tissues of the foot and leg.

The deep subinguinal nodes lie medial to the femoral vein and follow the course of this vessel into the pelvis where they join the external iliac

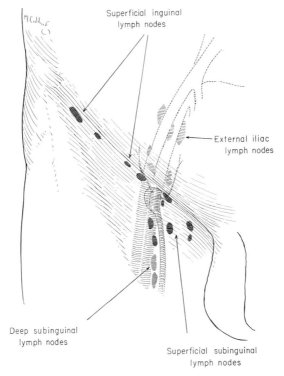

Figure 6–2. Lymph nodes of the groin.

Superficial inguinal lymph nodes receive lymphatic vessels from the integument of the penis, scrotum, perineum, buttock, and abdominal wall below the level of the umbilicus.

Superficial subinguinal lymph nodes receive the superficial lymphatic vessels of the leg and some from the penis, scrotum, perineum, and buttock.

Deep subinguinal lymph nodes receive the deep lymphatic trunks of the leg, and efferents from the penis, clitoris, and the superficial subinguinal nodes.

External iliac lymph nodes receive efferent vessels from the inguinal and subinguinal nodes, the deep lymphatics of the abdominal wall below the umbilicus, the glans penis, clitoris, membranous urethra, prostate, fundus of the bladder, cervix uteri, and upper part of the vagina.

nodes. The deep subinguinal nodes are involved in any extensive inflammation or neoplastic process involving the lower extremities.

The inguinal nodes lie along and parallel to the inguinal ligament. These drain the external genitalia, the perineum, and the anus.

Small, firm, nontender nodes are frequently palpable in the superficial subinguinal and inguinal group and represent the end result of previous episodes of mild infection. If enlarged and tender, they usually indicate a recent acute infection, but frequently the patient is not aware of the primary lesion.

Epidermophytosis is a common cause of relatively asymptomatic cracks and fissures of the feet which permit the entrance of virulent organisms into the tissues and lymphatics. This source of inflammation in enlarged, tender, superficial subinguinal nodes is often found by carefully separating the toes and inspecting the interdigital spaces. One should also scrutinize the genitalia, the perineum, and the anus for sites of infection when the superficial subinguinal chain of nodes is involved. The foreskin should be retracted and carefully inspected for ulceration or scarring. When no obvious site is found in the leg or perineum, a rectal examination may disclose either an inflammatory or a neoplastic lesion.

Extensive, painless inguinal adenopathy may be seen in *lymphoma, Hodgkin's disease,* and *lymphopathia venereum.* Metastases from minute, pigmented, *malignant melanomas* characteristically appear in the groin, and the primary lesion may be so small that detailed scrutiny of the entire extremity, especially the sole of the foot and toenails, is required. The hard, discrete nodules of *metastatic cancer* usually are the result of a primary source in the penis or anus. Biopsy may be required to establish the diagnosis.

III. HERNIA AND THE INGUINAL CANAL

Hernia: Some Definitions and General Considerations

Definitions

A *hernia* is a protrusion through a weak spot or cleft in the lining of a body cavity. An *abdominal hernia* is a protrusion of a sac lined with peritoneum through a defect in the abdominal wall. A *reducible hernia* is one in which the contents of the sac can be returned to the abdominal cavity. An *irreducible hernia* or *incarcerated hernia* is one in which the contents cannot be returned to the abdomen; there is no inflammation of the sac or contents and no interference with the blood supply. A *strangulated hernia* is one in which the blood supply to the contents of the sac has been obstructed. A *Richter's hernia* is a strangulated hernia in which only a portion of the wall of a loop of intestine is caught in the constricting ring. Gangrene may ensue without evidence of intestinal obstruction.

The Parts of a Hernia and the Nature of the Hernial Contents

All hernias consist of three parts: the sac, its contents, and its coverings. These will vary according to the location of a given hernia. In many instances it will contain no abdominal viscera. Omentum is most commonly encountered. Next in order of frequency are the ileum, the jejunum, and the sigmoid. The appendix, other segments of large bowel, the stomach, and even the liver have been reported within large hernial sacs.

The contents may be appraised upon physical examination. The omentum feels relatively plastic and slightly nodular. Bowel may be suspected when the sac is smooth and tense as in a hydrocele, but is not translucent. Occasionally, the examiner may feel gas moving within the loop or auscultation may reveal peristalis. A gas-filled loop of bowel will be tympanitic to percussion. In cases of strangulation the signs of inflammation may appear, but occasionally strangulated hernias are remarkably nontender.

Examination of the Inguinal Canal

The procedure is always uncomfortable for the patient and must be conducted with gentleness and consideration. It is performed by placing the examining finger at the lowermost portion of the scrotum and then invaginating the sac into the inguinal canal. If sufficient scrotum is invaginated, the palmar surface of the examining finger comes in contact with the external inguinal ring with enough play for the finger to be moved about freely without undue discomfort to the patient (Fig. 6–3). The following normal structures should be identified: the crest of the os pubis just lateral to the pubic spine, the arching fibers of the external inguinal ring, the cord as it passes into the inguinal canal, the tone and resistance of the posterior wall of the canal in Hesselbach's triangle, and the region of the internal ring.

If the ring is large enough to admit the finger, it may be introduced into the inguinal canal perpendicular to the abdominal wall where it somes into contact with the posterior wall of the inguinal canal in Hesselbach's triangle. The general tone and strength of this structure are noted. If there is a marked weakness or defect here, the finger may be introduced further so that it actually enters the abdominal cavity. Such relaxation presupposes the existence of a direct hernia.

If the finger is directed laterally and obliquely after entering the external ring, the spermatic cord can be followed upward toward the internal abdominal ring. The presence of a mass or impulse upon coughing should be sought with the finger in each of these locations. The following lesions must be distinguished during this part of the examination:

Indirect inguinal hernia. An indirect hernia appears as an elongated slightly elliptical mass which passes through the internal ring and de-

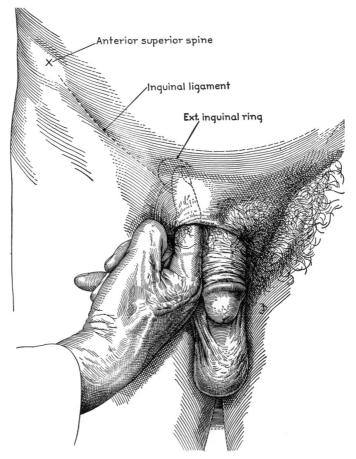

Figure 6–3. Technique of invagination of the scrotum to permit thorough palpation of the inguinal canal.

scends along the cord for a variable distance toward the scrotum (Fig. 6–4). The mass is often reducible and after reduction a distinct thickening in the canal may be felt at the upper edge of the scrotum. The manner in which a hernial sac descends through the canal when the patient coughs or strains may help to distinguish between a direct and an indirect hernia. If the finger is directed upward through the external ring toward the internal ring and the patient strains or coughs, the hernial mass can be felt to strike the tip of the finger. If the finger is pointed directly into Hesselbach's triangle, the sac of an indirect hernia will impinge on the side of the finger.

Direct inguinal hernia. A direct hernia appears as a globular swelling close to the pubis; it comes directly out of the region of Hesselbach's triangle (Fig. 6–4). It is almost always reducible and rarely enters the scro-

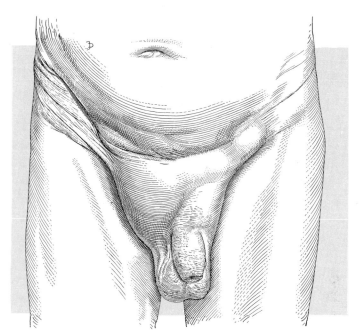

Figure 6–4. On the right, the elliptical swelling of an indirect inguinal hernia descending into the scrotum. On the left, the globular swelling of a direct inguinal hernia. The patient has been shaved in preparation for the operation.

tum. If the finger is directed toward Hesselbach's triangle, the sac will strike the tip of the finger when the patient coughs or strains. The location and direction of an indirect and a direct hernia are depicted diagrammatically in Figure 6–5.

With the patient supine and after reduction of the hernia mass, compression over the internal ring will prevent the appearance of an indirect hernia when the patient coughs. A direct hernia, however, will bulge out promptly.

A direct hernia coming through a very small defect in the transversalis fascia may be impossible to distinguish from an indirect hernia.

Scrotal hernia. If a scrotal hernia cannot be reduced it must be distinguished from lesions arising within the scrotum (Fig. 6–1) (see p. 118). If the hernia is reducible, it will then assume the characteristics of an indirect hernia, and as it is reduced, it can be traced upward along the inguinal canal toward the internal abdominal ring. When the patient coughs or strains the sac will be seen and felt coming down the inguinal canal rather than directly out of Hesselbach's triangle.

Hydrocele of the cord. A hydrocele of the cord appears as a small cystic mass anywhere along the course of the cord. It may be indistinguishable from an incarcerated hernia in the obese patient. The diagnosis

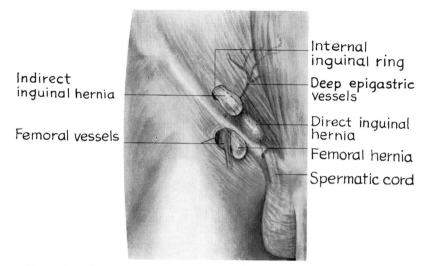

Indirect inguinal hernia

Femoral vessels

Internal inguinal ring

Deep epigastric vessels

Direct inguinal hernia

Femoral hernia

Spermatic cord

Figure 6-5. Diagrammatic projection of the sites of origin of a femoral hernia, and a direct and an indirect inguinal hernia.

becomes obvious if it can be transilluminated. The cyst should move with the cord if gentle traction is applied to the testicle.

The Reducibility of a Hernia

The reducibility of a hernia should always be ascertained with the patient in the recumbent position, since efforts to reduce a sac and its contents manually with the patient standing may induce incarceration or strangulation. In many instances, the hernia will immediately reduce when the patient assumes the reclining position and the musculature of the abdominal wall relaxes. If not, it is usually possible to bring about reduction by gentle pressure over the sac. If these efforts are not successful, the patient often is able to replace the hernia from previous experience. If difficulty is encountered, and there is question of incarceration or early strangulation, reduction may be accomplished by having the patient recline with his head lower than his feet. The leg on the affected side should be flexed, and the examiner should then gently manipulate the hernia with one hand and attempt to guide the contents of the sac through the ring with the other hand (Fig. 6-6). If these efforts are not successful, or if there are any associated signs of inflammation or strangulation, immediate operation is indicated.

If reduction has been successful but difficulty has been encountered, immediate and careful palpation of the hernial ring must be carried out in order to ascertain that the hernia has not been reduced "en bloc." In this situation the entire hernia and internal ring are reduced into the abdominal

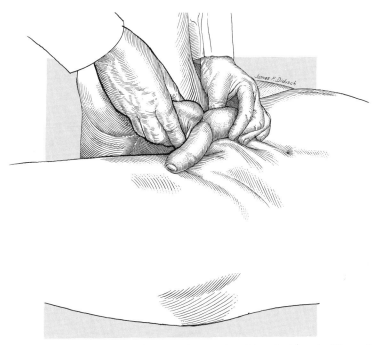

Figure 6–6. Technique of reduction of incarcerated inguinal hernia. The patient is in moderate Trendelenburg position. The leg is flexed to relax the abdominal musculature. The examiner grasps the hernial mass with one hand and gently guides it through the constricting ring with the other.

cavity without freeing the contents of the sac from the restricting effect of the internal ring. Symptoms of pain and signs of obstruction are accentuated. Continued pain and tenderness in the region of the ring require immediate surgical intervention.

IV. THE FEMORAL REGION

Palpation

The femoral region does not lend itself to such detailed palpation as the inguinal region. The external opening of the femoral canal is not distinctly palpable. It can be located in relation to the femoral artery and the inguinal ligament, which are the keys to an examination of this area. The inguinal ligament should first be outlined and the anterior-superior spine and the spine of the symphysis pubis identified. Midway between these two points the pulsations of the femoral artery will be felt just below the inguinal ligament. If the forefinger of the right hand is placed on the patient's right femoral artery, the index finger will lie over the femoral vein

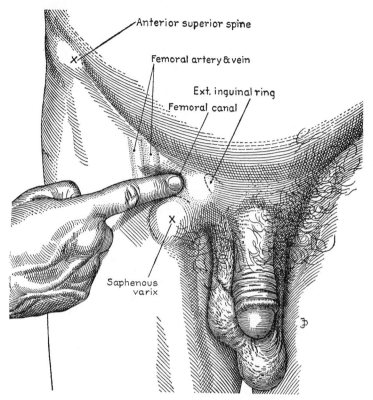

Figure 6–7. Palpation of the femoral canal. This point can be located with great accuracy by first identifying the femoral artery and the inguinal ligament. The femoral canal lies two fingerbreadths medial to the femoral artery just below the inguinal ligament.

and the ring finger over the femoral canal. The origin of the saphenous vein lies about one-half centimeter below this point (Fig. 6–7). In this region the following should be differentiated:

Femoral hernia. A reducible swelling lying directly in the femoral canal which transmits an impulse on coughing is unquestionably a femoral hernia. The diagnosis rests upon accurate localization of the femoral canal and distinguishing between the "impulse" transmitted by a hernia and the "thrill" transmitted by a saphenous varix (see p. 129).

Irreducible femoral hernia. A femoral hernia which has become incarcerated may stimulate an inguinal hernia, psoas abscess, or femoral adenitis. Large femoral hernias often push upward and overlie the inguinal ligament. They can be distinguished from inguinal hernias by precisely locating the neck of the sac. If the finger is placed on the spine of the symphysis pubis, the sac of a femoral hernia will be lateral and below it while the sac of an inguinal hernia will be above and medial to it.

Strangulated femoral hernia. Strangulation may develop in a femoral hernia without producing detectable local signs of pain, tenderness, or inflammation. The diagnosis of strangulation may depend upon systemic signs, such as an elevated pulse, leukocytosis, or fever. If bowel is involved, there will be peritoneal signs or evidence of intestinal obstruction. The local signs in the femoral canal, however, are frequently absent or minimal.

Saphenous varix. Since the saphenous vein arises about one-half centimeter below the femoral ring, a saphenous varix will be found lying a little below the usual site of a femoral hernia (Fig. 6–7). The varix will transmit a curious distinctive thrill rather than an impulse. A varix disappears when the patient assumes the supine position and reappears instantaneously on standing, while a femoral hernia reduces rather slowly or may have to be partially reduced with the aid of pressure. A venous hum may be heard with the stethoscope over a saphenous varix. There may be evidence of varicose veins in the thigh; percussion of such varicosities will transmit an impulse upward to a saphenous varix. An impulse cannot be elicited in this way over a femoral hernia.

Psoas abscess. The mass descends into the thigh well beyond the region of the saphenous ring. It is soft and fluctuant and often can be felt to extend above the inguinal ligament. If it is of pyogenic origin, signs of acute inflammation will be present. Retroperitoneal perforations of the colon from diverticulitis or ulcerative or granulomatous colitis may dissect below the inguinal ligament and present as a psoas abscess. If there are no inflammatory signs, tuberculosis or mycotic infections of the spine should be searched for by x-ray.

Femoral adenitis. This lesion usually can be recognized by the presence of low-grade inflammation and several irregular or matted nodes rather than a single discrete mass. A focus of infection may be discovered lower down in the leg or in the perineum. A small, broken-down, tender, fluctuant lymph node lying directly above the saphenous ring (gland of Cloquet) may be indistinguishable by palpation alone from a strangulated femoral hernia. Other factors in the history or signs of intestinal obstruction should make the distinction possible. If doubt exists, operation is necessary.

V. THE INGUINAL REGION IN THE FEMALE

Examination of the external genitalia in the female should be postponed and carried out as a part of the pelvic examination (see Chap. 13). Examination of the inguinal canal is carried out on the female at the same time as the abdominal examination and should precede it. The femoral canal may be appraised exactly as in the male. The inguinal region cannot be as satisfactorily palpated because the labia cannot be invaginated. By palpation of the inguinal ligament and the os pubis the exact site of the external ring can be located with the forefinger. When the patient coughs a sac may be felt and sometimes can be followed back a short distance into the canal. An incipient, indirect inguinal hernia is very difficult to detect in the female. Occasionally, if the palmar surface of the hand is placed over the internal ring, an impulse may be felt as the sac descends through the upper end of the canal. The same maneuver is occasionally of value in the male when a very small external ring prevents introduction of the finger into the canal. In both sexes small, indirect inguinal hernias can often be seen as distinct bulges upon coughing better than they can be felt on palpation. Emphasis is also placed on the need of repeating the examination in the supine as well as the standing position.

Hydrocele of the canal of Nuck. In the female the round ligament traverses the inguinal canal as the embryologic counterpart of the gubernaculum testis. In fetal life a vaginal process of peritoneum descends with the ligament and incomplete fusion of this process may result in a hydrocele which may lie anywhere between the internal ring and the labium majus. It presents itself as a cystic, irreducible, nontender swelling. It is translucent, but this is difficult to demonstrate unless the hydrocele is of considerable size.

chapter 7   # EXAMINATION OF THE ABDOMEN

The technique of abdominal examination varies with the nature of the patient's complaints and the suspected pathologic process under investigation. Many maneuvers of great importance in the evaluation of the acute abdomen or of a demonstrable or suspected lesion are properly omitted in the routine examination. Accordingly, *the elective examination, the appraisal of pathologic findings, the examination of the acute abdomen,* and *the examination of the postoperative abdomen* will be taken up separately.

I. THE ELECTIVE EXAMINATION

The principal objective of the examination is to ascertain that there is no abdominal tumor and that the viscera are not enlarged or abnormal in position.

The key to the examination is to have the patient relaxed and comfortable. The head and the knees should be supported in slight flexion; the hands should be at the sides. Appropriate draping, especially in female patients, is a significant factor in attaining complete relaxation (Fig. 7–1).

Inspection

Note the general contour of the abdomen, the presence or absence of dilated or distended veins, and the respiratory movements. The normal umbilicus is slightly retracted and inverted. Eversion of the umbilicus may be a sign of intra-abdominal fluid or distention. The presence, character, and position of abdominal scars are important. Ventral hernias or diastasis recti may become apparent if the patient is asked to raise his head or strain so as to increase intra-abdominal pressure.

131

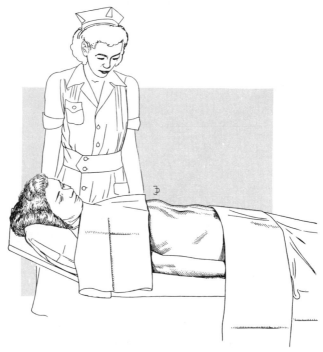

Figure 7–1. Appropriate draping is an important factor in obtaining abdominal relaxation.

Following a careful inspection of the abdomen, the inguinal and femoral canals and the male external genitalia should be examined (Chap. 6). Adherence to this routine guarantees that the examiner will not overlook an undescended testicle or a small nodule in the testicle as the clue to an otherwise baffling abdominal tumor, nor will he overlook a strangulated or incarcerated femoral or inguinal hernia as the cause of intestinal obstruction.

Auscultation

Routine auscultation of the abdomen is a good habit to acquire, since it familiarizes the examiner with the sounds of normal peristalsis.

Palpation

This is the essence of the routine abdominal examination. The cooperation of the patient and adequate relaxation are essential. First, one merely tests the tone of the rectus muscle by very gentle pressure with the hand resting flat against the abdomen. Gentle palpation of the four quadrants of the abdomen is then performed with the flexor surface of the palm of the hand and fingers in contact with the abdomen and with the forearm

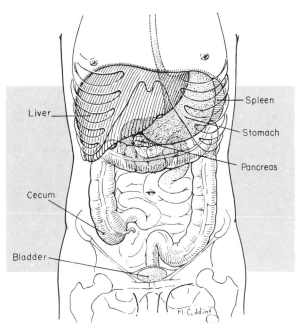

Figure 7–2. Normal location of the abdominal viscera.

and hand parallel to it. If the abdominal muscles are resistant and there is some question of involuntary spasm, the flat of the hand should be gently pressed against the rectus muscle while the patient is asked to breathe deeply with his mouth open. Voluntary spasm and rigidity will relax during expiration.

The normal location of the abdominal viscera is shown in Figure 7–2.

The Liver

Usually the liver cannot be palpated, but in thin individuals it may be felt at the costal margin. A palpable liver is not necessarily pathologic. Palpation is performed as follows: The examining fingers are placed flat against the abdominal wall just below the costal margin and are depressed by the fingers of the opposite hand. The patient is asked to take a deep breath and the palpating fingers are gently pressed inward and upward to impinge against the liver as it descends with respiration (Fig. 7–3). This procedure is repeated several times and if the edge is not felt, the liver is probably not enlarged. Palpation lateral to the rectus muscle will permit identification of a liver edge which otherwise is obscured by voluntary spasm of this muscle.

Percussion should begin in the axillary line about the fourth interspace and is carried downward until the resonant note of the lung is replaced by the dullness of the liver. The liver dullness is then traced until

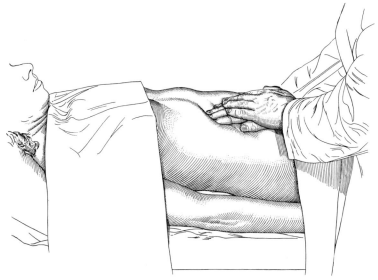

Figure 7–3. Palpation of the liver.

it is replaced by the tympany of the gas in the intestines. Ordinarily, the area of liver dullness extends from the fifth intercostal interspace to the costal margin. Percussion of the lower border is unreliable if there is abdominal distention. Occasionally, percussion will clearly demonstrate an enlarged liver although its edge cannot be identified by palpation.

The Gallbladder

The normal gallbladder cannot be palpated. A distended gallbladder may be felt just below the edge of the liver at about the outer edge of the rectus abdominis muscle.

The Spleen

The spleen is normally not palpable. It is sought by placing the left hand posteriorly in the flank below the costal margin in the midaxillary line. The patient is asked to breathe deeply and the fingers of the right hand are insinuated gently into the left upper quadrant of the abdomen (Fig. 7–4). This maneuver should be repeated two or three times, and if nothing is felt, the spleen is probably not greatly enlarged. If there is good reason to suspect slight enlargement of the spleen, palpation should be repeated with the patient turned on his right side. Having the patient lie with his left arm and fist under him rolls his left side forward, extends the spine and facilitates palpation of the spleen.

Percussion may be helpful. Normally, splenic dullness extends in the

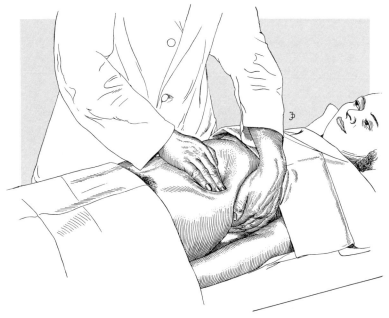

Figure 7-4. Palpation of the spleen.

midaxillary line from the ninth to the eleventh ribs; this area is often obscured by gas in the stomach or bowel so that percussion is usually not reliable unless the spleen is decidedly enlarged. An area of dullness extending above the ninth and below the eleventh ribs in the left midaxillary line is good evidence of an enlarged spleen.

The Kidneys

The left kidney is palpated with the right hand while the left hand is pressed into the flank posteriorly, lifting the kidney upward. The maneuver is similar to splenic palpation (Fig. 7-4), but the left hand is placed slightly lower and the right hand is somewhat more medial. This maneuver is duplicated on the right side (Fig. 7-5). The lower pole of the right kidney is frequently palpable as a smooth, slightly rounded mass which descends with respiration. The left kidney is not palpable unless it is enlarged or abnormally low in position.

The Urinary Bladder

If the urinary bladder is full, it may be palpable just above the symphysis as a smooth, ovoid, rather tense mass. Pressure on it will make the patient want to void. Percussion will outline the ovoid shape of a distended bladder, leaving little doubt as to its nature.

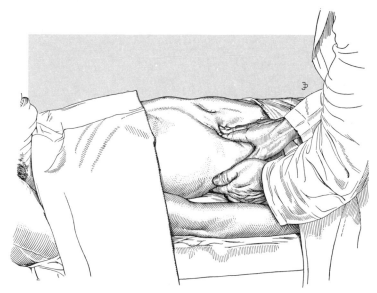

Figure 7–5. Palpation of the right kidney.

The Colon

The right colon, the cecum, and the descending colon and sigmoid are often palpable. The cecum and right colon are felt in the right lower quadrant as a soft, slightly tender, rounded mass. In the course of the palpation the patient may experience mild cramps, there may be audible peristalsis, and the palpable mass disappears. The sigmoid is often felt as a rather firm, narrow, tubular structure extending downward along the left lower quadrant into the pelvis.

Abdominal Reflexes

The routine examination is concluded by testing the abdominal reflexes. The skin is lightly scratched in each of the four quadrants. Contraction of the musculature is indicated by a sharp movement of the umbilicus toward the site of stimulation.

If the patient has no symptoms referable to the abdomen and no abnormalities have been detected, one may proceed with the remainder of the physical examination.

II. THE APPRAISAL OF ABNORMAL FINDINGS

The Appraisal of an Abdominal Mass

The examiner must be certain that what appears to be an abdominal mass is not a normal structure. There are several pitfalls (Fig. 7–6). The *distended bladder,* the *gravid uterus,* the *resistant edge* of the *rectus ab-dominus muscle,* the *promontory of the sacrum,* and the *dilated tortuous aorta* of the hypertensive patient—all have been mistaken for abdominal tumors of varied etiology. Catheterization may be required to exclude a distended bladder. Pregnancy should be considered in every midabdom-inal tumor in the female although the symptoms may be extremely vague. In thin patients the promontory of the sacrum may be palpated and mistaken for a midline abdominal tumor, particularly as it is sensitive to palpation. In such instances careful examination will reveal the aortic pulsations just above the supposed mass. A vaguely defined mass in this location has no significance unless there is reason to suspect a neoplastic lesion in the aortic nodes.

Voluntary tightening of the rectus muscle, particularly in obese pa-tients, often produces an apparent epigastric tumor. The fact that it does not move with respiration and that it conforms to the outer edge of the muscle should arouse suspicion as to its nature. Once adequate relaxation is obtained, the mass disappears.

Occasionally the *aorta is palpated* in the epigastrium and creates the impression of a middle pulsating tumor. It can be distinguished from a small aneurysm only by aortography. A large abdominal aneurysm not only pulsates but a distinct expansile character can be detected by placing a finger of each hand on opposite sides of the mass. The space between the fingers widens with each pulsation.

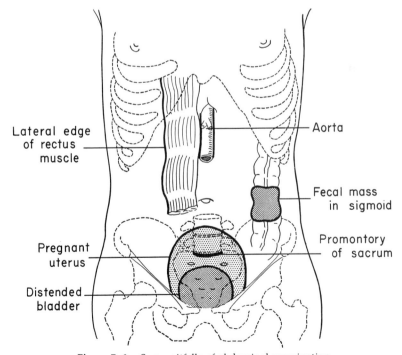

Figure 7–6. Some pitfalls of abdominal examination.

A pulsating mass at the level of the umbilicus or just below it is likely to be a *small abdominal aneurysm.*

A mass of *inspissated feces in the sigmoid* may simulate an abdominal tumor. If doubt exists, the abdomen should be examined after a cleansing enema has been given.

The mobility of a mass is of considerable significance. Lesions which descend with respiration are probably connected either with the liver, the kidneys, or the spleen. If the mass not only moves with respiration but also is movable by palpation, it probably is adjacent to, but not actually attached to, the liver or spleen. Gastric tumors usually have a moderate degree of mobility, while lesions in the ascending or descending colon are only slightly mobile. Complete fixation suggests a tumor of pancreatic or retroperitoneal origin or advanced malignancy with invasion of adjacent structures. Tumors of the small intestine or omentum are usually very freely movable. Pedunculated lesions, such as certain ovarian cysts or fibroids, also fall into this category.

The shape, consistency, and sensitivity of a mass are significant. Stony hard, nodular, nontender lesions suggest malignancy. A smooth, tense, rounded mass usually indicates a cyst. Tenderness suggests inflammation, hemorrhage, or necrosis.

The Detection of Fluid Within the Abdomen

Large amounts of fluid within the peritoneal cavity are usually readily detected by eliciting a "fluid wave." The conventional method of doing

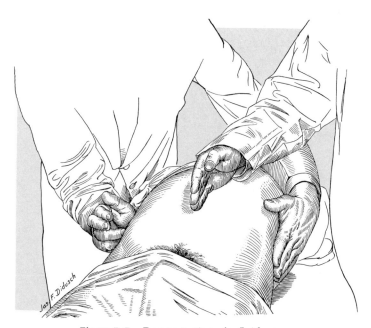

Figure 7-7. Demonstration of a fluid wave.

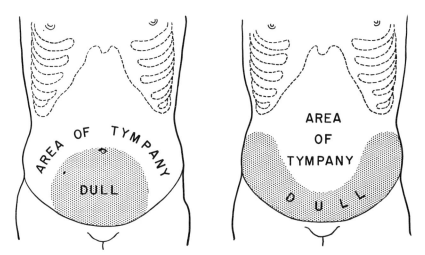

Figure 7–8. The distinction between an ovarian cyst (*left*) and ascites (*right*) by percussion of the abdomen.

this is shown in Figure 7–7. The examiner taps one flank with the finger of one hand and palpates the opposite flank with the other hand; at the same time an assistant prevents the abdominal wall from transmitting the impulse by placing the edge of his hand along the midline of the abdomen. If fluid is present, a distinct impulse will be transmitted to the palpating hand as the opposite flank is tapped with the finger. Unfortunately, this sign may be positive in the very obese patient due to transmission of the impulse by the abdominal wall even though the maneuver is correctly performed. It may be positive in the presence of encapsulated fluid as in a very large ovarian cyst.

The distinction between fluid in a large ovarian cyst and ascites. In ascites the abdomen is evenly distended with fullness in the flanks. There is tympany anteriorly, and the area of dullness in the flanks shifts on change of position. In an ovarian cyst there may be asymmetry in the abdominal swelling; there is dullness anteriorly and tympany in the flanks. There is no striking shift in the area of dullness on change of position. The characteristic areas of dullness in ascites and in large ovarian cysts are shown in Figure 7–8. The "ruler test" is useful (Fig. 7–9).

Ballottement. In the presence of ascites a mass may be difficult to feel, but its presence can often be detected by *ballottement*. The fingers are thrust rather quickly into the abdomen in the region where the mass is suspected, and as the fluid is displaced, the mass will float up against the palpating fingers.

Shifting dullness. It requires care to elicit this valuable sign of free fluid in the peritoneal cavity. The technique is shown in Figure 7–10.

Puddle sign. The puddle sign is an aid in the diagnosis of minimal ascites and is not influenced by obesity or the presence of intraluminal

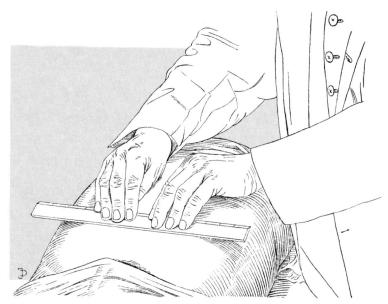

Figure 7–9. The ruler test for detection of an ovarian cyst. A ruler is laid across the abdomen just above the level of the anterior superior iliac spine and pressed firmly inward toward the vertebral column. In an ovarian cyst the pulsations of the abdominal aorta are transmitted to the ruler and can be seen and felt. In the presence of ascites the fluid is displaced into the flanks and no impulse is transmitted.

bowel fluid. The puddle sign is elicited as follows: the patient is requested to lie face down for five minutes and then to support his body on his hands and knees. The examiner places the Bowles stethoscope against the most dependent part of the abdomen. With his free hand the examiner repeatedly flicks one flank lightly with a constant intensity. At the same time the headpiece of the stethoscope is gradually moved to the flank opposite the percussion site (Fig. 7–11). A positive puddle sign is evidenced by a marked increase in the character and intensity of the percussion note as the stethoscope is moved toward the opposite flank. The patient then sits up and the maneuver is repeated with the instrument in the same position on the abdomen. If the percussion note becomes loud and clear the initial impression is confirmed.

The Enlarged Liver

Inspection may reveal the contour of an enlarged liver extending across the right upper abdomen and epigastrium. An enlarged liver is easily detected by palpation if relaxation is adequate and there is no abdominal distention. The characteristic diagnostic feature is the distinctly palpable edge of the liver. This may be somewhat blunted in the presence of cirrhosis, or irregular and nodular if the enlargement is due to car-

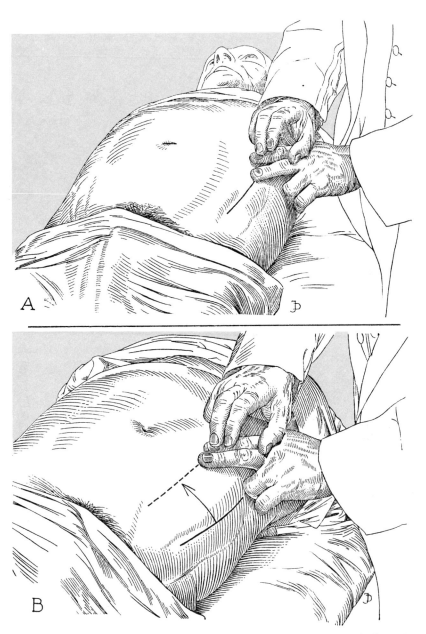

Figure 7–10. Detection of fluid within the abdominal cavity. *A,* With the patient supine the level of dullness in the flank created by the fluid is determined by percussion. *B,* The patient is then rolled on his side and the percussion is repeated. A shift in the level of the dullness on the dependent side is indicative of free fluid in the peritoneal cavity.

A

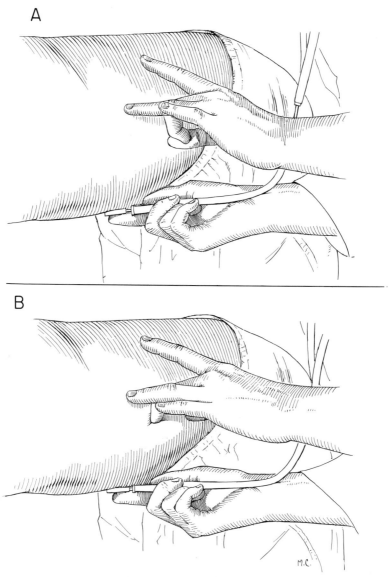

B

Figure 7–11. Position of patient for puddle sign. *A,* Position of examiner's hand before the abdomen is flicked. *B,* The flick completed.

cinoma. In thin individuals it is occasionally possible to outline the stony hard, nodular edge of metastatic cancer so accurately that there is little doubt about the diagnosis. The enlargement of the liver below the costal margin may be confirmed by percussion and outlined with a skin pencil. It is customary to estimate the distance between the edge of the liver and the costal margin in the nipple line in "fingerbreadths" as a rough index of the extent of liver enlargement.

If the liver is enlarged, one looks for traces of jaundice in the conjunctivae. The skin is carefully inspected for the characteristic scratch marks of pruritus, for jaundice, and for spider angiomata. Spider angiomata are seen over the anterior chest wall as delicate, bright red, branching vascular patterns which radiate from a central point. The hands may have the characteristic reddening of the thenar and hypothenar eminences, "liver palms," or there may be dilated veins in the abdominal wall.

A glass eye or an absent right breast may be the clue to unexplained jaundice or hepatomegaly, although the malignant lesions which required operation may have been removed long ago.

The Enlarged Gallbladder

The enlarged gallbladder is palpated as a smooth rounded tumor in the right upper quadrant. It is usually found just lateral to the outer edge of the rectus muscle, but there is considerable variation. It may be present quite far in the flank or more nearly in the epigastrium. Its lower border is distinct, smooth, and rounded; the upper border cannot be defined since it fades out either under the costal margin or appears to become confluent with the edge of the liver.

An enlarged, exquisitely tender gallbladder is characteristic of acute cholecystitis.

An enlarged nontender gallbladder in the presence of obstructive jaundice is characteristic of malignant obstruction of the bile ducts. This is based on the assumption ("Courvoisier's law") that in malignant disease of the pancreas the gallbladder is usually normal and is capable of marked distention after the obstruction of the common duct. In the presence of gallstone obstruction the gallbladder is often previously diseased from recurrent cholecystitis and is incapable of dilating. This is a useful guide, but there are many exceptions to it.

The Stomach

Normally the stomach cannot be felt, but if distended with air it can often be outlined by percussion.

Acute pyloric obstruction causes severe repeated vomiting, often without marked dilatation of the stomach. Electrolyte losses are large and rapid, with hypochloremia and hypokalemic alkalosis. Shock and collapse may occur.

In *chronic, slowly progressive pyloric obstruction,* enormous enlargement of the stomach may occur with only occasional intermittent vomiting. There may be very little disturbance of electrolyte and fluid balance. The enlarged air and fluid–filled organ may be palpated below the umbilicus. Even in less marked cases, a splashing sound (succussion) may be elicited if the patient is shaken.

Tumors of the stomach are often palpable: carcinoma, lymphoma, and leiomyosarcoma are the most common. The mass is often movable and is pushed down by the left lobe of the liver during inspiration.

A large palpable gastric mass may be slowly growing and is quite amenable to surgical removal.

Leiomyomas and leiomyosarcomas may reach enormous size with only minimal invasion or deformity of the gastric wall.

The Small Intestine

The small intestine can be localized in a general way by Monk's method. The root of the mesentery is projected on the abdominal wall by a line drawn half above and half below the umbilicus, extending from a point just to the left of the midline to a point to the right of the midline, midway between the umbilicus and the center of the inguinal ligament on the right. Two parallel lines drawn at right angles to this line divide the small bowel into upper, middle, and lower. This maneuver is of some use in localizing tumor masses and areas of tenderness.

Most pathologic lesions in the small bowel produce acute abdominal signs of intestinal obstruction, strangulation, perforation, hypermotility, or peritoneal irritation, and are more properly discussed under the "Acute Abdomen" (see below).

Carcinoma and lymphoma are the commonest tumors of the small bowel. Slowly growing tumors of the small bowel may become palpable before obstruction occurs. A freely movable firm abdominal mass associated with vague abdominal complaints is likely to be a tumor of the small bowel or its mesentery.

Chronic progressive obstruction of the small bowel from neoplasia may develop without abdominal pain or vomiting. Low grade distention, hyperactive peristalsis, and dilated, palpable loops of bowel are the presenting signs. The small bowel may actually thicken and hypertrophy in response to the slowly progressing stenosis. Symptoms may be more suggestive of a malabsorption syndrome than low small bowel obstruction.

Carcinoids of the small bowel rarely produce symptoms until metastases develop. Occasionally signs of obstruction, abdominal pain, or bleeding develop. Approximately 10 per cent of patients with carcinoid tumors of the small intestine present with the "carcinoid syndrome." This consists of cutaneous flushing, diarrhea, asthmatic wheezing with dyspnea, and in the late stages, right-sided heart failure. The syndrome is caused by biologically active degradation products of serotonin. 5-hydroxytryptophan kallikreins, or other histamine-like substances. Cardiac failure is related to deposits of collagen with subendothelial fibrosis and valvular incompetence.

The Enlarged Spleen

The only evidence of a slightly or moderately enlarged spleen may be an impulse which touches the tips of the palpating fingers as the patient inspires. Percussion may confirm the presence of some splenic enlargement. In marked splenic enlargement the organ is easily felt extending across the left upper quadrant. A distinct notch may be felt in the edge. This indentation of the edge of the spleen, the so-called splenic notch, is a significant diagnostic sign, but it frequently cannot be identified.

If splenic enlargement is suspected, one should search for physical signs of "hypersplenism." Scrutinize the conjunctivae, the mucous membranes, and the skin for pallor, purpura, or jaundice.

The Enlarged Kidney

The lower pole of the right kidney is frequently palpable. The left kidney is either enlarged or displaced downward if it is palpable. An enlarged kidney is identified by its posterior position; the palpating hand must be deep in the abdomen before the rounded edge of the kidney is appreciated. It descends well with respiration and then slips between the palpating hands as the patient exhales. At times one can make out the reniform shape of an enlarged kidney. If the hand in the flank is pressed upward, the impulse is transmitted to the kidney and can be appreciated readily by the abdominal hand. This sign is particularly helpful in distinguishing between an enlarged tender kidney with hydronephrosis and an enlarged tender gallbladder.

Bilateral enlargement of the kidneys suggests congenital polycystic disease. A distinctly anterior enlargement of the kidney is usually due to neoplastic disease. The organ seems to maintain its posterior position even with considerable enlargement due to hydronephrosis. In contrast to a splenic or hepatic lesion there is usually *tympany* over a renal mass due to the presence of the colon.

IS IT THE SPLEEN OR THE LEFT KIDNEY?

Confusion may exist between marked enlargement of the spleen and a markedly enlarged kidney. In general the spleen is an anterior organ; the kidney is posterior. The free edge of the spleen is sharper than that of the kidney and always points in a somewhat caudad direction. One may find a gap between the posterior edge of the spleen and the erector spinae group of muscles by careful palpation of the flank. This cannot be demonstrated in the presence of an enlarged kidney. The percussion note over the spleen is dull since the colon is usually displaced downward.

III. THE ACUTE ABDOMEN

A correct diagnosis in the "acute abdomen" requires a careful balancing of probabilities. Consequently, every bit of evidence must be obtained from the physical examination and, accordingly, a separate discussion is outlined.

Inspection

Note the position assumed by the patient. In severe colic he will be unable to lie quietly, while in the presence of peritoneal inflammation, he will remain quiet with his knees flexed even though in great pain. Note his facial expression and respiratory rate. Look particularly for splinting of the rectus muscles, the absence of the normal respiratory movements, and visible peristalsis.

Feel the pulse. The character and rate of the pulse are among the best indications of the gravity of an acute abdominal disease. A slow, full, regular pulse does not exclude a serious peritoneal infection, but it indicates that the patient is reacting well to it. A moderately elevated, quick, slightly bounding pulse is characteristic of progressing abdominal infection. It is a disturbing observation even when the abdominal findings are minimal. A rapid, thready pulse goes with advanced peritonitis.

Following inspection of the abdomen, the inguinofemoral region and male external genitalia should be examined, thus assuring that the examiner will not overlook an incarcerated strangulated hernia.

It is important to palpate the femoral artery during this part of the examination, since absent pulsation or discrepancy between the two sides in the presence of serious abdominal pain may be a clue to a dissecting aneurysm.

Auscultation

The examiner should have a clear conception of the sounds of normal peristalsis. Peristalsis may be increased, diminished, or absent in the presence of a suspected acute abdomen. Peristalsis may be said to be absent if no peritoneal sounds are heard over a period of several minutes. Absence of peristalsis means paralytic ileus due to diffuse peritoneal irritation. Increased peristalsis is commonly encountered in three forms:

(1) Fairly constant loud borborygmi which vary in intensity but have no definite pattern occur in *acute gastroenteritis* or *digestive upset* due to dietary indiscretion. This type of peristalsis has no definite rhythm and variations in its intensity occur without any alteration of the patient's abdominal discomfort.

(2) Less common, but far more important, are the sounds produced by the rhythmic contractures of the intestines in *acute mechanical ob-*

struction. In this condition the abdomen is silent between bouts of colic. Borborygmi of a gradually increasing intensity are then heard; these rise to a crescendo and then gradually die away until only a few faint tinkles are heard. The patient is aware of painful cramps which increase and subside with the peristaltic activity. The rhythmic peristaltic crescendo of acute mechanical obstruction is unmistakable when once heard.

(3) In *chronic partial obstruction of the lower small bowel* and in the recovery phases of a diffuse peritoneal inflammation, hollow gurgling and tinkling sounds are heard as dilated fluid-laden loops of bowel undergo periodic contractions. There is no rhythmic pattern to this type of peristalsis. It may or may not be accompanied by abdominal cramps.

(4) A bruit heard in the epigastrium may be an important sign of *chronic intestinal ischemia.* Bruits to one side or the other of the midline in the upper abdomen may indicate significant *renal vascular occlusion.* The detection of an abdominal bruit is of great importance in the appraisal of obscure episodic abdominal pain. (see Chap. 10).

Palpation

The patient should first be asked to cough. In the presence of acute peritoneal inflammation this usually elicits a sharp twinge of pain localized to the involved area. It is extremely valuable to elicit this "cough tenderness" and have the patient point with one finger to the exact area of pain. This localizes the area of inflammation before the examiner so much as touches the abdomen. He can thus avoid palpating this area until the remainder of the abdominal examination is completed.

The detection of spasm and the distinction between voluntary and involuntary spasm. It is vital not to hurt the patient. The hand of the examiner must be warm. The technique of testing for spasm is depicted in Figure 7–12. The extent of both recti muscles is palpated in this fashion; the area of marked tenderness (referred to in the cough test) is examined last. A faulty but commonly used method of palpating is shown in Figure 7–13.

Extensive rigidity of both rectus muscles indicates a diffuse peritoneal irritation. Segmental spasm of one rectus (spasm limited to one quadrant) is encountered in early peritonitis. However, since there is no compartment which limits the spread of peritoneal fluid to one side of the abdomen, extensive rigidity involving the length of one rectus muscle with complete flaccidity of the other cannot occur from peritonitis or peritoneal irritation. Extensive unilateral rigidity is reflexive in origin; it is sometimes seen in acute renal colic but the mechanism is not understood.

Palpation of both recti simultaneously is of value in assessing the extent and character of abdominal spasm.

Outlining the area of tenderness. The exact area of tenderness within the abdomen is now carefully mapped out by gentle one-finger pal-

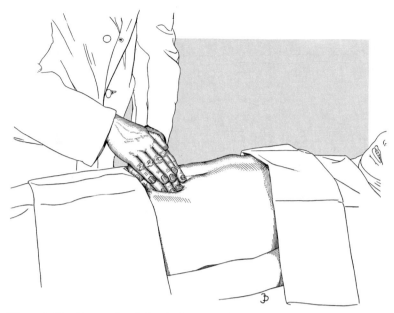

Figure 7–12. Testing for abdominal spasm. The flat of the entire left hand is placed on the abdomen in the quadrant farthest away from the area of pain and tenderness; it is held gently in this position long enough to assure the patient that he is not being hurt. He is then asked to breathe deeply and the fingers of the left hand, which are in contact with one of the rectus muscles, are gently depressed with the right hand. Voluntary spasm of the recti will always give way beneath the hand as the patient exhales; involuntary or true spasm will not yield. The muscle is felt as a rigid, firm, tense, boardlike structure. It is not necessary to push the hand deeply into the abdomen in order to elicit this sense of rigidity, and one should not produce pain.

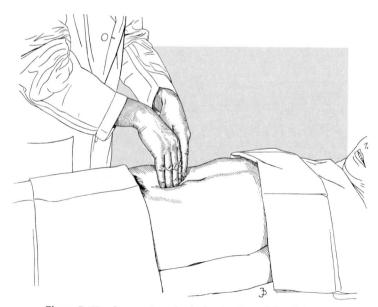

Figure 7–13. Incorrect method of palpation of the abdomen.

pation (Fig. 7–14). The tenderness of such conditions as acute appendicitis or acute cholecystitis is sharply localized to the immediate area of the organ involved unless there is a diffusing peritonitis. This observation can be made only by *careful, gentle palpation with one finger.* Palpation with the entire hand may give a false impression of the extent of the tenderness, since it does not permit accurate localization. Light percussion of the abdomen may also be used to localize tenderness.

Abdominal palpation is not complete without a careful examination of the flanks, the costovertebral angles and the lower portion of the costal cage. Use only one finger to explore these areas carefully. Firm, one-finger palpation of the lower intercostal spaces will sometimes reveal exquisite tenderness and thus provide an important clue to a lesion above the diaphragm which is simulating abdominal disease. In testing for costovertebral tenderness one should place the finger precisely in the angle between the spine and the twelfth rib (Fig. 7–15). Tenderness localized in this area is diagnostic of an inflammatory process in the kidney while tenderness more laterally over the ribs or over the flank may be indicative of a variety of conditions.

The detection of a mass. The examiner has now located the exact site of the tenderness without causing pain. He has also determined the presence and extent of muscle spasm. He next attempts to palpate the abdomen more deeply. True rigidity of the musculature will make this impossible. It may be exceedingly difficult to identify organs or masses even

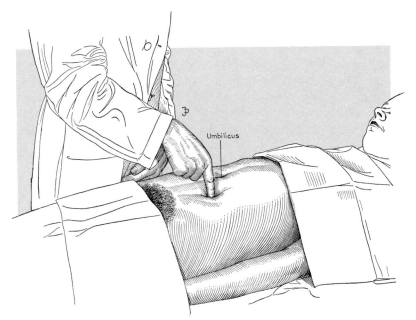

Umbilicus

Figure 7–14. Gentle systematic palpation of the entire abdomen with one finger is an essential step in the accurate localization of an area of tenderness.

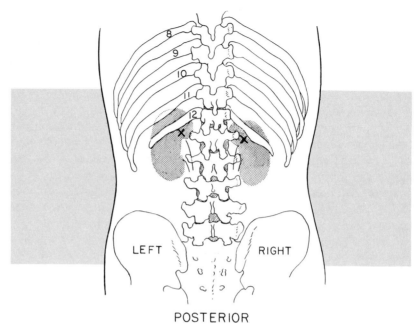

POSTERIOR

Figure 7–15. In testing for costovertebral angle tenderness the examiner's finger must be placed precisely in the angle between the twelfth rib and the vertebral muscles.

without rigidity if exquisite tenderness is present. However, by very gentle palpation without hurting the patient sufficiently to produce voluntary spasm, the experienced clinician may distinctly outline the borders of tender masses such as a tense gallbladder or an appendiceal abscess.

It is always wise to *palpate the acute abdomen a second time* after the patient has been given morphine and once again in the operating room after the induction of anesthesia. Rigid observation of this rule will frequently reveal masses which have been overlooked. It also permits a far more accurate appraisal of the nature of previously detected masses.

Percussion of the Abdomen

Gentle percussion is of value in localizing an area of tenderness. It also occasionally reveals an unexpected area of dullness coinciding with an area of tenderness; this gives a clue to a hitherto unrecognized mass which is displacing the intestines. Signs of shifting dullness within the abdomen may establish a diagnosis of intra-abdominal bleeding following abdominal injuries. The extent of liver and bladder dullness must be carefully appraised.

The Pelvic and Rectal Examinations

The technique of these examinations is described in Chapters 13 and 14. These are done last, but must never be omitted. Lesions in the pouch of Douglas are more readily felt in the lithotomy position than in the lateral position. Systematic palpation of the rectum and of the pouch of Douglas should be performed; the exact location of the tenderness may thus be determined and may prove to be a significant point in establishing the diagnosis. The prostate and seminal vesicles deserve particular attention because inflammation in these organs may simulate an acute abdomen. In the female, gentle, sensitive palpation may detect the increased pulsations of the uterine vessels characteristic of pregnancy, or the crepitation of the broad ligament which occurs in gas bacillus cellulitis following a septic abortion. The correct diagnosis, and sometimes life itself, may depend upon such details. The rectal and pelvic examinations should be repeated after anesthesia has been induced if there is reason to suspect a pelvic lesion.

Special Tests

There are a number of special tests which may be helpful in elucidating the diagnosis in particular cases.

The sign of cough tenderness has already been described.

Rebound tenderness. This sign is elicited by pressing fairly deeply into the abdomen on the side away from a suspected acute inflammatory process and then quickly releasing the pressure. As the abdominal wall snaps out to its normal position, a twinge of pain is felt by the patient either at the site of pressure or at the site of the inflammatory process. Rebound tenderness referred to the opposite side, which is the side of the lesion, is useful contributory evidence of acute peritoneal irritation localized to the painful area. It is of the same significance as cough tenderness and is more reliable, since it is present when cough tenderness is absent.

Rebound tenderness referred to the point of pressure anywhere in the abdomen indicates a diffuse peritoneal irritation. It is not necessary to employ this maneuver in the presence of an obvious diffuse peritonitis, since it is painful to the patient. In doubtful cases, particularly in obese patients who are heavily muscled and have a thick omentum, this sign is of considerable value in determining the extent of an inflammatory process.

Iliopsoas test. Have the patient attempt to flex his thigh against slight pressure of the examiner's hand (Fig. 7–16). Pain will be elicited if there is an inflammatory process in contact with the psoas muscle. Minor degrees of irritation may be detected by having the patient lie on the opposite side and extend the thigh on the affected side to its full extent.

Obturator test. The thigh is flexed to a right angle and is then rotated both externally and internally (Fig. 7–17). Hypogastric pain may be elicited if there is an inflammatory mass lying in contact with the *obturator internus muscle*. It may be positive in the presence of pelvic appendicitis or an accumulation of fluid or blood in the pelvis.

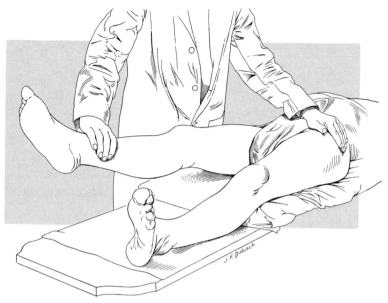

Figure 7–16.   Iliopsoas test.

Fist percussion of the lower anterior thoracic wall (Fig. 7–18).   A positive result may be obtained in a variety of conditions, including acute hepatitis. This sign is positive in the presence of an acute gallbladder. It is a useful adjunct and, when negative, the examiner should be very hesitant to make a diagnosis of an acute upper abdominal inflammation.

The sign of contralateral tenderness.   It may be difficult at times to distinguish between thoracic disease which is causing abdominal pain and rigidity and an acute inflammatory process in an upper quadrant of the ab-

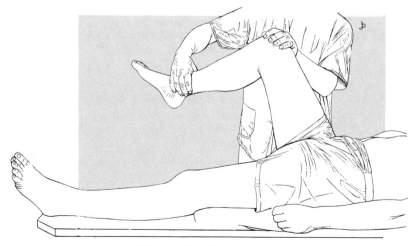

Figure 7–17.   Obturator test.

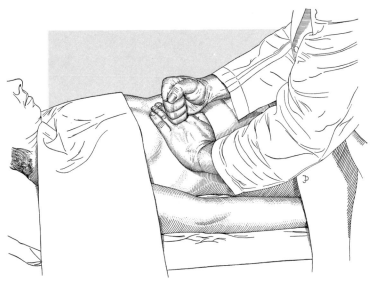

Figure 7–18. Fist percussion of lower anterior thoracic wall. The intensity of the blow can be well controlled and it is possible to carry out this maneuver with great gentleness. The patient experiences a sharp twinge of pain in the presence of an acute inflammatory process beneath the diaphragm or liver on the right side, or around the spleen and stomach on the left side.

domen. Pressure on the opposite side of the abdomen carried in rather deeply toward the affected side will often cause pain if the disease is intra-abdominal; it will not cause pain if the disease is above the diaphragm.

Inspiratory arrest (Murphy). This is a valuable sign of acute cholecystitis. The patient is asked to take a long breath, while at the same time deep pressure is made against the abdominal wall in the region of the gallbladder. As the liver descends, the gallbladder is brought in contact with the examining fingers. The patient experiences a sharp twinge of pain and the inspiration is immediately arrested. It may be positive in acute hepatitis or in the congested liver of acute cardiac failure.

Discoloration of the umbilicus (Cullen). A faintly bluish hue to the skin of the umbilicus may be noted in the presence of an extensive hemoperitoneum. This was originally described as an indication of a ruptured ectopic pregnancy. The sign may be encountered in any condition in which there is an extensive amount of free blood in the peritoneal cavity. Its absence does not exclude intraperitoneal bleeding.

IV. DIFFERENTIAL SIGNS IN THE ACUTE ABDOMEN

The differential diagnosis of acute abdominal diseases is manifestly beyond the scope of this volume. However, since a correctly performed physical examination determines the advisability of operation, the classic findings and the more frequently encountered variants of some important abdominal emergencies are presented.

Acute Appendicitis

The manifestations of this disease are legion. It may simulate most other acute abdominal conditions. Differences in the location of the appendix and in the extent and rate of progression of the inflammatory process account for the extraordinary variety of clinical syndromes.

CLASSIC ACUTE APPENDICITIS (THE APPENDIX BEING IN THE RIGHT LOWER QUADRANT)

Inspection

The patient may not appear ill in the early stages. He will be aware of persistent pain which usually is aggravated by motion; he may prefer to lie quietly; on rising or walking he may guard his right side. No abnormalities will be detected on inspection of the abdomen.

Auscultation

Peristalsis may be diminished, but is often normal.

Palpation

Pain elicited by coughing will be referred to the right lower quadrant. One finger palpation of the abdomen will demonstrate tenderness well localized to the right lower quadrant in the region of McBurney's point (Fig. 7–19). It often corresponds closely to the reference point of the "cough tenderness." There may be voluntary spasm of the right rectus muscle, but no true spasm. Rigidity is indicative of peritoneal inflammation and is not a sign of early appendicitis.

Rectal and pelvic examinations will be negative in the early stages. The only consistent physical finding in early appendicitis is *localized tenderness*. This observation is so reliable that generalized or diffuse tenderness may be regarded as evidence against the diagnosis of early uncomplicated appendicitis.

Variants of Acute Appendicitis

Because localized tenderness is the only consistently reliable finding in early appendicitis, the condition is frequently overlooked when the appendix lies in a protected or unusual position (Fig. 7–20).

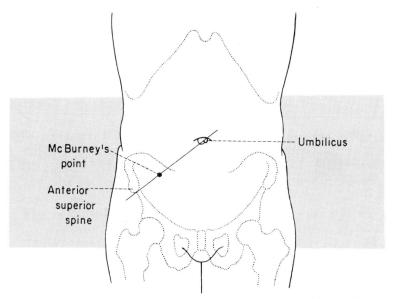

Figure 7-19. McBurney's point is of historical interest only. The localization of tenderness in appendicitis depends entirely on the position of the appendix (see Fig. 7-21).

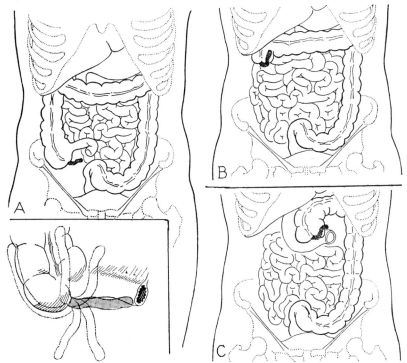

Figure 7-20. Positions of the vermiform appendix. The physical findings in acute appendicitis depend upon the position of the cecum and the relation of the appendix to the cecum. *A*, The cecum is in the right lower quadrant. The appendix may lie behind the ileum, free in the peritoneal cavity, in the iliac fossa, or in the pelvis. *B*, The cecum is in the right upper quadrant. The appendix may be in front of or behind the ileocecal junction. *C*, The malrotated cecum is in the left upper quadrant. Because of failure of attachment of the cecum, the appendix is usually free.

Retrocecal appendicitis. The point of localized tenderness will be found well lateral in the flank. Abdominal signs may be absent and cough tenderness is frequently not demonstrable. Rigidity may not be present in the rectus muscle in advanced retrocecal appendicitis, but will be found laterally in the muscles of the flank. A high retrocecal appendix may simulate cholecystitis or renal disease. In palplating the flank it is essential to distinguish carefully between flank tenderness and costovertebral angle tenderness (Fig. 7–15).

Pelvic appendicitis. This most dangerous and baffling form of the disease is characterized by the remarkable normality of the abdominal examination. Since diarrhea and vomiting are prominent symptoms in this form of appendicitis, a diagnosis of gastroenteritis is easily entertained unless the physical findings are properly interpreted. Early in the course of the disease, tenderness may not be demonstrable by either abdominal, rectal, or pelvic examination. *It is essential to repeat both pelvic and rectal examinations at frequent intervals, as they will provide the earliest clue to the diagnosis.* Exquisite tenderness in the pouch of Douglas appears when the abdominal examination reveals little variation from the normal. Abdominal signs become striking as the disease progresses and pelvic peritonitis develops. The *iliopsoas test* and *obturator test* may be positive in pelvic appendicitis.

Iliac appendicitis. The physical findings may be fairly classic when the appendix lies just over the brim of the pelvis, or the point of tenderness may be quite low in the abdomen just above the inguinal ligament. The appendix is frequently in contact with the iliopsoas muscle in this location; a positive iliopsoas sign is helpful confirmatory evidence.

Obstructive appendicitis. Complete obstruction of the appendix by a fecalith may lead to vascular occlusion, gangrene, and early perforation. Pain may be so severe that mesenteric thrombosis or volvulus is mimicked.

Bizarre forms of acute appendicitis. Because of the variable position of the appendix, appendicitis may simulate most any other acute abdominal disease. An inflamed appendix in the right upper quadrant may simulate acute cholecystitis or perforated ulcer. A long appendix with perforation at its tip may reach across the abdomen and produce all the manifestations of diverticulitis.

For these reasons it is generally maintained that in the differential diagnosis of acute abdominal inflammation, appendicitis should never be lower than second on the list.

Acute Cholecystitis

Inspection

The respiratory rate is frequently elevated and at times is so rapid that pneumonia may be suspected. This elevation of the respiratory rate is partly attributable to the fact that the enlarged, acutely inflamed gallbladder comes in contact with the anterior parietes with normal breathing and accentuates the pain. Short, rapid breathing prevents this and gives the patient considerable relief.

Slight distention of the upper abdomen is frequently an early sign and is not due to peritonitis. This distention is attributable to the air which the patient has swallowed in the mistaken belief that he has "gas on his stomach." This reaction is quite common in patients with acute cholecystitis.

Auscultation

Peristalsis is practically always present; it may be quite active. A silent abdomen is a late sign and indicates perforation of the gallbladder. If encountered at an early stage, one should suspect perforated duodenal ulcer rather than acute cholecystitis.

The signs of fist percussion and *inspiratory arrest* are *generally positive.* Both of these signs may be positive in the presence of a tender liver from acute cardiac failure or acute hepatitis. These signs indicate that there is an acute inflammatory process in the upper abdomen, and considerable doubt should be cast on the diagnosis of acute cholecystitis if they are negative.

Palpation

One-finger palpation will localize tenderness to the gallbladder in the early stages of the disease. Rigidity is not present, but voluntary spasm is often so marked that care must be taken to exclude true muscular spasm. Careful, gentle palpation will usually disclose the tense, pear-shaped, exquisitely tender mass of the enlarged gallbladder. *Identification of the tender gallbladder by palpation* is the most reassuring diagnostic physical finding in acute cholecystitis.

JAUNDICE AND THE ACUTE ABDOMEN

Jaundice may occur in acute cholecystitis. If mild (bilirubin below 5 to 7 mg. per 100 ml.), it may be only a consequence of edema and pressure from the distended gallbladder on the common duct. If marked (bilirubin above 7 mg. per 100 ml.), an associated obstruction of the common duct by a gallstone is likely.

Cholangitis. Chills, fever, abdominal pain, and jaundice are characteristic of cholangitis or pylephlebitis.

Suppurative cholangitis. Chills, fever, jaundice, abdominal pain, and hypotension, with lethargy and mental confusion, are manifestations of suppurative cholangitis—a critical, surgical emergency. Jaundice may be mild and abdominal signs minimal.

Gallstone ileus. Abdominal pain and transient jaundice followed hours or days later by signs of intestinal obstruction suggest gallstone ileus. Physical signs are usually those of low grade partial intestinal obstruction. An x-ray will show air in the biliary tract and may show the offending gallstone. The initial attack may be so mild that the patient does not seek medical care, with the result that the presenting picture is one of intestinal obstruction unless a very careful history is taken.

Rarely, erosion of a gallstone into the duodenum is manifested by massive hemorrhage.

Perforated Gastric or Duodenal Ulcer

The physical signs vary with the stage of the illness. A state of collapse may dominate the picture if the patient is seen shortly after the onset. The patient is ashen in color, faint, sweating, and complains of severe epigastric or substernal pain. Hypotension is common, but the pulse rate is usually below 100. Retraction of the epigastrium, boardlike rigidity of the abdominal musculature, generalized tenderness, rectal tenderness, and absent peristalsis are outstanding features of the physical examination.

The patient's general condition may seem improved if he is seen somewhat later in the disease or after pain has been relieved by medication. His color returns, the syncopal state passes off, and the blood pressure returns to normal. The pulse rate may not be markedly elevated, but the pulse is usually full and bounding and more rapid than at an earlier period when the patient appeared to be in collapse. A very rapid thready pulse is not characteristic of early peritonitis; it is a late sign. The physical signs in the abdomen will remain unchanged despite the patient's appearance of improvement. At this stage it is most important that the physician be not misled by the apparent well-being of the patient; he must place proper emphasis on the physical examination. Late in the disease (after 12 to 18 hours) the signs of generalized peritonitis appear. These are discussed elsewhere.

Certain points must be emphasized as manifestations of free anterior perforation of duodenal or gastric ulcer. The *rigidity is boardlike. Retraction of the epigastrium* due to contraction of the recti abdomini and the diaphragm is frequently seen in the thin individual. The abdomen appears to have a band around it. There may be diminished or *absent liver dullness.* Tympany over the anterior portion of the liver is of little value since it frequently is caused by gas in loops of the small bowel. Tympany over the liver in the midaxillary line two inches or more above the costal margin is reliable evidence of free air in the peritoneal cavity (Fig. 7–21). The sign is useful if positive, but there may be no change in the area of liver dullness in the presence of gross contamination of the peritoneal cavity

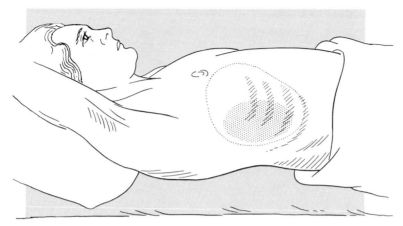

Figure 7–21. Demonstration of significant area of tympany (shaded area) over the liver with free air in the peritoneal cavity. Tympany anteriorly is of no significance, as it may be produced by distended loops of bowel.

from perforated gastric or duodenal ulcer. Indeed, an x-ray film taken in the upright position may fail to reveal free air beneath the diaphragm.

Perforated Duodenal Ulcer with a Slow Leakage of Duodenal Contents

Occasionally the contents of the bowel escape slowly and in such small quantity from a perforated duodenal ulcer that contamination of the free peritoneal cavity does not occur. The colon and omentum act as a watershed and direct the fluid into the right iliac fossa; the physical findings are predominantly those of an inflammatory lesion in that area. The history of pain arising in the epigastrium and shifting to the right lower abdomen may lead the examiner to suspect appendicitis. The differential diagnosis can usually be made by a careful one-finger palpation of the abdomen. The diagnosis of perforated ulcer is to be favored if a rather diffuse area of tenderness extending into the epigastrium is demonstrable. It is most unusual for acute appendicitis to produce clear-cut signs in both the upper and lower abdomen without other evidence of spreading peritonitis. Sometimes the differential diagnosis can be established only at operation.

Posterior Perforation of Duodenal Ulcer

A duodenal ulcer may perforate posteriorly into the pancreas or into the retroperitoneal tissue. The abdominal findings may be slight or may resemble acute pancreatitis. A subphrenic abscess may be the first manifestation of a posterior perforation of a duodenal ulcer.

Acute Pancreatitis

The abdominal findings in pancreatic disease may be minimal or absent because of the protected position of the pancreas behind the stomach, colon, and gastrocolic ligament. In *mild acute pancreatitis* the patient looks ill, but examination of the abdomen may show only vaguely localized tenderness in the epigastrium. In *acute necrotizing pancreatitis* the patient may go into collapse with cardiac irregularities which are suggestive of coronary occlusion. The signs of peritonitis may be lacking at first; when present they indicate the disease is well advanced. Deep tenderness over the pancreas and in the left upper quadrant is the most reliable early physical finding. Edema in the flanks is frequently present in the more advanced cases. Abdominal distention is usually found and peristalsis is diminished or absent. As a rule abdominal rigidity is not an early sign.

Jaundice, hypotension, and oliguria are grave signs.

Intensive shock therapy with massive fluid replacement is essential. Recently, peritoneal dialysis has proved beneficial.

Acute Diverticulitis

Diverticulitis of the colon is as protean in its manifestations as appendicitis. At times it may closely simulate appendicitis, but the findings are on the left side. Usually the tenderness in diverticulitis is more diffuse and frequently there is evidence of a local peritonitis even in the early stages of the disease. A palpable mass often is found in the left lower quadrant or in the pelvis. Diverticulitis less commonly produces acute large bowel obstruction and these signs and symptoms may be indistinguishable from those seen in carcinoma of the colon. An inflammatory mass in the flank or groin may be produced by perforation of a diverticulum. The diverticulum may perforate retroperitoneally or into the bladder or vagina without producing severe abdominal pain or major signs of sepsis. When a silent perforation involves the bladder, the passing of bubbles of air in the urine is an experience which the patient never forgets.

Early uncomplicated diverticulitis often responds to conservative treatment. Perforation, abscess formation, obstruction, or recurrent attacks require operation.

Perinephric Abscess

Perinephric abscess is usually insidious in onset, with fever and vague back pain. Deep tenderness in the flank may be elicited. Spasm of the iliopsoas muscle causes the patient to flex the hip; some scoliosis is present. A mass may become apparent as the disease becomes full blown. Differentiating this condition from renal tumors and cysts, leaking abdominal aneurysm, lymphoma, and pancreatitis involving the tail of the pancreas is not always easy.

Mesenteric Vascular Occlusion

Mesenteric vascular occlusion, either venous or arterial, is characterized by a remarkable contrast between the severity of the patient's symptoms and the paucity of the abdominal signs. Severe and persistent abdominal pain associated with varying signs of a gastrointestinal disturbance, such as vomiting, diarrhea, or an alteration of bowel function, is the usual presenting syndrome. The physical signs in the abdomen, however, are not unlike those seen in acute pancreatitis, with which mesenteric vascular occlusion is often confused. In the early stages there is no peritoneal irritation. Tenderness on deep palpation is often the only abnormality. Peristalsis may be normal or hyperactive. Spasm and distention are late manifestations and appear only after gangrene of the bowel and peritonitis have occurred.

The course of the disease depends upon the location and extent of the occlusion. An occlusion of the main venous trunk allows the patient to bleed massively into the mesentery with the rapid onset of shock and collapse. Large arterial occlusions are also associated with considerable shock. It is more common, however, with either venous or arterial occlusions to find the patient with severe, persistent abdominal pain, intractable to the usual measures for its relief and with few detectable abnormalities on the abdominal examination. A progressively rising pulse rate and leukocytosis are better guides to the gravity of the condition than are the abdominal signs. Later the signs of peritonitis appear.

Early diagnosis followed by surgical intervention with resection of the infarcted bowel is often lifesaving. The paucity of physical signs despite severe abdominal pain is an important clue to the diagnosis.

Mesenteric Ischemic Syndromes

Severe abdominal pain with essentially no abnormal physical findings suggestive of peritoneal irritation may result from mesenteric ischemia.

Arteriosclerosis of the celiac and superior mesenteric arteries is the more common cause but compression of the celiac artery by a congenital malformation of the arcuate ligament has been described and documented in a number of cases. There may be weight loss and in some cases severe malnutrition due to malabsorption.

The diagnosis is established by arteriography.

Dissecting Aneurysm of the Aorta

The underlying lesion is a degeneration of the media with initial rupture of the intima of the aorta near the aortic valves or in the descending aorta near the left subclavian artery. The patients usually have marked hypertension.

Death may occur from rapid dissection and rupture within a few hours. In subacute cases the process may continue over a period of days or weeks.

The onset is sudden with agonizing pain in the chest or epigastrium. Radiation to the neck, back, or into the abdomen is common. Shock and loss of consciousness often follow.

Varying signs of arterial insufficiency to the brain, arms, or legs suggestive of multiple embolization are important diagnostic clues. Roentgenograms may show a widening of the thoracic aorta. Angiocardiograms are diagnostic. There may be no electrocardiographic changes.

Prompt recognition is essential, as the condition can now be dealt with surgically.

Rupture of an Abdominal Aneurysm

Premonitory symptoms of pain and indigestion may lead to the diagnosis of an abdominal aneurysm prior to rupture. Careful physical examination will detect a number of aneurysms which are relatively asymptomatic and thus permit elective corrective surgery.

Rupture occurs into the retroperitoneal space, but there is often bleeding into the peritoneal cavity or rarely into a viscus or the vena cava. The signs are those of a major abdominal catastrophe with excruciating pain and shock. Peritoneal irritation may be minimal. A pulsating mass extending into the flank and lower abdomen combined with signs of shock and blood loss is diagnostic. In contrast to dissecting aneurysm the peripheral pulses are not obliterated as a rule and disappear only as a manifestation of profound shock.

The prognosis is grave, placing great importance on recognition of the lesion prior to rupture. However, emergency operation in experienced hands has greatly improved salvage in recent years.

The Signs of Obstruction of the Small Intestine

Simple Obstruction of the Small Bowel

The physical findings depend upon the cause and location of the obstruction. The most reliable single finding in early acute simple mid–small bowel obstruction due to an adhesive band or an internal hernia is the characteristic pattern of the peristaltic sounds. Inspection will indicate that the patient is suffering from intermittent bouts of colic between which he is quite comfortable. Occasionally a peristaltic wave may be seen if the abdominal wall is thin and flaccid. Early in the disease auscultation will reveal the classic rhythmic peristaltic pattern rising to a crescendo as the patient experiences his colic. As the pain subsides peristalsis will also die away. This observation of hyperactive peristalsis synchronous with the colic is the most significant early physical finding. The abdomen will be silent between seizures of pain or a few tinkles of normal peristalsis may be heard. Palpation may reveal tenderness over the involved loop of bowel. This is significant, but is by no means a constant finding. The involved loop of bowel may be so protected from the palpating hand that clear-cut tenderness cannot be elicited early in the disease. At this early stage a plain roentgenogram of the abdomen will usually provide confirmatory evidence of a distended loop of small intestine. Abdominal distention and tenderness appear later. The characteristic ladder pattern of visible peristalsis is also a late sign. Marked generalized tenderness is a sign of peritoneal irritation; it indicates perforation of the bowel or impending gangrene.

The manifestations vary with the level of the obstruction. In very high or very low obstruction the classic pattern of pain and peristalsis may not appear. In high obstruction, vomiting is a prominent feature but distention will not be present until peritonitis and ileus develop. In low obstruction, distention is early and progressive but vomiting is late. When it appears, it is likely to be feculent.

In all patients with intestinal obstruction the sites of hernia must be examined and re-examined.

Strangulation Obstruction of the Small Bowel

Strangulation and gangrene may be present without obvious clinical signs other than those of the intestinal obstruction. Consequently, early operation is the only way to exclude early gangrene. In advanced gangrene and strangulation, the patient appears critically ill. The pulse is rapid and full. There may be intermittent waves of colic, but between seizures of pain the patient will be aware of a persistent dull ache and discomfort in the abdomen. This may become agonizing, particularly in arterial occlusions. The characteristic crescendo pattern of peristaltic activity ceases with the onset of gangrene. The bowel may continue to be active and peristalsis may be heard for a time, but gradually the abdomen becomes silent.

Peritonitis is manifested by tenderness and rigidity. Shock and collapse may ensue, especially in venous occlusion in which blood may be lost in great quantity into the bowel and mesentery.

Chronic Incomplete Obstruction of the Small Bowel

Chronic partial obstruction of the small bowel from tumor or slowly progressive inflammation or adhesions is characterized by intermittent episodic abdominal cramps. Marked distention of the small bowel with muscular hypertrophy may occur. The bowel compensates for the partial obstruction so that vomiting does not occur and distention is often mild. There may be occasional episodes of diarrhea, simulating a malabsorption syndrome. X-ray will show the dilated hypertrophied bowel but the area of stenosis is easily overlooked. Decompression of the bowel with a long nasogastric tube followed by the introduction of contrast material through the tube will establish the diagnosis.

The condition must be distinguished from pseudo-obstruction of the small bowel which results from disturbances of motility either idiopathic or associated with scleroderma, amyloid disease, or chronic use of tranquilizing drugs. In these conditions barium x-ray will exclude mechanical obstruction.

The Signs of Obstruction of the Colon

Obstruction of the colon is usually due to *carcinoma, diverticulitis, intussusception,* or *volvulus.* Each of these conditions has certain physical signs which are peculiar to it. Diverticulitis has been discussed earlier in this chapter.

INTUSSUSCEPTION

Intussusception commonly occurs in children but is seen in adults, particularly in the presence of a benign tumor which acts as the leading point of the intussusception. The physical signs vary to some extent with the stage of the disease. Pain is usually severe, but is not continuous. The patient tends to lie quietly with his knees flexed between bouts of pain. Some degree of syncope and collapse is usually present, especially if the pain is severe and prostrating. Occasionally peristaltic waves may be seen.

Palpation

A striking physical feature which usually establishes the diagnosis beyond doubt is a sausage-shaped abdominal mass; it will be found somewhere along the course of the colon, depending upon the stage of the disease. A mass will always be present if bloody fluid has been passed by rectum; it may be difficult to demonstrate if it lies under either hypochondrium at the flexures of the colon. Frequently confirmatory evidence may be found by careful palpation of the right lower quadrant which will seem empty because of the absence of the cecum and ascending colon. In more advanced stages, the tip of the intussusception may be palpable by rectum. The combination of colicky abdominal pain, passage of blood by rectum, and the finding of a sausage-shaped mass within the abdomen is classic.

ACUTE OBSTRUCTION DUE TO CARCINOMA OF THE COLON

Sudden, acute colonic obstruction is produced occasionally by carcinoma. Usually there are premonitory signs due to the presence of the tumor; these include a change in bowel habits or the passage of blood per rectum, but they may not have occurred or may have escaped the attention of the patient. Once complete occlusion of the colon occurs, the subsequent course is dependent to some extent upon the competency of the ileocecal valve. Fluid will not regurgitate into the ileum if the valve is competent. The colon becomes enormously distended with great rapidity. Vomiting may not occur, and the pain is often not severe, but obstipation will be present. Physical findings include marked generalized distention of the abdomen, tympany to percussion, loud irregular borborygmi with peristaltic rushes and gurgling, and tenderness over the course of the colon. A mass may or may not be palpable. Perforation of the colon may occur, with signs of rapidly disseminating peritonitis. Usually the cecum or right colon is the site of perforation.

The signs are less rapidly progressive if the ileocecal valve is incompetent. Vomiting will occur, and the degree of distention is less marked and better tolerated by the patient.

VOLVULUS OF THE SIGMOID

Acute sigmoid volvulus is more common in countries in which the diet is of high residue. In the Western world this condition is most commonly seen in elderly patients, psychiatric patients, and residents of nursing homes. The clinical picture is striking, with severe abdominal pain, rapid distention of the abdomen, nausea, and vomiting. The pain is persistent with colicky exacerbations. The abdominal distention may appear asymmetric but is always massive. It may be possible to outline the huge distended loops of sigmoid by palpation and percussion.

In volvulus of the sigmoid, the loop rotates to the right of the midline. The x-ray picture is striking and will show a narrow beaklike deformity (Fig. 7–22).

In early cases the obstructive loop can be decompressed by gently passing a well lubricated rectal tube through a sigmoidoscope into the area of torsion. If this is unsuccessful or if the condition is an advanced case with signs of peritonitis, emergency operation is indicated.

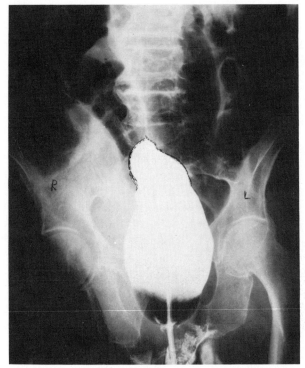

Figure 7–22. Sigmoid volvulus. The column of barium shows the "bird's beak" deformity. The proximal bowel is greatly distended.

VOLVULUS OF THE CECUM

Volvulus of the cecum is less common. It also occurs in the elderly and may be precipitated by low grade ileus secondary to systemic illness such as pneumonia or renal failure. There must be some degree of incomplete fixation of the cecum which rotates medially and upward. The distended loop may extend to the left side of the abdomen (Fig. 7–23). The thin wall of the cecum is prone to early gangrene and perforation; therefore, early emergency operation is indicated as soon as the diagnosis is made.

The Signs of Peritonitis

Acute diffuse peritonitis is manifested by signs of such importance that they are properly described as an entity.

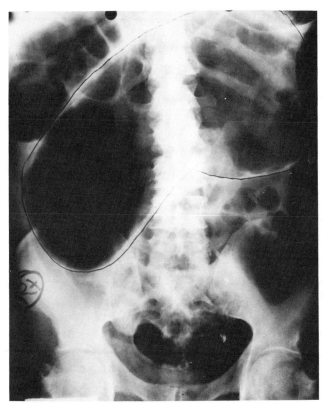

Figure 7–23. Volvulus of the cecum. The greatly distended cecum extends far into the left side of the abdomen.

Inspection

The patient appears ill and anxious. The astute observer will detect a pallor in the facies and a little movement of the alae nasi even in the early stages; a sober anxious look in the eye or a feigned appearance of well-being will indicate at a glance that the patient has a serious disease. The pulse is usually elevated, above 100, and is full and bounding. In advanced peritonitis it becomes weak, rapid, and thready. There are exceptions and one must not be misled by a slow pulse. The circulatory system may not be disturbed in the rugged, heavy-set well conditioned individual by infection and a loss of plasma into the peritoneal cavity, which would produce shock in a small, asthenic individual. A striking exception to the usual appearance of a patient with peritonitis is that seen in association with acute gonorrheal salpingitis. Here the general appearance of brightness and well-being of the patient is in decided contrast to the extent of the abdominal signs.

The patient with peritonitis lies quietly, preferably on his side with the hips slightly flexed in order to relax the abdominal musculature. Motion is painful. This posture is the opposite of that seen in patients with colic or intestinal cramps, for they cannot remain quiet during seizures of pain.

Observation of the abdomen is most important. Early in the disease it is scaphoid and retracted, particularly across the epigastrium. This appearance is occasioned by spasm of the rectus muscles and limitation of motions of the diaphragm. Normal respiratory movements of the abdomen are absent. Later the abdomen will appear full, with slight pouting of the umbilicus as distention develops. Extreme distention is rare and should be regarded as a very late sign or as evidence of an associated intestinal obstruction.

Palpation

The degree of muscular rigidity varies. The rigidity will be boardlike and completely unyielding to firm pressure if the anterior wall of the peritoneal cavity is involved by a generalized inflammatory process; this is true even when the patient breathes deeply with his mouth open. Extreme rigidity is characteristic of free anterior perforations of a duodenal or gastric ulcer. It may also occur in obstructive appendicitis with early gangrene and perforation. Rigidity is not a prominent early sign in peritonitis associated with acute pancreatitis, becuase the inflammatory process arises in the lesser peritoneal cavity and later the omentum protects the anterior abdominal wall from the extravasated peritoneal fluid. One may generally expect less rigidity in the obese patient, regardless of the etiology of the peritonitis, because of the protecting action of a large fatty omentum. Marked muscular rigidity may not occur in the elderly or debilitated individual even in the presence of a free perforation simply because the muscle tone is poor.

Tenderness distributed throughout the abdomen, with rebound tenderness referred to the point of pressure, is characteristic of a diffuse or generalized peritonitis. Cough tenderness is diffuse but the patient feels it most in the midabdomen. It may cause severe pain to elicit this sign.

Palpation of the abdomen should always be repeated after sedation has been given and again after the induction of anesthesia, whether or not the diagnosis has been clearly established.

Percussion

This should always be gently and carefully performed since it may outline a mass which cannot be palpated because of the tenderness and spasm. Percussion of the area of liver dullness may indicate the presence of free air in the peritoneal cavity.

Auscultation

The abdomen rapidly becomes silent. The finding of normal peristalsis in what appears to be an acute peritonitis should lead the examiner to consider severe gastroenteritis or acute dysentery, both of which may present with diffuse abdominal tenderness. Systemic causes of abdominal pain and tenderness, such as impending diabetic coma or porphyria, should be excluded. Acute diaphragmatic pleurisy or acute coronary thrombosis may also closely stimulate an acute peritonitis. In these situations gentle firm pressure with the flat of the hand against the abdominal musculature will be well tolerated by the patient, while in the presence of peritonitis it will be persistently painful. Re-examination of the abdomen after relief of excruciating pain by sedation will enable the examiner to perceive that the abdominal examination is not abnormal and will direct his attention to the thorax.

Rectal and vaginal examinations cannot be omitted and will confirm the presence of an acute generalized inflammatory process, since pressure against the pouch of Douglas will elicit pain. There may be a sense of fullness on pressure in the pouch of Douglas.

Stage of Toxemia and Shock

Profound toxemia in the very late stages is manifested by the dusky pallor of the skin, the sunken eyes, the pinched nose, the dry coated tongue, and the silent distended abdomen. The weak, thready, running pulse indicates that the end is near. Pain is usually alleviated, but consciousness often remains to the last.

The Effect of Antibiotics on the Clinical Picture of Peritonitis

The liberal use of the antibiotics greatly alters the signs of peritonitis. There may be very little abdominal tenderness, rigidity, or distention. Peristalsis may continue actively in the face of a spreading peritonitis. If the cause of the peritonitis is self-limited, this alteration of the abdominal signs is a favorable omen. In the presence of continued contamination of the peritoneal cavity, however, the amelioration of the physical signs does not mean that the infection is effectively controlled. Sudden profound shock and toxemia may occur with renal failure and death without the more classic signs of peritonitis appearing.

V. THE POSTOPERATIVE ABDOMEN

The examination of the postoperative abdomen is comparable in many ways to the examination of the acute abdomen. The detection of complications and the care of the patient are governed by a correct interpretation of pain, tenderness, spasm, peristalsis, distention, and changes in the temperature, pulse, and respiration. The serious sequelae of major abdominal surgery are common to the acute surgical lesions, namely, peritonitis, abscess formation, and intestinal obstruction. There are also certain complications more or less peculiar to the trauma of surgery, such as urinary retention, postoperative distention, hemorrhage, and acute gastric dilatation. Space does not permit a discussion of postoperative care following abdominal surgery, but the importance of physical signs in the evaluation of the postoperative abdomen merits emphasis.

The Uncomplicated Postoperative Abdomen

There is amazingly little reaction to a well performed major abdominal operation. If the bowel has been handled gently, tissue has not been traumatized, and a careful peritoneal toilet has been performed prior to closure, the most extensive operation results in no untoward physical signs.

Pain should be minimal and clearly related to the wound in that it is aggravated by moving or coughing and is readily controlled by medication. Severe constant pain, not readily controlled by sedation, is very unusual. It is a disturbing sign and suggests peritoneal irritation or vascular damage to the bowel. It warrants a very careful appraisal of all related signs. It may be caused by urinary retention without the patient's being able to recognize or localize the character of his pain.

The pulse should be slow, below 100 per minute, if blood loss has been replaced and if there is no sign of a pulmonary complication. A slow, regular, quiet, full but not bounding pulse is one of the most gratifying physical signs after major abdominal surgery. It clearly says that all is well. A moderate elevation of the pulse is often explained by a pulmonary complication or by apprehension and pain. A moderately elevated but bounding pulse is slightly disturbing. It may merely indicate the extent of the surgery, but it is also an early sign of peritoneal contamination. A rapid, thready pulse is distinctly abnormal. It almost invariably signals the presence of a significant complication or indicates that blood loss has not been adequately replaced. A progressively rising pulse within a few hours of completion of an operation should arouse a suspicion of hemorrhage.

Fever is not a reliable sign in the early period after operation. Temperature should be normal or only slightly elevated but frequently is high within the first 48 hours because of what may be a relatively minor pulmonary complication. It may be low or only slightly elevated in the presence of serious peritoneal infection. The liberal use of the antibiotics has rendered fever in the postoperative period a particularly unreliable sign. However, a progressively rising staircase type of fever requires detailed investigation. It is characteristic of a progressing abscess. A rare but significant fever is one which swings from very high to subnormal with associated chills and sweats. It is characteristic of pylephlebitis and multiple liver abscesses, but here again the typical pattern may be altered greatly by antibiotic therapy.

The respiratory rate is often slightly elevated because of wound pain. An abdominal binder too tightly applied or placed so as to restrict the costal cage is an avoidable cause of elevated respirations. Quiet, easy respirations are almost as reassuring as a quiet pulse. Very rapid respiration or dyspnea in the absence of a definite pulmonary complication is most alarming. When the abdominal signs are minimal and no clear-cut evidence of a pulmonary complication can be found, an acute gastric dilatation should be suspected. A gastric tube will clarify the cause better than the stethoscope.

Inspection of the abdomen tells a good deal. If it is flat and the normal respiratory movements can be seen, there is little likelihood of serious difficulty. Slight fullness of the abdomen and mild distention are fairly common, particularly about 48 hours after operation. Obvious distention of the abdomen requires thorough investigation.

Palpation of the abdomen may be restricted in the uncomplicated case merely to testing for tenderness and noting the general tone of the musculature. This should be done at some distance away from the wound. If it is gently performed, there should be no rigidity or tenderness. Percussion need not be carried out unless there is evidence of distention or one suspects gastric dilatation. Percussion then may be of great help in localizing areas of distended bowel or stomach.

Auscultation is most important and should invariably be performed. Within the first 48 hours after an operation peristaltic sounds are usually diminished. The casual observer may think them to be absent, but a careful long listen will disclose an occasional normal tinkle which is most reassuring. Although normal peristaltic sounds may be heard within 24 hours of an operation, they do not exclude the possibility of a slowly developing peritoneal complication. If there is reason to fear the development of peritonitis, auscultation must be carefully repeated at 6 to 12 hour intervals. Complete absence of peristalsis over a period of several minutes is an ominous sign.

Danger Signals After Major Abdominal Surgery

The danger signals after major abdominal surgery are persistent pain, a rapid pulse, elevated respirations or dyspnea in the absence of a pulmonary complication, early distention, and a silent abdomen on auscultation. The presence of any of these requires a detailed appraisal of the situation. The essential steps will be pointed out under the discussion of each of the major complications.

A word of caution is necessary. The liberal use of the antibiotics renders the appraisal of the postoperative abdomen exceptionally difficult. Complications may develop under cover of the antibiotics and sedation, with minimal evidence of pain, tenderness, or muscular rigidity.

Urinary Retention

It is an essential part of postoperative care to determine whether or not the patient has voided following operation. If he has not done so within six to eight hours, the physical signs of a distended bladder should be sought. Frequently the diagnosis is easily made because the patient has a painful desire to void but cannot do so. Palpation and percussion of the lower abdomen will disclose the oval-shaped mass of the distended, tender bladder. However, the picture is not always cut so clearly. Not infrequently the bladder distends so slowly that the patient experiences little or no discomfort and the only evidence of urinary retention is the huge distended bladder. Occasionally after major procedures the bladder becomes distended without the patient's being able to localize the source of his discomfort. Medication may be given to quiet the patient and thus permit further distention of the bladder. Eventually, agonizing, poorly localized pain develops. If the patient is obese, the signs of a distended bladder may not be readily detected. Gentle pressure just above the symphysis pubis will usually accentuate the pain and render its character evident, but catheterization may be necessary to establish or exclude the presence of a distended bladder.

Postoperative Distention

A curious type of functional ileus follows many abdominal operations. It is characterized by abdominal distention and crampy pains which the patient identifies as "gas pains." It makes its appearance about 36 hours or more after operation and in most instances promptly subsides as soon as the patient begins to pass flatus by rectum. It is attributable to many factors, of which excessive swallowing of air is among the most important. The handling of the intestines during an operation may be a factor, but is not the principal one since the condition frequently occurs following hernial operations or renal operations in which the peritoneal cavity is not greatly disturbed. The bowel is not paralyzed and the term "paralytic ileus" should not be applied to this condition. There is a functional defect in peristalsis which permits the accumulation of gas in both the small and the large bowel. In extreme cases there may be great dilatation of both intestines and stomach.

The physical findings are variable. Slight distention and moderate tympany on percussion over the lower abdomen are sufficient to make the diagnosis in mild cases. Peristalsis may be diminished or it may be hyperactive. The activity of peristalsis is not synchronous with the patient's cramps. A rather high-pitched, continuous peristalsis frequently is encountered. If peristalsis is diminished, the question of paralytic ileus immediately enters the equation. Usually the benignity of the operation and the generally excellent condition of the patient excludes this possibility. After major intestinal or gastric surgery, however, one may have to listen to the abdomen for a long time before the reassuring sounds of peristalsis are heard. Tenderness is an important sign. It is not found in simple, postoperative distention and if it is present, particularly at some distance away from the wound, it is indicative of peritoneal irritation. An absolutely silent abdomen through which the sounds of the aortic pulsations are clearly heard is not consistent with a diagnosis of simple postoperative distention.

It is an interesting fact that postoperative distention is less common after major procedures on the gastrointestinal tract, probably because in these instances gastric suction is maintained for 24 or 48 hours after operation, thus preventing the swallowing of air which is the principal source of the gas in postoperative distention. Distention which develops despite the use of continuous gastric suction is not likely to be due to a functional ileus.

Acute Gastric Dilatation

Acute dilatation of the stomach may be a complication of either postoperative distention or peritonitis. In its milder forms it may be a consequence of excessive swallowing of air and intake of fluids prior to the resumption of normal intestinal activities. It may reach such extreme proportions that there is interference with respirations. *Hiccough is a frequent symptom.* The patient may vomit, but usually repeatedly regurgitates a small amount of dark, brownish black fluid. The astute clinician will recognize the development of gastric dilatation before hiccough, regurgitation, or marked distention with respiratory distress appear. In the early stages there is a slight fullness in the upper abdomen. This asymmetric distention of the abdomen is very suggestive of gastric dilatation. The patient looks and feels uncomfortable. Despite a sense of fullness, he is frequently thirsty and continues to drink, thereby worsening his condition. Palpation will confirm the impression of fullness in the upper abdomen. Usually there is sufficient gas as well as fluid in the stomach so that the dilated viscus can be outlined by percussion. The diagnosis is established by passing a Levin tube and aspirating the stomach. Great quantities of air and fluid are obtained, with immediate decompression of the abdomen and marked relief to the patient. If there is the slightest doubt about incipient gastric dilatation, one should immediately pass an aspirating tube. The condition is encountered much less frequently after major gastrointestinal surgery because of the frequent use of a gastric tube.

Acute gastric dilatation may be a feature of peritonitis, in which case other signs of peritonitis and paralytic ileus will be present.

Peritonitis

A progressive peritonitis following abdominal surgery rarely follows mere contamination of the peritoneal cavity. It is caused by necrosis of bowel, leakage from an anastomosis, seepage of bile, or acute pancreatitis. Fortunately, proper preoperative preparation, improved surgical techniques, and a liberal use of antibiotics have made this a rare condition.

The classic manifestations of peritonitis are seldom seen in the postoperative period. Many factors are responsible for this. The initial stages of the disease may be obscured by the recovery phase of anesthesia. Pain dulled by morphine is readily attributable to the wound, moderate alterations of temperature or pulse to a pulmonary complication, and early distention to functional ileus. Because of the presence of a wound, spasm, rigidity, and tenderness are difficult to evaluate. If antibiotics are being given in large doses, the physical signs may be extraordinarily slight. Extensive peritonitis may develop without spasm, rigidity, or exquisite tenderness. Moreover, peristalsis sufficient to mislead the examiner may continue fitfully for many hours or even days. Indeed, continuous gastric suction and the antibiotics may so mask the usual signs of peritonitis that the stage of collapse and toxemia may abruptly develop while the physical signs are equivocal.

Patients do so well today following major gastrointestinal surgery that any untoward sign should suggest the possibility of a serious intraperitoneal complication. A rising pulse rate or a full, bounding, rapid pulse, when taken together with slight but progressive deep tenderness on palpation, markedly diminished peristalsis, and the siphonage of large amounts of dark fluid from the stomach will indicate the diagnosis to the careful observer when a casual examination of the abdomen might make a diagnosis of peritonitis seem impossible. More important than the physical findings at any given moment is the progression of changes. Increasing, deep abdominal tenderness when associated with a steadily rising pulse and diminished to absent peristalsis may be the only signs on which the diagnosis can be made.

It is of the utmost importance to recognize a steadily progressing peritonitis because, with modern methods of resuscitation and the antibiotic control of infections, re-operation for such complications can be readily undertaken. Following operations on the biliary tract or stomach, signs of peritoneal irritation may represent a complicating acute pancreatitis. Confirmation of this diagnosis may be obtained by a blood amylase determination.

Finally, because of the paucity of abdominal signs which may accompany postoperative peritonitis during heavy antibiotic therapy, hypotension and shock appearing several days following an operation may be due to peritonitis despite equivocal abdominal signs.

Residual Abscess

Intraperitoneal abscesses are a consequence of peritoneal infections, localized or diffuse. Frequently the peritonitis has been obvious, as in acute perforated appendicitis or duodenal ulcer. On other occasions, particularly following clean abdominal surgery, a localized peritonitis is often overlooked, and the development of a residual abscess is the first indication that all has not gone well.

Abscesses may occur anywhere in the peritoneal cavity. The pelvis and the immediate operative field are the most usual sites, but abscesses may develop among loops of small bowel, in the peritoneal gutters, along the course of the colon or in the subdiaphragmatic spaces. As a result of antibiotic therapy residual abscesses which progress to the point of requiring drainage are less frequent than formerly. They are also much harder to detect, and a progressing intraperitoneal abscess may drag a patient down before making its presence obvious by local signs.

If antibiotics are not being given, fever is usually the first sign of a residual abscess. It generally makes its appearance toward the end of the first week after operation at a time when convalescence is apparently progressing well. *A staircase type of fever, rising slightly higher each day and not returning to normal at any time, is typical of a progressing abscess.* If the abscess is in the pelvis, it may be detectable at this early date as a slightly tender, indurated mass in the pouch of Douglas. As it progresses it enlarges and softens, and the patient usually suffers from an irritative diarrhea. Elsewhere than in the pelvis, carefully repeated physical examinations of the abdomen may be necessary to locate the site of the infection. Increasing tenderness localized to a given area and slight resistance and fullness on palpation are early signs. Later a well defined mass may appear.

If the patient is recovering from an extensive peritonitis and is receiving large doses of antibiotics, the presence of a residual abscess is less easily detected. Fever is not a reliable sign; it may be normal, irregularly elevated or it may show the more characteristic staircase type of elevation. *Anorexia, failure to gain in weight and strength, vague abdominal pain, and a moderate elevation of the pulse rate are frequently the only presenting manifestations of sizable abscesses.* The physical examination of the abdomen may be exceedingly misleading. Here again, comparative examinations repeated from day to day are much more informative than any single appraisal of the abdomen. The general peritoneal cavity, the pelvis, and the subdiaphragmatic spaces must be examined and re-examined. If the related circumstances indicate a definite probability of a residual abscess and the patient is slowly losing ground, exploration of the most probable site of infection is indicated. At times, the most extraordinary collections of pus may be encountered when the physical signs remain equivocal. Plain x-ray films of the abdomen may disclose opacities between gas-filled loops of bowel suggesting collections of fluid, or rarely may indicate gas and a fluid level in a large abscess. The use of ultrasound is proving to be of great value in detecting peritoneal and retroperitoneal abscesses.

Postoperative subphrenic abscesses have the same manifestations and pose the same problems in diagnosis as has been discussed earlier (see page 85).

Hemorrhage

Postoperative intraperitoneal bleeding has become an extraordinarily rare complication; so rare, in fact, that the surgeon finds it difficult to believe. It is an early complication, generally developing within 24 hours of operation. Delayed hemorrhage is almost never seen following elective abdominal surgery, although it may be a complication of abdominal wounds. The physical signs are those of acute blood loss and are described in more detail elsewhere (Chap. 19). The precise levels of the blood pressure and pulse rate may be misleading. Pallor, sweating, anxiety, and air hunger may indicate the diagnosis better than the level of the pulse and blood pressure. The course of the pulse and blood pressure is more reliable than the exact level. Tachycardia and hypotension suddenly developing some hours after operation should arouse suspicion of bleeding. Blood may issue from drains or, in the case of a gastric operation, be aspirated or vomited, but extensive bleeding may occur without this happening.

The abdominal findings are difficult to interpret because of the presence of a very fresh wound. Progressive deep abdominal tenderness some distance away from the wound is perhaps the most reliable sign. Shifting dullness may be demonstrable, but usually it is not. Laboratory data may be quite misleading, since following operation there may be moderate dehydration, and a normal hematocrit may be obtained despite extensive loss of blood. Re-operation is a better course than hopeful observation.

There are many operations performed today in which extensive blood loss is unavoidable, such as excision of a ruptured aortic aneurysm or an extensive aorto-iliac thromboendarterectomy. Massive blood replacement is essential and despite all forms of monitoring it may be difficult to tell at any given moment the adequacy of blood replacement. In the postoperative period, intra-abdominal bleeding may continue, but the systemic signs of blood loss are masked by continuing replacement. Very often the patient is removed from the operating table with continuing tachycardia and an unstable blood pressure. Under these circumstances, progressive enlargement of the abdomen may be the most reliable sign of a continuing, major postoperative intra-abdominal hemorrhage. Tying a string around the abdomen to measure progressive enlargement is a very useful maneuver.

Laboratory data may be quite misleading. Following operation there may be moderate dehydration or overhydration, and the level of the hematocrit fails to reflect the degree of blood loss.

In straightforward, uncomplicated elective operations in which postoperative hemorrhage should not occur, immediate re-operation is required for signs of blood loss. On the other hand, in extensive intra-abdominal operations of necessity associated with extensive loss of blood, continuing blood replacement and careful monitoring may avoid re-operation even though it is evident that there is continuing bleeding. If the bleeding is chiefly retroperitoneal oozing, even though it may be considerable and spontaneous, clotting or tamponade usually occurs.

Intestinal Obstruction

The signs of intestinal obstruction in the postoperative period follow the patterns described in the section on the acute abdomen. If there has been peritoneal inflammation and ileus, the distinction between a mechanical obstruction and continued ileus is at times exceedingly difficult. Repeated examinations of the abdomen when correlated with the x-ray data, especially after the passage of an intestinal tube, usually clarify the situation. Persistent distention, localizing tenderness, sometimes a little fullness or a questionable mass when corroborated by continued dilation of a particular loop of bowel on the x-ray film, point to a mechanical obstruction. The classic pattern of rhythmic peristalsis and colicky pain may be absent because of the associated partial ileus.

A straightforward mechanical obstruction of a loop of small bowel is quite obvious in the postoperative period. Early after operation it may be overlooked momentarily because of the patient's general discomfort and what may at first appear to be postoperative distention, but the colicky nature of the pain, the characteristic peristaltic pattern, and the onset of obstipation and distention soon make the differentiation easy. One must not be misled by a lack of distention if the abdomen is being decompressed by continuous intestinal suction. Frequently the nature of the operation provides a clue to the site of a postoperative obstruction, such as a colostomy or ileostomy around which a loop of bowel may have rotated. Total colectomy for ulcerative colitis is frequently complicated by partial or complete postoperative obstruction of the small bowel.

chapter 8   # EXAMINATION OF THE ABDOMEN OF INFANTS AND CHILDREN

It has been said that the adult may be safely treated as a child, but the converse can lead to disaster. The child is not a little man, and the physical examination must be modified accordingly. It cannot be hurried; it must be gently performed, and the child's confidence must be gained. Provided the child is old enough, the examiner must be willing to explain what he is going to do and give honest answers to the child's questions. At times it is advisable to have the parents remain outside the examining room, since their presence may encourage a child to be uncooperative. A genuine fondness for children is a great asset to the examiner.

I. GENERAL CONDUCT OF THE EXAMINATION

The examination of the head, neck and chest should be postponed until after the abdominal examination. The manipulations of these examinations are apt to upset infants and children and render an evaluation of the abdominal findings more difficult. Laboratory studies which require drawing of blood should also be postponed until the entire physical examination is completed. The following sequence is recommended:

Inspection

Every detail of the child's behavior and physical characteristics must be carefully noted. The rate of respiration, the color of the skin, the position which the patient assumes with special reference to his legs, indications of pain or restlessness, and the presence of sunken eyes, visible peristalsis, or distention are especially important.

178

Auscultation

If the bell of the stethoscope is warm, ausculation is painless. It tends to intrigue rather than upset the child. It should be performed prior to palpation. The abnormalities of the peristaltic sounds which may be heard have been described in Chapter 7.

Palpation

It is particularly important to divert the child's attention (if he is old enough to speak) by light conversation during palpation. Keep a sharp lookout for changes in the child's facial expression, since they are more accurate indications of the presence or absence of tenderness than is direct questioning. Deep palpation and the other details of the visceral examination are similar to that employed in adults. Bimanual palpation of the kidneys is essential. The liver and spleen are normally palpable at the costal margin in infants and young children.

The general physical examination follows the abdominal examination. Particular attention is given to the ears, sinuses, throat, and chest, since infections in these areas are often the cause of abdominal complaints. In young infants the fontanelles should be inspected and palpated, since they indicate dehydration if they are sunken and increased intracranial pressure if they are bulging. A rectal examination should be performed last. The fifth finger should be used in infants, but the index finger can be used in older children in the usual manner. The maximum amount of information can be gained from the physical examination if this sequence of events is followed.

II. ABDOMINAL SYNDROMES IN INFANTS AND CHILDREN

Some of the more common abdominal syndromes in infants and children are described below.

Infantile Hypertrophic Pyloric Stenosis

This disease appears most frequently between three and six weeks of life and is more common in males. Non-bilious projectile vomiting is the cardinal symptom. The vomiting will be less forceful in weak or premature infants. If the disease is of more than a few days' duration, the infant becomes markedly dehydrated and looks like a "little old man." The baby will be described as having constipation because few, dry stools will be passed. Waves of gastric peristalsis can be seen moving from the left cos-

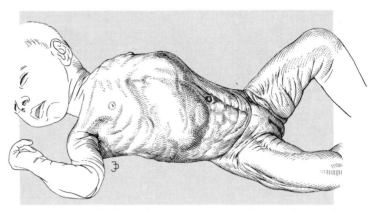

Figure 8–1. Visible peristalsis in an infant with pyloric stenosis.

tal margin to the right epigastrium (Fig. 8–1). The upper abdomen is full, and the lower abdomen is sunken. The hypertrophic pyloric muscle can be located where the peristaltic waves stop. Usually the pyloris is in the right upper quadrant, but it may be in the mid-epigastrium or possibly below the level of the umbilicus, depending on its mobility. The pyloric "tumor" is palpated best when the examiner is on the left side of the patient. The examiner and the infant must be completely relaxed. Relaxation of the infant's abdominal wall is accomplished by feeding the baby sweetened water, or the abdomen may become relaxed immediately after the infant has vomited. The index and long fingers are used to fix the tumor to the posterior abdominal wall. The mass will feel like a firm, cartilaginous "olive," even though the actual pyloric hypertrophy is 1.5 × 2.5 cm. in size. The mass tends to slip freely from under the finger. The typical history and physical findings are sufficient to establish the diagnosis, and the baby may be prepared for a pyloromyotomy without further diagnostic study. Occasionally a gastrointestinal contrast study will be necessary to show the narrow pyloric canal.

Intussusception

Intussusception typically occurs in otherwise healthy, plump babies under 2 years of age. The infant suddenly cries out in obvious severe pain and draws up his legs. Such an episode lasts for a short time, and the child then relaxes and returns to normal activity or remains quiet and withdrawn, only to cry out again minutes later. There is non-bilious vomiting initially, but with time, the distal bowel obstruction results in vomiting of green bile. In 95 per cent of the cases the ileum telescopes into the right colon and the bowel may intussuscept to the transverse or distal colon. The intussusception may be palpable in the mid-epigastrium or under the costal margins as a "sausage-shaped" mass when the child is completely relaxed. Occasionally, the right lower quadrant feels empty when the intussusception has advanced beyond the transverse colon. Later in the course, bloody mucus or "currant-jelly" clots may be passed. Advanced intussusception is palpable by rectal examination, and the intussusceptum feels like the cervix uteri.

A barium enema is performed to establish the diagnosis, and the hydrostatic pressure is used to reduce the intussusceptum. If barium enema fails, surgical reduction is necessary.

Congenital Obstruction of the Duodenum and Intestine

Obstruction of the duodenum in newborn infants may be produced by atresia, stenosis, annular pancreas, or intestinal malrotation with adhesive bands. When the duodenal obstruction is distal to the ampulla of Vater, the infant vomits bile. With duodenal obstruction, the upper abdomen is distended and the lower abdomen is scaphoid.

Obstructions of the jejunum, ileum, and colon may result from atresia, stenosis, meconium ileus, or congenital megacolon (Hirschsprung's disease). The distended bowel with peristalsis may be outlined on the abdominal wall. The intestinal segments may be palpated, and in cases of meconium ileus, the meconium-filled bowel may be palpable. Except in cases of intestinal stenosis, very little if any stool will be encountered in the rectal examination.

Hirschsprung's disease is caused by the absence of intramural ganglion cells in the bowel wall. It begins at the anus and extends a varying distance proximally. The rectum and distal colon are collapsed and tonic contraction prevents normal emptying of the proximal intestine. In 80 per cent of the cases, the transition zone of normal but dilated and hypertrophied bowel is located in the sigmoid colon. In 10 per cent of the infants the entire bowel is aganglionic, and in 15 per cent only the rectum is affected.

The stool-filled, dilated colon is usually palpable through the chronically distended abdominal wall. Rectal examination generally reveals an ampulla without stool. However, in short-segment Hirschsprung's disease, stool may be palpable down to the anus. Anal sphincter tone may or may not be appreciated as greater than normal. Barium enema shows abnormal contraction waves in the rectum and a normal caliber bowel to the transition zone where the colon becomes greatly dilated. Rectal biopsy is used to show the absence of ganglion cells.

Anomalies of the Biliary System

Congenital obstruction of the bile ducts may be due to biliary atresia or choledochal cyst. The salient finding is jaundice. In newborn infants, the jaundice may develop shortly after birth or there may be a jaundice-free interval of several weeks before icterus is noted. The abdomen is full, owing to the enlarged liver, and after several months accumulation of ascitic fluid develops. The spleen is frequently enlarged. A choledochal cyst may be identified as a mass palpable beneath the enlarged liver. Choledochal cysts in older children present with intermittent jaundice, right upper quadrant pain, and a palpable mass.

Duplications of the Alimentary Tract

Duplications may be spherical or tubular and are located on the mesenteric side of the intestine. They may produce symptoms of intestinal bleeding, perforation, or obstruction. If large enough, an elusive, mobile mass will be palpable. Tubular duplication of the distal colon and rectum may be palpable as a soft, sausage-shaped mass on abdominal and rectal palpation.

Colon and Rectal Polyps

Polyps of the colon and rectum in infants and children are most commonly the inflammatory, "juvenile," or retention type. Isolated adenomatous polyps are rare. Adenomatous polyps associated with familial polyposis may develop very early in childhood. Peutz-Jeghers syndrome associated with hamartomatous polyps in the colon of children is very rare. Multiple polypoid formation due to lymphoid hyperplasia also occurs in infancy. Each of these lesions may produce bright red rectal bleeding located on the surface of stool, or the lesion may prolapse through the anal canal. Eighty per cent are within reach of the examining finger and 90 per cent can be detected by sigmoidoscopy. A general anesthetic is required for proctoscopy or sigmoidscopy in infants and small children.

Appendicitis

The child's appendix is longer in relation to the abdominal cavity than is that of the adult. The cecum and right colon are very mobile and the mesoappendix is also correspondingly longer and less fixed. For these reasons the point of maximal tenderness varies more in location than it does in adults. It may appear near the midline, well down in the pelvic region, or in the right flank. When the pain is accompanied by involuntary muscle spasm, it is evidence of inflammatory involvement of the parietal peritoneum. Localized tenderness and guarding are essential findings to make the diagnosis. Rectal examination of a low-lying pelvic appendix may cause exquisite tenderness which is not elicited by abdominal palpation. Elicitation of rebound tenderness is undesirable in children because the element of surprise and pain is difficult to evaluate and strains the examiner's rapport with the patient. A better technique for eliciting local peritonitis is to use gentle percussion of the abdomen. The psoas and obturator signs are also difficult to detect in infancy and childhood. Irritation of the psoas muscle by an abscess or inflamed appendix is more apt to be recognized in a child by noting the position he assumes when left undisturbed; he will tend to lie on the right side, partially flexed. Retrocecal appendicitis is difficult to diagnose because the inflammatory process may not affect the anterior abdominal wall. Consistent, localized tenderness to deep palpation within the right lower quadrant and in the right flank, associated with ileo-psoas muscle spasm, should be identified. The general appearance of the child, his temperature, and his pulse are often better indications of the severity of appendicitis than are the abdominal findings, which are often minimal, even in the presence of a ruptured appendix. Generally, the child with appendicitis will tend to have a higher pulse rate and temperature than will an adult.

Differentiation of the abdominal spasm of the acute abdomen from pneumonia of pleural effusion is important. Abdominal spasm due to disease in the chest will gradually disappear if the examiner's hand takes over the function of splinting the lower chest wall. Any spasm which remains in spite of continual manual pressure on the abdomen is an indication of peritoneal irritation.

Primary Peritonitis

Children with nephrosis are especially prone to primary peritonitis caused by streptococci or pneumococci. The infant or child appears extremely ill, with a high fever and rapid pulse. The abdomen is diffusely tender, distended, and may be rigid. In some instances the abdomen may be soft and doughy. Peristalsis is present in the early stages of the disease, but later disappears. Clinical differentiation between primary peritonitis and peritonitis due to a ruptured appendix may be difficult.

Acute Mesenteric Adenitis (Nontuberculous)

Acute mesenteric adenitis must be distinguished from acute appendicitis in childhood. It usually accompanies or follows a respiratory infection. The pain may be generalized but tends to be more marked in the right lower quadrant. Fever is of low grade or absent, and abdominal tenderness is not as severe or well localized as in appendicitis. The white blood cell count is seldom above 10,000. The disease is not progressive, and repeated clinical observation may serve to rule out appendicitis. If a reasonable doubt exists as to the diagnosis, laparotomy should be performed.

Diseases of the Umbilical Region

Omphalomesenteric remnants. Persistence of yolk sac remnants may leave an intact *omphalomesenteric fistula* between the umbilicus and the distal ileum. If the tract adjacent to the ileum becomes obliterated, the remnant is an umbilical sinus. Such omphalomesenteric fistulas or sinuses will be recognized by a mucoid or mucopurulent discharge at the umbilicus. When the mucosal lining of the omphalomesenteric tract is obliterated, leaving a fibrous band between the umbilicus and ileum, the intestine may twist around the band, producing intestinal obstruction.

In 85 per cent of cases, the umbilical end of the omphalomesenteric duct atrophies, leaving a *Meckel's diverticulum* on the antimesenteric border of the ileum. Meckel's diverticula are usually lined by ileal mucosa and remain asymptomatic. However, massive bleeding from the lower gastrointestinal tract may be due to ulceration of the ileum from ectopic gastric mucosa in the Meckel's diverticulum. Generally, the physical findings are unremarkable, unless the ulcer perforates and produces peritonitis.

When the lumen of the diverticulum becomes obstructed, or when a foreign body lodges in it, chronic or acute inflammation will mimic appendicitis. Pain, guarding, and tenderness usually remain in the mid-abdomen, rather than localizing in the right lower abdomen as in appendicitis.

Omphalitis. Infection in the umbilicus of the young infant may produce no more than edema, redness, tenderness, and a serous discharge. Gentle pressure above or below the umbilicus may expel a drop or two of pus. Edema, tenderness, and redness or duskiness appear in the upper abdominal skin when cellulitis extends along the fascial planes or lymphatics. If the process produces thrombophlebitis of the umbilical vein and ductus venosus and propagates to the intrahepatic portal veins, extrahepatic portal hypertension may develop. Liver abscess, high fever, and jaundice may overshadow the local findings if a blood stream infection exists, and peritonitis may occur.

Patent urachus. Patent urachus is identified by the escape of urine at the umbilicus. The red, pouting bladder mucosa may be seen at the umbilicus. Granulation tissue developing after the dried cord has separated may be confused with a patent urachus, but the umbilicus will heal quickly after local application of silver nitrate. If the umbilical portion of the urachus is closed, a urachal cyst may form. Urachal cyst is manifested by a deep midline swelling below the umbilicus. It has a broad attachment to the deeper portions of the abdominal wall. Abscess frequently becomes the initial manifestation of urachal cyst.

Omphalocele and gastroschisis. An omphalocele is a defect in the mid-abdominal wall in which the intra-abdominal organs are covered only by amnion and peritonium. There are two types of omphalocele. In the first type, there is a relatively small fascial defect, and bowel herniates into the umbilical cord, producing a variable sized protrusion from the abdomen. The larger omphaloceles are flat, contain liver, spleen, stomach, and intestine, and the umbilical cord is at the caudal edge of the defect. The latter defect is usually associated with multiple anomalies.

Gastroschisis is probably caused by a rupture in utero of the membranes covering an omphalocele. The bowel herniates into the amniotic cavity and the amniotic fluid produces an inflammatory reaction on the serosal surfaces of the bowel wall. The junction of umbilical cord and the abdominal wall is normal, and most of the defects in the abdominal wall are to the right of the umbilicus.

Umbilical hernia. Delayed closure of the umbilical fascial ring about the umbilical vessels produces umbilical hernia. There is a rounded protuberance of the navel when the child strains (Fig. 8–3). The peritoneal sac is covered only by subcutaneous fat and skin, and the hernial ring is easily palpable as an edge of firm connective tissue. The herniation of bowel may be very large, but the size of the fascial defect is more important to assess. Most of these fascial defects close spontaneously before the child is 5 years old. Incarcerated hernia is rare, and repair can be delayed until it is certain that spontaneous closure will not occur.

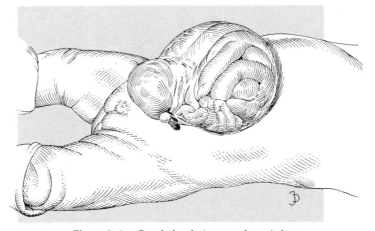

Figure 8–2. Omphalocele in a newborn infant.

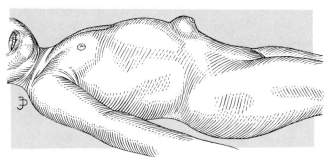

Figure 8–3. Umbilical hernia in a four-year-old girl.

Congenital Posterolateral Hernia of the Diaphragm

When the pleuroperitoneal folds fail to fuse with the septum transversum, a defect remains in the posterolateral portions of the diaphragm. The intra-abdominal viscera herniate into the chest and compress the lungs. If herniation occurs early in gestation, the lungs will be hypoplastic. At birth, the infant may be deeply cyanotic with severe respiratory distress and tachycardia, or he may have few symptoms, depending upon the degree of lung development and compression. Posterolateral diaphragmatic hernia occurs four times more frequently on the left side. The infant has a scaphoid abdomen. Heart sounds are heard best over the right side of the chest, and dullness with poorly transmitted breath sounds are heard over the left side of the chest. Conversely, with right-sided diaphragmatic hernia, the bowel and the right chest will displace the heart to the left, and dullness and poor breath sounds will be on the right side.

Intra-abdominal Hernia

Congenital defects may occur in any part of the mesentery, but are especially common in the terminal ileum. Similar openings may appear in the ascending mesocolon or just below the ligament of Treitz (paraduodenal hernia). These hernias are rare, but when they do occur the child appears acutely ill and has signs of intestinal obstruction. A localized tender mass can often be felt if the dilated bowel proximal to the herniated portion does not obscure it.

Inguinal Hernia

The examination for inguinal hernia in children differs materially from the same examination in adults. Inguinal hernia in childhood practically always originates at the internal ring. Direct inguinal hernia and femoral hernia are extremely rare. The hernia presents itself as a bulge in the groin which may extend beyond the external ring and into the scrotum or labia majora. It is useless to invert a child's scrotum with the finger to search for the external ring or to palpate the inguinal canal. The scrotum and the external ring are so small that no information is gained, and the child is greatly disturbed.

Inspection is carefully done before the child is touched. If he is old enough, this should be done with the child in the standing position. The appearance and disappearance of an inguinal swelling during coughing, crying, or straining will establish the diagnosis (Fig. 8–4).

If an inguinal mass does not appear after the child strains, a history of recurrent inguinal swelling from a reliable observer is sufficient reason to proceed with surgical repair.

Signs such as increased thickness of the spermatic cord or the sensation of silk gloves when rubbing the groin or cord with the finger are not sufficiently reliable to make the diagnosis unless a bulge is seen.

The oblique direction of the inguinal canal and the small size of the internal and external inguinal rings make incarceration of a hernia very frequent. The younger the patient, the more likely that incarceration will occur.

In girls, the ovary, fallopian tube, and even the uterus will be the her-

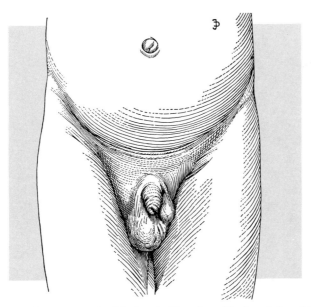

Figure 8–4. Appearance of a right inguinal hernia and hydrocele in a child. Note the inguinal hernia descending into the scrotum with the hydrocele below it. The left testicle is in its normal position.

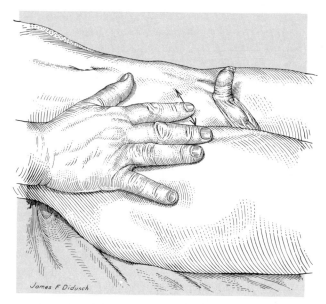

Figure 8–5. Palpation of the inguinal canal in a child. The examiner slides the skin and subcutaneous tissue over the canal with his finger. The two sides are compared. Thickening of the canal can be detected in the presence of a hernial sac. A sensation similar to rustling together two surfaces of silk is frequently imparted to the examining finger if a hernial sac is present.

niated organ in more than one-half of cases. Usually, an asymptomatic firm lump will be palpable at the external ring which represents the herniated ovary.

A recurring inguinal hernia makes a child fretful, and an incarcerated hernia is very painful. Incarceration produces a tense, tender mass and signs and symptoms of intestinal obstruction quickly occur. An incarcerated hernia should be reduced by gentle pressure. This may require using a narcotic to relieve the child of pain and to gain abdominal relaxation. Inguinal adenitis will produce a tender mass in the groin but it is usually below the level of the inguinal ligament. A hydrocele of the cord is painless and may be identified by transillumination. If the mass is not reducible, the internal ring may be palpated intra-abdominally by rectal examination to detect bowel which has herniated through the internal ring.

Hydrocele

In infants and children, hydrocele almost always develops from a persistently patent processus vaginalis. The processus vaginalis may be obliterated anywhere from the internal ring to the scrotum or labia. Intra-abdominal fluid extends into the processus vaginalis, and when trapped by narrowing along the tract, it will produce a bulge in the labium or scrotum and groin, or it may be confined to the groin only. A hydrocele is usually larger at the end of the day than in the early morning. The diagnosis is confirmed by noting that it transilluminates when a flashlight is placed against it. Most hydroceles resolve spontaneously when the processus vaginalis becomes obliterated with time.

Undescended Testicle

Cryptorchidism must be carefully differentiated from retractile testicles. Infants and young children have very active cremaster muscles, and they can readily draw the testicles into the groin. If the child is in a warm environment and relaxed, usually a retracted testis can be gently "milked" into the scrotum. A truly undescended testis will be arrested intra-abdominally or in any position along the inguinal canal, or it may be ectopically located beyond the external ring in the groin, thigh, or perineum. A testis arrested in the inguinal canal is often difficult to palpate. The scrotum on the involved side will be poorly developed and lack rugal folds. A patent processus vaginalis occurs in 95 per cent of undescended testes, but recurrent hernia may not be a frequent problem.

Torsion of the Testis and the Appendix Testis

Remnants of the mesonephros produce little pedunculated nodules, which most commonly occur in the upper pole of the testis in the groove adjacent to the epididymis. The appendix testis may become twisted, resulting in an exquisitely tender, pea-sized nodule. Shortly after the onset of torsion, the testis is in the normal position, and the tenderness and redness are localized in the upper pole of the testis. Pain may extend from the scrotum to the groin and abdomen. In time the scrotum will become greatly edematous, and extension of the tenderness and redness may make it impossible to distinguish this condition from torsion of the spermatic cord and testicle.

Torsion of the Testicle

Torsion of the spermatic cord may occur above the tunica vaginalis or within the tunica. Intravaginal torsion occurs when there is no fixation of the testis and epididymis to the tunica; it is suspended by a narrow pedicle much like a bell clapper. Torsion of the spermatic cord results in ischemia of the testis, and produces severe pain and vomiting. The testis is drawn up toward the external ring and the scrotum becomes red and edematous.

Epididymo-orchitis must be differentiated from torsion of the testis or appendix testis; it also produces a painful, red, and edematous scrotum. Pus and bacteria are usually seen in the urine. When the scrotum is elevated, the pain of epididymitis may be relieved but the pain of torsion is exaggerated. Torsion of the spermatic cord is a surgical emergency.

Anomalies of the Anus and Rectum

When the uro-rectal septum of the fetus incompletely divides the cloaca into the urogenital sinus and rectum, a variety of anomalies occur. The rectum usually communicates with the prostatic urethra or bladder in males and with the upper vagina in females. Meconium may be seen at the urethral meatus or vagina.

In low-type anomalies, the distal rectum has developed and has extended below the levator ani muscles. The anal canal will be ectopically located in the lower vagina or fourchette in girls, and in the anterior perineum in boys.

A covered anus consists of a normally placed or slightly anterior anus which is covered by skin. Meconium or epithelial inclusions may be seen in a track along the scrotal raphe.

Congenital anal stenosis is a normally placed but abnormally small anal canal.

Abdominal Masses in Infants and Children

The frequency of the various types of abdominal tumors found in newborn infants differs from that in older children. Most of the abdominal masses in infants are benign, and 75 per cent originate in the kidney. Most abdominal masses in older children are malignant.

Newborn infants. In infants, a mass in one or both flanks and upper abdominal quadrants may be due to hydronephrosis, or to multicystic, polycystic, or solitary cystic kidney. These masses will be irregular, soft, and somewhat mobile, and they will demonstrate transillumination. Renal vein thrombosis will produce a hemorrhagic mass, and ecchymoses will be noted in the flank, scrotum, or labia. Wilms' tumor will produce a solitary smooth, hard, rounded mass confined to one side of the abdomen. A horseshoe kidney will produce a mass in the mid-abdomen.

Other retroperitoneal masses include neuroblastoma, adrenal hemorrhage, and teratoma. A neuroblastoma in infancy usually causes liver enlargement from hepatic metastases, and the primary tumor is not usually palpable in the newborn.

Tumors of the liver may be due to solitary or diffuse hemangioma-

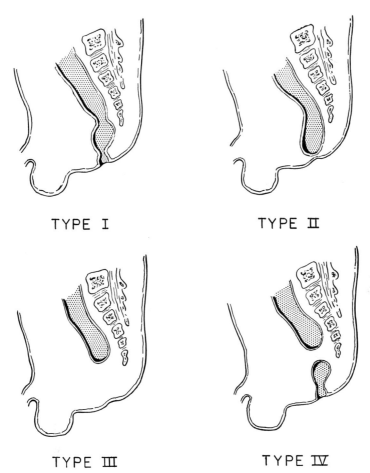

TYPE I   TYPE II

TYPE III   TYPE IV

Figure 8–6. Types of anal and rectal congenital anomalies. Type I, Stenosis of the anus and rectum. Type II, Imperforate anus. A membrane persists and obstructs. Type III, Imperforate anus. Rectal pouch ends blindly several centimeters above the anus. Type IV, Normal anus and anal pouch. Rectal pouch ends blindly. (After Gross, R. E.: The Surgery of Infancy and Childhood. Philadelphia, W. B. Saunders Co., 1953.)

tosis, hepatoblastoma, or hamartoma. Metastases to liver are usually multiple in infants and produce diffuse hepatomegaly rather than a solitary lesion. The relatively large liver of infants extends far to the left side of the abdomen, and a tumor arising in the left lobe may be confused with splenomegaly. The liver is suspended from the diaphragm, and masses in the liver will move with respiration, whereas retroperitoneal masses usually do not. A bruit may be heard over the liver from turbulent blood flow through hemangiomatas with large arteriovenous shunts.

Abdominal masses in the lower midline may be due to an obstructed bladder, urachal cyst, hydrometrocolpos, or an ovarian tumor. Urachal cysts are usually tense and fixed to the abdominal wall. The distended bladder will be relieved by compression and voiding, or by catheteriza-

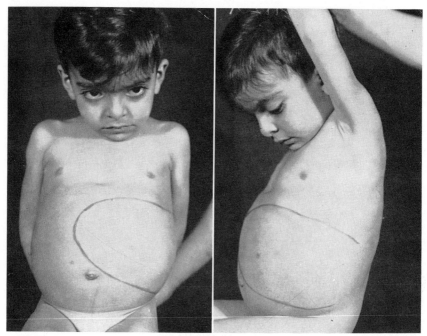

Figure 8–7. Wilms' tumor of the kidney. The mass can often be seen as well as palpated. (Children's Hospital case, courtesy of Dr. Robert Gross.)

tion. A chronically obstructed bladder will have a palpably thick wall. In girls, a bulging intact hymen or a distal vaginal atresia will identify a midline abdominal mass resulting from hydrometrocolpos. Ovarian tumors are usually displaced out of the small pelvis and are detected in the abdominal cavity as soft, smooth, mobile tumors. Most of the ovarian tumors are large cysts or teratomas.

Older children. Except for hepatosplenomegaly resulting from numerous local and systemic diseases, most abdominal masses in older children are neoplasms. The upper abdominal masses include neuroblastoma, Wilms' tumor, and hepatic tumors. Neuroblastoma presents as a large, hard, irregular and commonly tender tumor that frequently extends across the midline of the abdomen. Wilms' tumor is usually very large, firm, and smooth, but it is confined to one side of the abdomen. Retroperitoneal teratoma may be confused with Wilms' tumor, but if it contains large cysts, it will be transilluminated. Hepatic tumors are usually large, firm, smooth masses that blend with the projected normal liver edge, and they move with respiration. Duplications of the bowel and mesenteric tumors such as lymphangiomas and mesenteric cysts are mid-abdominal in location and are soft or cystic. Because of their mobility, they may be very elusive and difficult to define clearly. The clinical impression gained from physical examination is confirmed by intravenous pyelogram, liver scan, arteriogram, echograms, and gastrointestinal contrast studies.

chapter 9

EXAMINATION OF THE EXTREMITIES

Diseases of the extremities may be peculiar to a particular extremity or may be an expression of a systemic disease. Their multiplicity makes this examination of critical importance. It is easily and quickly performed. More detailed and specific examinations are required if there are complaints referable to an extremity or if abnormalities are detected.

JOINT, BONE, AND MUSCLE PAIN

Because of the frequency of various forms of arthritis, joint pain is a common complaint. Joint pain is intensified by motion, passive or active. Swelling and deformity of the joint may or may not be present. *Bone pain* is the most common symptom of osseous disease; it is usually more severe at night and may be referred to the nearest joint. Localized tenderness and swelling may be present over the bone. *Muscular pain* may be differentiated from joint, bone, and neuritis pain by eliciting tenderness through compression of the muscle between the examiner's thumb and index finger. Muscle pain, like articular pain, is increased by movement. Prompt radiologic examination is indicated for the symptom of bone or joint pain.

I. THE ELECTIVE EXAMINATION

The Upper Extremity

Position

The patient should be sitting upright, the shoulders and arms completely exposed and the arms somewhat dependent.

Inspection

Compare the arms for asymmetry, deformity, atrophy, or swelling. Note the color of the skin; scrutinize it on both surfaces for blemishes of any kind, and carefully appraise the condition of the fingernails. Count the digits during this part of the examination so that any missing digit or a congenital syndactylism or polydactylism will be noted. Ask the patient to extend his fingers and to spread them widely and hold his hands steady so that any degree of tremor may be noted. A fine tremor may be brought out by placing a piece of paper on the extended hand. Compare the color and prominence of the veins of the hands and arms in both the elevated and dependent positions.

Palpation

Feel the radial, ulnar, brachial, and axillary pulses. The *radial* and *ulnar arteries* are palpable just medial to the radial and ulnar styloid processes, respectively, on the volar surface of the wrist (Fig. 9–1). The *compression test* is an excellent means of testing the patency and blood flow through these vessels. Ask the patient to close his fist tightly in order to empty the superficial tissues of blood. Normal pink color returns in a few seconds when the fist is opened with the arm slightly elevated. The

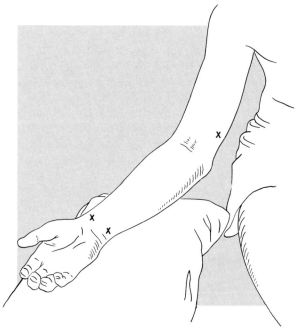

Figure 9–1. Sites of palpation of the radial, ulnar, and brachial pulses.

maneuver is then repeated, but the examiner occludes the radial artery by pressure with his finger. The rapidity with which normal color returns to the hand is an excellent index of the rate of flow through the ulnar artery. The procedure is repeated with occlusion of the ulnar to test the flow through the radial artery.

The *brachial artery* is felt on the medial aspect of the middle third of the upper arm and in the midportion of the antecubital space (Fig. 9–1). The *axillary artery* is best felt in the apex of the axilla with the arm in 90 degree abduction at the shoulder.

Feel the palms of the hands and note their temperature and moisture.

Now ask the patient to put his arm through the normal range of motion involving the wrist, elbow, and shoulder joints.

Check the biceps, triceps, and radial reflexes (see Fig. 17–1, p. 321).

All major disorders affecting the upper extremities can be excluded if there are no complaints referable to the extremity and if no abnormalities are noted during the above examination.

The Lower Extremity

Position

The legs should be examined in both the supine and standing positions.

Inspection

First scrutinize the skin; note its color and search it for ulceration or pigmentation. The toes must be separated and the interdigital spaces inspected for evidence of epidermophytosis. The color of the skin in the elevated, horizontal, and dependent positions is of great importance; blanching of the skin in the elevated position and suffusion in the dependent position is one of the earliest manifestations of peripheral arteriosclerosis. Examine the patient in a standing position for varicosities.

Edema is recognized by pitting of the tissues resulting from firm pressure with the tip of the forefinger against the lower aspect of the tibia just above the ankle.

Palpation

Compare the temperature of the skin of the feet, lower leg, and thigh. Feel the pulsations of the femoral, popliteal, posterior tibial, and dorsalis pedis arteries. The patient must be recumbent. The *femoral artery* is palpated midway between the anterior superior iliac spine and the symphysis pubis just below the inguinal ligament. The *popliteal artery* is best pal-

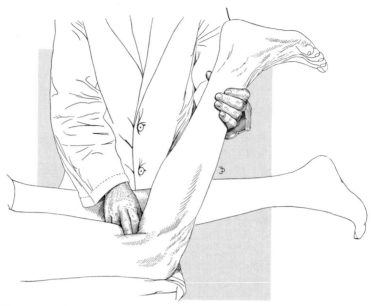

Figure 9–2. Position of the patient for palpation of the popliteal artery. The examiner supports the patient's leg in approximately 90 degrees flexion with one hand and palpates the popliteal space with the other. The popliteal pulse can be consistently felt only in this position.

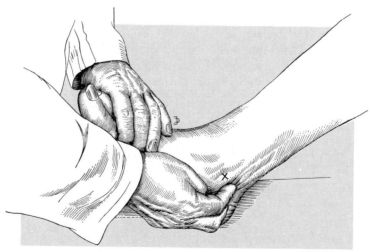

Figure 9–3. Palpation of the posterior tibial artery. The cross identifies the internal malleolus.

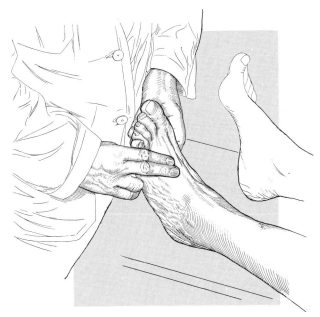

Figure 9–4. Palpation of the dorsalis pedis artery. The artery usually lies just lateral to the tendon of the extensor hallucis longus, which can be seen when the patient dorsiflexes his great toe.

pated slightly to the lateral side of the popliteal space deeply between the hamstring tendons; the patient is positioned face down with the knee flexed at 90 degrees (Fig. 9–2). The *posterior tibial artery* is palpable halfway between the tendon of Achilles and the internal malleolus (Fig. 9–3). The *dorsalis pedis artery* is felt midway between the ankle and the base of the toes. This is just lateral to the tendon of the extensor hallucis longus, which is identified when the patient dorsiflexes his great toe (Fig. 9–4). Occasionally the dorsalis pedis is constituted by the perforating branch of the peroneal artery; it will then be found in a more lateral position. The *anterior tibial artery* can be felt in lateral relation to the tendon of the extensor hallucis longus midway between the malleoli.

Ask the patient to put the extremity through the normal ranges of motion. Test the plantar, patellar, and Achilles reflexes (see Fig. 17–1, p. 321).

II. THE INFECTED HAND

The hand is exposed in an unusual degree to bacterial invasion. Trauma in some form is responsible for the origin of most of these infections, but in many instances there has been no obvious injury. Some infections of the hand are distinct clinical entities, but all may be complicated by the intricate anatomy of the part. Therapy to prevent the devastating effects of inflammation in the tissues of the hand depends on precise diagnosis. The sole method by which an accurate diagnosis of hand infections can be made is a careful physical examination.

Basic Signs of Inflammation

The classic signs of inflammation, *redness, swelling, heat,* and *tenderness,* to which must be added *loss of function,* all are present in the infected hand. These signs, however, may be modified by the anatomy of the part. For example, the tough connective tissue of the fingers and palm tends to limit swelling and by doing so produces excruciating pain. *Fluctuation* is probably the oldest physical sign in clinical surgery but is seldom present in hand infections. Indeed, in examination of the infected hand it provides little information to the examiner, and to attempt to elicit this sign unnecessarily hurts the patient.

The patient, depending upon the virulence of the infection, may react to an infection of the hand with only a degree or so of fever or may have shaking chills and a high fever. The presence or absence of lymphangitis, manifested by red streaks going up the volar surface of the arm, and the presence or absence of lymphadenitis in the epitrochlear and axillary regions should be determined in all hand infections. The local signs of inflammation of the hand may be modified considerably by the use of anti-

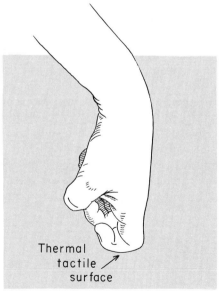

Thermal
tactile
surface

Figure 9–5. The back of the hand, particularly over the middle phalanges, is very sensitive to differences in temperature.

biotic therapy, but owing to the structure of the hand the tension and resultant pain associated with infection in closed spaces are not abolished. Systemic signs may be completely abolished by vigorous antibiotic therapy although the local process may be progressing.

Redness and swelling are obvious on inspection and comparison of the infected with the normal hand. *Local heat* can be ascertained by gently touching the inflamed skin with the dorsum of the examiner's flexed finger (Fig. 9–5). This is the optimum thermal tactile surface, and normal skin is always available for comparison. However, if the part is red, it can be assumed that there is increased local heat. *Local tenderness* is sought for gently but firmly. The examiner's finger tip is too broad for accurate localization of the tenderness in hand infections. The blunt end of a pen or the eraser tip of a pencil is an excellent probe to determine the extent of areas of tenderness along a tendon sheath. Sudden stabbing exploration for suspected areas of tenderness is to be condemned. *If there is an open wound, no matter how small, strict aseptic technique should be followed and only sterile probes or instruments should be used for the examination.*

Special Entities

Felon. This is an acute suppurative inflammation confined to the closed pulp space of the finger tip (Fig. 9–6). Infection is commonly carried to this closed region by puncture wounds or trivial injuries. The walls of this space are so tough that tension within the space rapidly increases and results in intense throbbing pain which is accentuated when

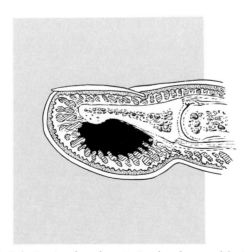

Figure 9–6. The infection involves the anterior closed space of the terminal phalanx.

the patient lowers the involved finger. The pulp of the finger appears tense and swollen. Tenderness is best elicited by gentle pressure with a pen or pencil on the distal tip of the finger. It is severe in the early stages, but in neglected cases may become minimal. Fluctuation is not found unless the infection is advanced and the fibrous tissue septa have been ruptured. At that stage the terminal phalanx is almost certainly destroyed.

Paronychia. This infection usually starts from a hangnail. There is swelling and redness of the skin around the side and the base of the nail. It is red, puffy, and quite tender (Fig. 9–7). If the lesion becomes chronic, the skin becomes dull red and exudes a small amount of purulent material from the margin of the cuticle. Granulation tissue may grow at the margin of the cuticle.

Carbuncle of the hand. Carbuncles occur on the hairy surface of the back of the hand or fingers. The appearance of a carbuncle is unmistakable. There is a central necrotic core from which pus is discharging through several openings. This is surrounded by a violaceous zone beyond which there is a rim of induration and redness. Furuncles occur in the same region, but have only one central opening or area of necrosis (Fig. 9–8).

Subcutaneous abscess. Subcutaneous abscess may occur on the dorsum of the fingers or in the fat pads on the palmar aspect of the fingers. Sharply localized signs of inflammation are found.

Collar-button abscess of the palm. These infections usually originate in the palmar calluses at the base of the fingers. The signs of inflammation are first noted at the palmar base of the fingers, but the infection extends into the web between the fingers and may penetrate to the dorsum of the hand.

Infections from human bites. Mouth organisms produce foul progressive anaerobic infections. Unless promptly recognized and treated, a trivial wound may result in loss of the entire hand and arm from a spreading gangrenous anaerobic cellulitis. The infection often arises over the

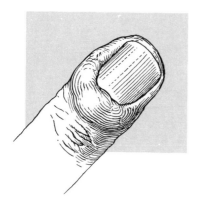

Figure 9–7. Paronychia. (From Homans, J.: Textbook of Surgery. Springfield, Ill., Charles C Thomas, 1945.)

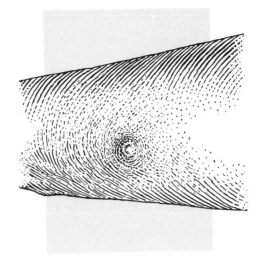

Figure 9–8. Furuncle of the forearm.

proximal portion of the knuckle where teeth have been struck with the fist and the infection has entered the joint. The initial laceration of the skin may appear trivial. However, after one or two days of pain, swelling and tenderness become apparent. The signs of lymphangitis may be present, and a putrid discharge may exude from the original wound. The skin has a peculiar violaceous hue, indicative of the undermining necrotizing character of the infection.

Tenosynovitis and Fascial Space Infections

In general there are three major pathways infection can travel in the hand: (1) the palmar fascial spaces, (2) the tendon sheaths, and (3) the lymphatic system. Each form of infection may run an uncomplicated course or may involve one or more of the other systems. Thus infection may spread from fascial space to tendon sheath or vice versa, and from the deep lymphatics to the sheaths or the fascial spaces.

Tenosynovitis. The tendon sheaths of the little finger and the thumb have a relatively constant connection with the proximal portion of the two divisions of the tendon sheaths or bursae which pass beneath the annular ligament to a point just above the wrist joint (Fig. 9–9). The sheath of the little finger usually communicates with the ulnar bursa, and the sheath of the thumb is continuous with the radial bursa, so that pus in one can easily break into the other. Pus in the tendon sheaths of the remaining fingers, while not in direct communication with fascial spaces of the palm, can rupture into them. Infections from the index finger break into the thenar space and those from the middle and ring fingers break into the midpalmar space (Fig. 9–9).

Digital tendon sheaths

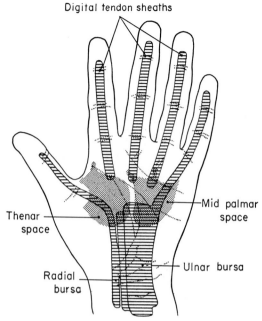

Thenar space

Mid palmar space

Radial bursa

Ulnar bursa

Figure 9–9. Diagram of the fascial spaces and tendon sheaths of the hand.

The cardinal physical signs of infection in a tendon sheath are as follows: (1) The finger is held in slight flexion. (2) It is uniformly swollen. (3) Any attempt to straighten the finger actively or passively causes exquisite pain. (4) Tenderness is confined to the area of the tendon sheath.

In a localized infection of the finger there is no characteristic deformity; the swelling is asymmetric and tenderness is not uniformly limited to the tendon sheath. A diffuse subcutaneous cellulitis may simulate a tendon sheath infection, but the characteristic position of flexion and pain on motion are lacking. Palpation will show that the tenderness is not confined to the tendon sheath. The localization of tenderness to the tendon sheath can be demonstrated only by the use of a narrow dull-pointed instrument such as a match stick or pencil. The examiner's finger tip covers too wide an area to permit accurate localization.

Infection of the midpalmar space. The temperature is often elevated to 103 or 104 degrees. The patient may be restless and extremely irritable. Pain in the palm is extreme. The hollow of the palm is obliterated. The strong palmar fascia, however, restricts bulging and prevents brawny induration, so characteristic of most inflammatory processes, from showing at the surface. The fingers are held in flexion but less rigidly than in the case of infection of the flexor sheath, and there is less pain on motion of the fingers. Fluctuation is difficult to distinguish. The dorsum of the hand is rounded and puffed, but not indurated. There is also considerable edema of the thenar eminence and dorsum of the hand. Pain and tenderness may be greatly ameliorated by antibiotic therapy.

Infection of the thenar space. The thenar eminence is markedly enlarged and tense, and the thumb is held in abduction with the distal joint flexed. The edema of the dorsum and swelling of the palm are not so obvious, owing to resistance offered by the strong palmar fascia. The systemic reaction of the patient may be marked.

When infections of the thenar and midpalmar spaces exist together, the physical signs of the thenar space infection will predominate since greater swelling is permitted by the tissues in that region. Extension from the thenar to the midpalmar space is uncommon since thenar space infections are seldom neglected.

The subaponeurotic space on the dorsum of the hand often appears to be infected when in fact it is not. The back of the hand is red and swollen in association with almost all suppurative processes of the palm or fingers. Actual suppuration need not be suspected unless induration and fluctuation are present. Knowledge of the location of the original infection and of its probable anatomic spread is of assistance in making the distinction.

Lymphangitis. The origin of infection may be obvious or so indefinite that it cannot be found; it may be a scratch or a blister or it may be a full-blown infection of the hand. The patient may be quite ill with chills and fever, and red lines may be seen extending up the arm. The epitrochlear and axillary lymph nodes are enlarged and tender. The lymphatic channels may be palpable (tubular lymphangitis).

Summary of Physical Signs Associated with Infections of the Hand

1. *Paronychia* is an infection of the skin around the base of the fingernail and is recognized by the redness and swelling along the edge and base of the nail.

2. *Felon* is an infection of the closed space of the pulp of the tip of the finger and is recognized by the intense throbbing pain which it causes and by the uniform swelling and exquisite tenderness of the pulp of the finger.

3. *Carbuncles* and *furuncles* occur on the dorsum of the hand and fingers. Their appearance is so characteristic that they are recognized by inspection alone.

4. *Collar-button abscess* of the hand originates in the palmar callus at the base of the finger and extends into the web and to the dorsum of the hand. It can be recognized by inspection and palpation.

5. *Human bite infections* of the hand are recognized by the history of

the injury, the location of the skin laceration on a knuckle and the appearance of the infection.

6. *Tenosynovitis* is recognized by flexion of the involved finger, uniform swelling of the finger, intense pain on attempts to extend the flexed finger, and tenderness confined to the inflamed tendon sheath.

7. *Midpalmar space infections* are characterized by systemic reaction, loss of the hollow of the palm, flexion of the fingers but less pain on motion of the fingers than in tendon sheath infection, and swelling of the dorsum of the hand.

8. *Thenar space infections* are recognized by the systemic reaction and the prominence of the thenar eminence accompanied by abduction and flexion of the thumb.

III. MISCELLANEOUS LESIONS OF THE EXTREMITIES

Since many lesions of the extremities are difficult to place in any particular category, a description of the physical characteristics of some of these will be given in this section. The majority can be recognized on inspection without any particular maneuvers on the part of the examiner.

Syndactylism (web fingers). Two or more digits are united by a web which may be very thin in some instances or the full thickness of the fingers in others.

Polydactylism (supernumerary digits). The congenital anomaly is characterized by the presence of extra digits or toes. There is a familial tendency. The diagnosis is made by simply counting the number of digits (Fig. 9–10).

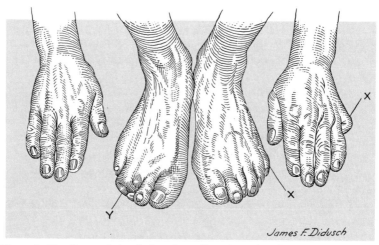

Figure 9–10. Congenital polydactylism (X) and syndactylism (Y) in the same patient.

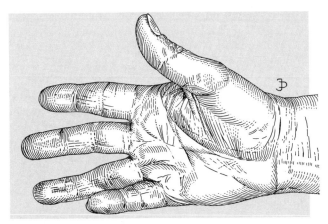

Figure 9–11. Early Dupuytren's contracture. Note the slight flexion of the little finger. The thickened palmar fascia is best appreciated by palpation.

Callus. A callus is an acquired thickening of the skin caused by prolonged pressure or friction upon the skin over a bony prominence. It is common upon the hand on the palmar aspect at the base of the fingers. It may occur on any portion of the hand constantly used in work or play.

Melanomas. These tumors may occur on the hand or foot as well as anywhere on the body. Occasionally they are found on the digits or beneath the finger- and toenails. They appear as flat or slightly raised tumors ranging from blue-black to brown in color. Melanocarcinoma is the commonest malignant tumor of the lower extremity. A subungual melanoma usually occurs on the thumb between the matrix of the nail and the cuticle. If neglected it becomes a dark, fungating, painful swelling (melanotic whitlow). It is highly malignant, with early metastases to the regional nodes. (See p. 17, Fig. 2–6.)

Dupuytren's contracture. This remarkable state is characterized by a flexion contracture, usually of the ring and little fingers, with thickening of the palmar fascia over the tendons of the involved finger. The skin eventually becomes wrinkled and drawn into marked creases by the thickening and contracture of the palmar fascia (Fig. 9–11).

Mallet finger (drop finger). This lesion results from the sudden and violent hyperflexion of the tip of the finger, as when a baseball hits the end of the finger. The extensor tendon is torn so that the patient cannot extend the distal interphalangeal joint.

The *buttonhole* or *boutonniere deformity* results if the extensor tendon is cut or ruptured over the middle interphalangeal joint.

Ganglion. A ganglion is a collection of mucinous fluid in a delicate sac attached to a joint or tendon sheath and is commonly found upon the back of the wrist. When the joint is hyperflexed, the cyst becomes more prominent. It is smooth, nontender, and encapsulated. It is only slightly movable but is not attached to the skin.

Stenosing tenosynovitis. The fibrous sheaths over the flexor tendons of the hand may undergo a chronic inflammatory change and thickening so as to interfere with motion of the tendons. The lesion commonly occurs at the base of the middle finger or thumb, or over the radial styloid. The term "trigger finger" or "snapping thumb" is given to the condition. Once seen, it is easily recognized. The patient closes the hand and then is asked to open it. The involved finger cannot be extended without assistance. A mere touch directed toward unflexing the finger causes it to snap back immediately in line with the other fingers.

When stenosing tenosynovitis occurs at the radial styloid it has been referred to as "de Quervain's disease."

Glomus tumors. A glomus tumor, or glomangioma, appears as a small pinkish blue mass, painful to the touch. Occasionally it is the source of severe spontaneous pain. It may form on any part of the extremity, but it more commonly occurs beneath the fingernail.

Volkmann's ischemic contracture. A deforming flexion contracture may follow an injury of the upper extremity when the blood supply has been impaired by edema. The fingers tend to be flexed, but can be partially extended when the wrist is flexed. In extreme cases a claw hand may result.

Subacromial bursitis (subdeltoid bursitis). The bursa under the deltoid muscle is inflamed and may be the site of adhesions and deposits of calcium. Abduction and outward rotation of the upper arm are limited. The patient can barely move the arm at the shoulder joint. If fluid is present in the bursa, it cannot be detected with the arm in adduction, but when the arm is abducted, the fluid is forced back into the bursa from the shoulder joint and causes an appreciable swelling beneath the deltoid muscle. If the supraspinatus tendon is torn, abduction will be weak. If this tendon is completely torn, abduction cannot be initiated while the patient stands erect, arm at side, nor once passively obtained can the abducted arm be held against the slightest downward pressure. Atrophy of the deltoid muscle is usually present.

Olecranon bursitis. An olecranon bursitis is readily recognized as a tender, constant swelling over the olecranon process. If secondary infection has occurred, the overlying skin is hot and red.

Tennis elbow (radiohumeral bursitis). Tenderness seemingly is present over the external condyle of the humerus but in reality it is over the radiohumeral joint. Pronation, especially with extension of the wrist, is limited and painful.

Rupture of the biceps tendon. Usually the tendon of the long head of the biceps is ruptured, and this allows the muscle to sag downward and inward. When the patient contracts the muscle, a characteristic deformity is produced (Fig. 9–12).

Winging of the scapula. Lesions of the long thoracic nerve produce paralysis of the serratus magnus muscle. This can be demonstrated

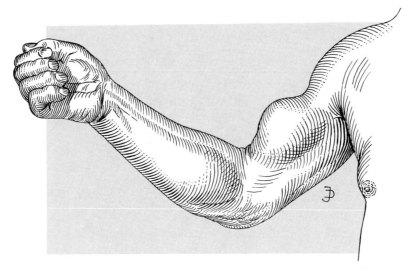

Figure 9–12. Rupture of the biceps tendon.

by having the patient push against the wall with his outstretched hand. When this is done, the scapula stands out like a wing (Fig. 9–13). Congenital elevation of the scapula is usually evident on inspection. The scapula in those instances is smaller than the normal side.

Axillary abscess. An axillary abscess is fairly common. The lesion is often secondary to furunculosis. It may follow the use of a depilatory. Occasionally an axillary adenitis will suppurate and form an abscess (Fig. 9–14).

Lesions of the popliteal space. The popliteal space should be inspected for swelling with the patient standing. The common swellings seen in this region are semimembranous bursa, Baker's cyst, ganglion, abscess, and aneurysm.

Palpation of the space is performed with the patient lying face down and with the knee flexed (Fig. 9–2). The pulsation of the popliteal artery is searched for, and if a mass is present, it should be determined whether it has an expansile impulse. If the mass is cystic, it should be compressed to determine if it communicates with the knee joint. A Baker's cyst originates as a pressure diverticulum of the synovia, whereas ganglia and bursae do not have an open connection with synovia of the joint.

Prepatellar bursitis. The prepatellar bursa is situated between the patella and the skin. This bursa is traumatized repeatedly by those who work in a kneeling position. The injured bursa is swollen and is identified as a prominent encapsulated mass overlying the patella (Fig. 9–15). Secondary infection is common.

Osgood-Schlatter's disease. The disease is usually seen in boys just before puberty. The tibial tubercle is partly avulsed before the

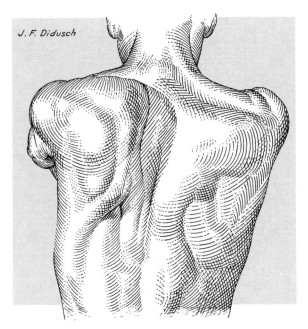

Figure 9–13. Winging of the left scapula due to paralysis of the long thoracic nerve.

epiphysis has become completely ossified. There are swelling and tenderness over the tubercle. Extension at the knee is painful and limited.

Epidermophytosis. The most familiar manifestations of this ubiquitous disease are a soft white thickening of the skin between the toes, a sealing eruption of the plantar skin, and small deep cutaneous blisters.

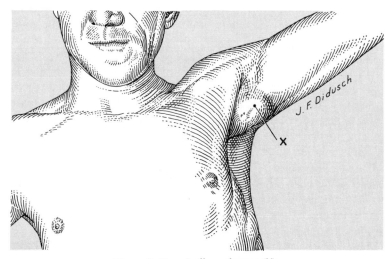

Figure 9–14. Axillary abscess (X).

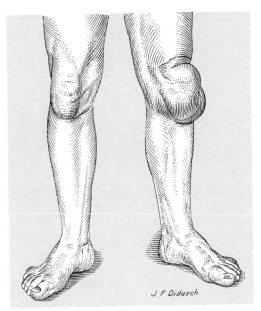

Figure 9–15. Prepatellar bursitis. Both knees are involved. On the left knee the lesion is unusually extensive.

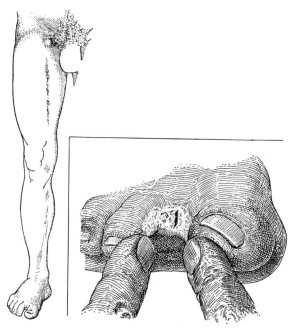

Figure 9–16. On the left, a tubular lymphadenitis. Note the enlarged lymph node in the groin. On the right, the toes are separated to show the area of epidermophytosis which formed the portal of entry of the streptococcal lymphangitis. (From Homans, J.: Textbook of Surgery. Springfield, Ill., Charles C Thomas, 1945.)

Marked itching is the prime symptom. Secondary infection and lymphangitis are common complications (Fig. 9–16). Thickening and discoloration of the toenails are frequently present.

Ingrown toenail. Ingrown toenail is confined to the great toe. The soft parts are pushed over the curved edge of the nail and become red, swollen, and infected. Granulations and a foul discharge are frequently present.

Infections of the foot. Most deep infections of the foot are associated with arterial insufficiency and some degree of gangrene, except the sepsis introduced by puncture wounds or other trauma. The systemic signs of deep infection of the foot are fever and local pain. Edema and redness of the dorsum are present, and local tenderness to pressure may be extreme. Gangrene of the toes may be present if the patient suffers from poor arterial supply (see Chap. 11).

Painful Foot

Pain in the foot is a common complaint. When this symptom is encountered, the following conditions should be searched for during the examination.

Foot strain. The pain is referred to the inner side of the foot and is burning in character. The patient may also complain of pain in the knee and back because of the faulty posture that frequently accompanies foot strain. The foot is pronated and everted, and the longitudinal arch is lowered or gone. The transverse arch may also be weakened. Painful calluses may be present in the region of the lowered transverse arch (metatarsal heads). There may be tenderness and swelling along the course of either the longitudinal or the transverse arches.

Metatarsalgia (Morton's disease). This condition is characterized by collapse of the transverse arch, which is formed by the heads of the metatarsal bones. The resultant pressure on the plantar nerves results in intense cramplike pain which is referred to the base of the fourth toe. It often compels the sufferer to remove his shoe to obtain relief. Transverse pressure exerted across the transverse arch will reproduce the pain. The longitudinal arch may be perfectly normal.

Stress fracture (march fracture). This fracture usually occurs in the shaft of the second or third metatarsal without history of injury. Pain in the foot is the only symptom, and the fracture may be betrayed only when there is evidence of repair seen in the x-ray film. On examination thickening and tenderness may be found on the dorsum of the foot in the region of the affected bone.

Osteochondritis. Aseptic necrosis in the tarsal scaphoid (Köhler's disease) or in the head of the second metatarsal (Freiberg's infraction) is an obscure cause of foot pain. The diagnosis is established by x-ray.

Plantar warts. This painful lesion is found on the sole of the foot ei-

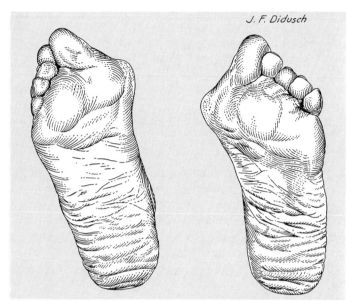

Figure 9–17. Plantar view of bilateral hallux vulgus. Note the calluses on the soles of the feet.

ther on the heel or in the region of the metatarsal heads. It is distinguished from a callus by its sensitivity and the fact that a callus can be easily shaved off, whereas a plantar wart or a corn extends deeply into the skin. Minute brownish specks are present on the shaven surface of a wart, whereas a callus has a homogenous pearly gray color.

Hallux valgus. There is a characteristic appearance due to the marked turning out of the great toe (Fig. 9–17). When the bursa over the first metatarsal becomes inflamed in this condition a "bunion" is said to exist.

Hammer toe. The toe, usually the second or third, is sharply angulated in plantar flexion. A painful callus develops over the dorsum of

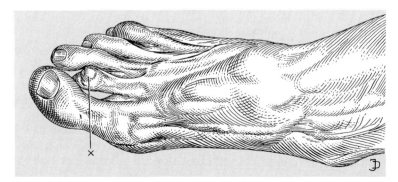

Figure 9–18. Hammer toe. Note the callus (X) on the dorsum of the second toe.

the first interphalangeal joint and sometimes on the tip of the toe (Fig. 9–18).

Painful heel.   Pain in the heel may be disabling. Localized tenderness may be found by pressure over the plantar surface of the heel. X-ray examination should be made to search for a bony spur arising from the os calcis.

Clinical Manifestations of Inflammatory and Specific Diseases of Joints

Suppurative inflammation of the joints.   The onset of disease is characterized by heat and swelling, usually sufficient to obliterate the bony landmarks of the joint. The systemic symptoms may be very marked, and chills and fever are common. The joint is protected by muscle spasm, usually in some degree of flexion. Pain is severe, and tenderness is frequently so exquisite that the slightest movement will cause excruciating pain. The joint may have become infected from trauma, penetrating wounds, or septic processes arising near them.

Gonococcal infection of the joints may occur at any stage of a gonorrheal infection; more than one joint may be involved.

Tuberculosis of the joints.   Tuberculous arthritis usually is insidious in onset, and it may be weeks or months before the disease becomes full-blown. Lameness of the joint is frequently the first symptom. Swelling is not as marked as it is in suppurative inflammation. Atrophy and contracture develop as the disease progresses.

Syphilis of the joints.   Syphilis produces a chronic arthritis and has to be differentiated from tuberculosis. It may produce arthralgia, gumma, or synovitis.

Charcot's disease.   Joint insecurity, false motion, and swelling of the joints are the earliest signs. It usually occurs late in the course of tabes dorsalis. When the disease is well established, the joint is markedly deformed and swollen. It feels boggy.

Hemophiliac joints.   The patients are always males, usually under fifteen years of age. The knees are the most common joints affected, but the elbows, ankles, hips, and shoulders also may be involved. The initial hemorrhage into the joint may appear to be spontaneous or may follow a known injury. The joint rapidly becomes tensely swollen and painful, and the temperature is elevated. There is no external sign of bleeding. The blood is absorbed over a long period of time.

If there is only one bout of bleeding, very little damage may result, but if it is recurrent, the result is chronic arthritis. In these instances fluid is constantly present in the joint, the capsule is thickened, and the surface markings are obliterated. The joint motion may be limited, and acute pain and lameness may come and go. If the disease progresses with repeated hemorrhages, deformity results.

chapter 10

EXAMINATION OF THE SPINE AND HIPS

I. EXAMINATION OF THE SPINE

In the course of the elective examination the area of the back need only be examined with reference to the patient's posture, the manner in which he climbs on and off the examining table, and the mobility of the spine. Any complaints referable to the back or abnormalities of posture or mobility indicate the need for a detailed examination. An x-ray cannot substitute for a careful physical examination of the back. The essential steps in the examination of the back are outlined in Figure 10–1.

Inspection

Note the stance and general habitus of the patient. Have the patient walk about in order to observe his gait. Check the levels of the shoulders, scapulae, iliac crests, and gluteal folds. Note the anterior posterior curve of the spine and the presence or absence of lateral curvature. Have the patient bend forward and note any asymmetry of the soft tissues of the back. A soft tissue neoplasm may only be apparent in this position.

Palpation

With the patient still standing, palpate the musculature of the back. Using both hands, feel for tenderness and tension over the trapezius muscle and over the entire course of the erector spinae group of muscles. Palpate the iliolumbar angle, which is the space between the spine and the crest of the ilium posteriorly. Press gently but firmly against the spinous process of each vertebra, testing for tenderness or accentuation of existing pain. Palpate the sacroiliac joints. They may be located just medial to

```
┌─────────────────────────────────────────────────────┐
│  I. INSPECTION                                        │
│         A. STANCE                                     │
│         B. GAIT                                       │
│         C. LEVELS OF THE SHOULDERS, HIPS,             │
│            AND GLUTEAL FOLDS                          │
├─────────────────────────────────────────────────────┤
│  2. PALPATION                                         │
│         A. MUSCLES                                    │
│         B. SPINOUS PROCESSES                          │
│         C. ILIOLUMBAR ANGLES                          │
│         D. SACROILIAC JOINTS                          │
│         E. SACROSCIATIC NOTCHES                       │
├─────────────────────────────────────────────────────┤
│  3. MOTIONS                                           │
│       ACTIVE                                          │
│         A. STANDING                                   │
│         B. SITTING                                    │
│         C. LYING                                      │
│       PASSIVE                                         │
│         A. STRAIGHT LEG RAISING                       │
│         B. FLEXED LEG RAISING                         │
│         C. HYPEREXTENSION OF THE HIPS                 │
│         D. HYPEREXTENSION OF THE BACK                 │
├─────────────────────────────────────────────────────┤
│  4. REFLEXES                                          │
│         A. QUADRICEPS                                 │
│         B. ANKLE JERKS                                │
│         C. PLANTAR RESPONSES                          │
│         D. SENSATION TO PIN PRICK                     │
├─────────────────────────────────────────────────────┤
│  5. MEASUREMENTS                                      │
│         A. CHEST EXPANSION                            │
│         B. CIRCUMFERENCE OF THIGHS 10                 │
│            CM. AND 20 CM. ABOVE MIDPATELLA            │
│         C. CIRCUMFERENCE OF MIDCALF                   │
│         D. LEG LENGTH                                 │
└─────────────────────────────────────────────────────┘
```

Figure 10–1. Steps in examination of the back.

and below the dimples over the posterior spine of the ilium (Fig. 10–2). Palpate the sacrosciatic notch, which is the point of exit of the sciatic nerve. This point may be identified as a slight depression in the central portion of the buttock in the region of the gluteal fold.

Ask the patient to bend forward and gently percuss with a rubber hammer each intervertebral space and spinous process. Palpation should be repeated later with the patient in the prone position, as will be described.

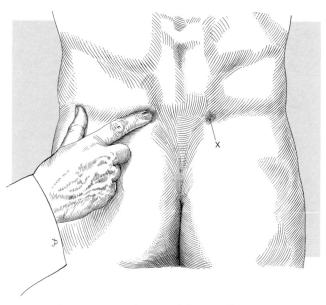

Figure 10–2. Palpation of the sacroiliac joints.

Motions

With the patient still standing, test the mobility of the spine by having him bend forward and backward from the waist and then to each side. The motions of lateral bending can best be judged if the patient places his hands behind his neck when the movements are executed (Fig. 10–3). Rotation of the spine is best determined with the patient seated, since the pelvis is fixed by resting the buttocks on the chair. Have the patient place his hands behind his head, and using his arms as a lever, check the rotary movements by swinging the trunk around on a vertical axis to the right and left.

Now ask the patient to get on the examining table, noting the manner in which he does this and the position he assumes on the table. The following special tests of mobility should be performed with the patient supine.

Straight leg raising. The examiner slowly raises one of the patient's legs with the knee fully extended and with the patient relaxed. Flexion is gradually increased passively until the maximum angle is obtained at the hip or until the patient complains of pain. The range of motion should be observed for comparison of the two sides. The procedure is now repeated with the opposite leg. The location, character, and radiation of pain should be carefully recorded. This maneuver places a strain on the sciatic nerve, hamstring muscles, and the sacroiliac joint.

Straight leg raising plus dorsiflexion. A distinction can be made between pain caused by tight hamstring muscles and that caused by a

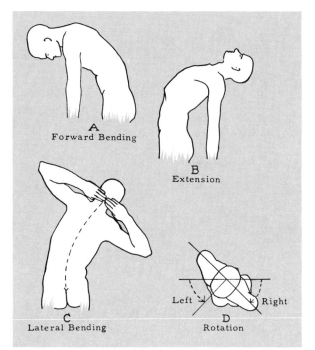

Figure 10–3. Motions of the spine. (From Cave, E. F. and Roberts, S. M.: J. Bone Joint Surg., *18*:455–465, April, 1936.)

lesion of the sciatic nerve by raising the straightened leg to the point just below the first indications of pain and then dorsiflexing the foot. This presumably tenses the sciatic nerve without increasing tension on the hamstring muscles; if the pain is accentuated by this test, the lesion is localized to the nerve.

Flexed leg raising. With the knees in flexion, both legs are then flexed at the thigh until the knees rest upon the chest. This maneuver places the strain primarily on the lumbosacral area of the spine and the hip joints. Flexion of the thigh upon the hip is painless in lesions of the sciatic nerve, and such flexion is easily accomplished when the knee is flexed, thus distinguishing painful lesions of the sciatic nerve from disease of the hip joint, in which marked flexion is painful or impossible.

Hyperextension of the hip. The patient should now be asked to assume the prone position, and the motions of hyperextension are tested as follows: With the knees flexed the examiner lifts the leg in order to produce hyperextension of the hip, which in turn produces hyperextension of the lumbar spine and sacrum and indicates the presence or absence of flexion contracture.

Hyperextension of the back. Ask the patient to place his hand behind his head and then raise it from the table in order to hyperflex the entire spine. This maneuver may be helpful in accurately localizing pain to a particular vertebra.

Palpation in Prone Position

While the patient is in the prone position palpation should be repeated for the detection of painful nodules of fibrositis, lipomas, or fatty herniations. If a pillow is placed beneath the abdomen, the musculature of the back will relax and permit a more satisfactory palpation than can be obtained in the standing position. Common locations for lesions are just lateral to the posterior superior spine of the ilium, along the course of the sciatic nerve, in the gluteal muscles, along the transverse processes of the vertebrae, and over and around the scapula and in the neck. Careful, systematic palpation of these areas may reveal painful nodules, which are a principal source of confusing back pain. Palpation is carefully performed for tenderness over the spinous processes, intervertebral spaces, and laterally over the foramina. Care should be taken not to mistake the transverse processes of the vertebrae for abnormalities.

Reflexes

With a patient sitting and the legs hanging free and completely relaxed, a careful comparison of the reflexes of the lower extremities should be made. A diminished knee jerk or ankle jerk may be of considerable significance, particularly with reference to nerve root compression.

Measurements

Measure the chest expansion, the circumference of each thigh 10 cm. and 20 cm. above the patella, the circumference of the midcalves, and the length of each leg.

Limited chest expansion is an early sign of arthritis of the spine. Atrophy of the vastus medialis is indicated by a loss in circumference of the lower thigh. A diminished circumference of the upper thigh reflects a general atrophy of all the musculature.

The true length of the legs is measured as follows: With the patient flat on his back and the legs parallel and extended, the measurement of each leg is taken from the tip of the anterior superior spine of the ilium to the medial malleolus. *Apparent shortening* or *lengthening of the leg* is obtained if it is measured from the umbilicus to the medial malleolus.

II. EXAMINATION OF THE HIP JOINT

The function of the hip joints should be tested in conjunction with the examination of the back. Conversely, pain referred to the hip warrants a detailed examination of the back.

The patient's gait and stance should be observed. Flexion contractures of the hip tend to produce lordosis. Flattening of the buttock indicates atrophy in relation to hip joint disease.

Measurement

The length of the leg should be measured as described above.

Motions

Flexion of the hip is tested with the patient supine, the knee bent, and the pelvis maintained flat on the table. An unsuspected lordosis will

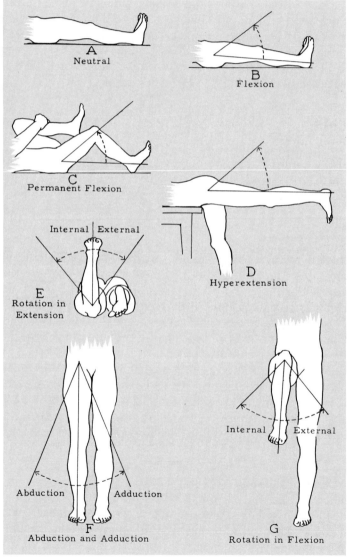

Figure 10–4. Motions of the hip. (From Cave, E. F. and Roberts, S. M.: J. Bone Joint Surg., *18*:455–465, April, 1936.)

mask permanent flexion of the thigh. To exclude or measure permanent flexion, fix the pelvis to the table by flexing the opposite thigh and flattening the lumbar spine. If there is a permanent flexion, the other thigh will rise from the table (Fig. 10-4 *C*).

Abduction and adduction are tested with the patient supine and the pelvis flat on the table; the leg is gently carried medially and laterally by the examiner, who grasps it just above the ankle (Fig. 10-4 *F*).

Rotation is now tested; the thigh is gently rotated internally and externally to ascertain that the movement is free and painless. The full range of rotation in flexion is now tested by flexing the thigh and knee to an angle of 90 degrees and then rotating the hip (Fig. 10-4 *G*).

Hyperextension is tested with the patient prone and preferably with the opposite thigh over the end of the examining table at an angle of 90 degrees (Fig. 10-4*D*).

Rotation in extension is tested with the patient prone and the knee flexed to 90 degrees (Fig. 10-4*E*).

The complete evaluation of symptoms referable to the back and hips will also require a careful motor and sensory examination of the extremities and an examination of the knees, ankles, and feet. These examinations will not be described here, but emphasis is placed upon their importance in the examination of the patient with complaints referable to the back.

III. DISORDERS OF THE SPINE

The differential diagnosis of diseases of the spine and hip joint is not within the scope of this volume. However, the following conditions will serve as examples of how the foregoing examination may be utilized in the appraisal of symptoms referable to these areas.

Scoliosis

Scoliosis is a common and often serious deformity which is readily detected on physical examination. Distinction must be made between a postural and a structural scoliosis.

Postural Scoliosis

Inspection. Inspection reveals a lateral deviation of the vertebral column to one side or the other, usually the left. There is little rotation of the spine, but if there is any, it inclines toward the concave side of the curve so that the trunk on that side may be a little more prominent. There is no limitation of motion on testing mobility. The scoliosis disappears

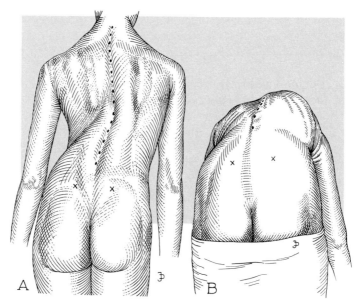

Figure 10–5. Structural scoliosis. *A*, Deviation of the spine occurs in more than one direction. *B*, On flexion the rotation is accentuated and the trunk is prominent on the convex side.

completely in recumbency. The remainder of the examination may be negative. A slumping posture or shortening of one leg may be found as the basic cause of the curvature.

Structural Scoliosis

Inspection.   The curvature is ordinarily multiple so that deviation of the spine from the midline occurs in more than one direction. Rotation of the spine is the striking finding, and it is always toward the convex side of the curve (Fig. 10–5 *A*). This rotation is exaggerated when the spine is flexed, and a prominence of the trunk may be noted on the convex side (Fig. 10–5 *B*).

Mobility of the spine is greatly restricted, and the curvatures will not disappear on motion or recumbency. The remainder of the physical examination may reveal other structural abnormalities such as congenital defects, muscular weakness due to poliomyelitis, or a thoracic deformity from previous surgery or chronic emphysema.

Kyphosis

Inspection

Inspection discloses an angular curvature of the spine in an anterior-posterior direction; the convexity is always posterior. In advanced cases

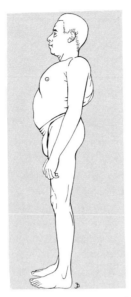

Figure 10–6. Kyphosis. A case of tuberculosis of the spine.

the familiar "hunchback" appearance develops (Fig. 10–6). Minor degrees of kyphosis may be overlooked unless inspection is carefully performed. Sometimes palpation will reveal a kyphosis which has been missed in inspection. It should be determined whether the spine is normally mobile or not. Tuberculosis may be present in other areas of the body if it is the cause of the kyphosis.

Lumbar and Lumbosacral Strain

Inspection

There may be an increase in the normal lumbar lordosis. The lower spine will be held rigid; the patient bends forward from the hips rather than from the waist. Lateral motions in the lumbar regions are restricted, and rotation may produce pain referable to the lumbar spine. Palpation and percussion may elicit tenderness over the lumbar spine.

Special Tests

Straight leg raising may be relatively free but flexed leg raising will produce pain and may be markedly restricted. Hyperextension of the spine may produce pain in the lumbar region. Final evaluation of the nature of the process will require x-ray study of the spine.

Ruptured Intervertebral Disk

This diagnosis should be considered in all instances of back pain, particularly when associated with radicular pain. The manifestations of a ruptured cervical disk are discussed in Chapter 2.

The physical findings in rupture of a nucleus pulposus in the lumbosacral region are variable. Pain may be present in early cases, but objective changes may not be demonstrable. In advanced cases the patient's posture may suggest a structural deformity of the spine. A lateral list of the lumbar spine, a so-called sciatic scoliosis, is quite common if the symptoms are acute. Usually the list is away from the side of the lesion. Flexion of the lumbar spine to open up the spine posteriorly is common. These deformities persist on motion and may make it difficult, if not impossible, for the patient to climb on or off an examining table. The position of supine recumbency is often impossible for the patient to assume. In other instances the findings are predominantly neurologic and simulate a tumor of the spinal cord. The following signs are especially characteristic, although all may not be present:

1. Diminished or obliterated lumbar curve.

2. Limitation of motion of the spine, especially flexion. Hyperextension of the lumbar spine is painful.

3. Asymmetric limitation of straight leg raising from pain and muscle

Disk Involved	L₃- L₄ (3-5%)	L₄- L₅ (45%)	L₅- S₁ (50%)
Leg Pain	Anterior thigh	Posterior thigh, calf dorsum of foot	Posterior thigh, calf, ankle
Paresthesias	Antero-medial surface of thigh	Medial-dorsal surface of foot; great toe	Lateral-dorsal surface of foot; little toe
Tenderness	Over femoral nerve trunk	Over sciatic nerve trunk	Over sciatic nerve trunk
Motor Weakness	Quadriceps	Tibialis anterior and dorsi-flexors of toes	Gastrocnemius group and plantar flexors of toes
Atrophy	Maximal in thigh	Maximal in lower leg	Maximal in calf
Reflexes	Knee jerk diminished to absent	Normal often K.J. may be hyperactive A.J. may be hypoactive slightly	Ankle jerk usually diminished to absent
Sensation	Hypalgesia over L₄ dermatome	Hypalgesia over L₅ dermatome	Hypalgesia over S₁ dermatome

Figure 10–7. Location of herniated intervertebral disk.

spasm with a positive dorsiflexion sign. Crossed reference of pain occurs when the unaffected leg is raised.

4. Percussion tenderness over the affected intervertebral space.

5. Increase of pain on *jugular compression.*

6. Measurable atrophy of the calf and thigh.

7. A neurologic defect—depending upon the level of the lesion, one may find motor weakness, sensory loss, diminished or absent patellar or ankle reflexes.

8. The level of the extruded disk can often be determined by the physical findings (Fig. 10–7).

Tuberculosis of the Spine

Tuberculosis may affect any portion of the spine, but it is most common in the thoracolumbar region. In advanced stages a characteristic kyphosis makes the diagnosis readily detectable. In early tuberculosis, however, the process is insidious. Stiffness of the spine is a classic sign. The disease attacks the body of the vertebrae, and the musculature tightens and holds the spine rigid in an attempt to shift the weight posteriorly to the neural arches. Motions of the spine are markedly restricted. Children with tuberculosis hold the spine erect in stooping to pick up an object from the floor; they flex their knees and legs and then bend laterally to reach the object. The psoas muscle may be involved, and the resulting spasm limits hyperextension of the hip or spine.

Neoplasms of the Spine

Neoplasms of the spine may produce no manifestations and be undetectable upon physical examination until the disease process interferes with the function of the involved vertebrae. Resulting pain, limitation of motion, and local tenderness will direct attention to the vertebrae in question; whenever the physical examination discloses pain and tenderness sharply localized to one vertebra, x-rays should be taken to search for primary or secondary neoplasms. In advanced cases sensory and motor defects may be found. Complete paralysis may develop. A painful kyphosis in the adult should always arouse suspicion of neoplastic disease.

Spondylolisthesis

Spondylolisthesis is a forward displacement of the fifth lumbar vertebra upon the sacrum. There is a lack of support between the arch and the body. The signs and symptoms are chronic low back pain and sometimes a noticeable deformity.

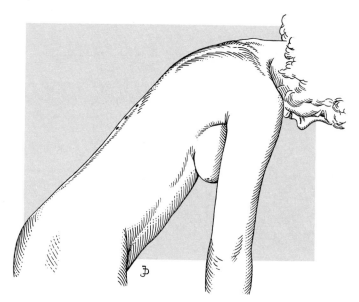

Figure 10–8.   Strümpell-Marie disease.

On physical examination the diagnosis may be suspected by a marked accentuation of the lumbar lordosis. A palpable "jog" at the spinous processes at the level of the lesion may be present. The sacrum tends to stand out posteriorly, and the back appears to be telescoped.

Arthritis of the Spine

Various and sundry physical deformities may be produced by arthritis, and the early manifestations may be similar to those seen in lumbar and lumbosacral strain. Certain forms of arthritis produce characteristic deformities, as in the rigid "poker-back" of spondylitis deformans (Strümpell-Marie disease) (Fig. 10–8). Decrease in chest expansion is an early sign of arthritis of the spine.

IV. DISORDERS OF THE HIP

Congenital Dislocations

Prior to weight-bearing, this condition is often overlooked because of failure to examine the hips as part of a routine pediatric examination. The findings are characteristic if carefully elicited.

Inspection

The affected leg is shorter, and the gluteal skin folds are asymmetric; the fold on the involved side is more proximal. The level of the knee on the affected side is lower with the legs flexed and the feet on the table. Measurement will confirm the presence of shortening. If weight-bearing has begun, there is considerable limp, manifested by a lurch toward the affected side. The Trendelenburg test is positive.

Trendelenburg's test for movements of the gluteal fold is performed as follows: The patient is stripped and stands with his back to the examiner; he is told to lift one foot and then the other. The position and movements of the gluteal fold are observed. Normally when the patient stands on one leg, the opposite gluteal fold rises. The test is positive when the patient stands on the affected leg and the opposite gluteal fold falls due to instability of the affected hip joint.

Motion

The range of abduction is restricted. With the knee bent and the thigh flexed there is abnormal mobility between the femur and the pelvis, which has been described as "telescoping of the hip."

Palpation

The head of the femur cannot be felt in its normal position at the intersection of the femoral artery and the inguinal ligament.

In *bilateral dislocations* the diagnosis prior to weight-bearing is more difficult because there is no discrepancy between the two limbs. The limitations of abduction, failure to feel the head of the femur beneath the inguinal ligament, and increased posterior mobility are the most important signs. Once weight-bearing begins, however, there is a severe lordosis. The child walks with a waddling gait.

Tuberculosis of the Hip

The disease may be insidious at onset, with very little pain; a limp is the principal sign, and pain may be referred to the knee.

Inspection

Muscle atrophy is often striking in comparison with the normal thigh. The leg is held in a position of outward rotation owing to joint effusion and muscle spasm.

Mobility

Pain and limitation of hyperextension are early signs, but if the disease is at all advanced, motion is limited in all directions, owing partly to reflex spasm. In advanced cases flexion, abduction, internal rotation, and apparent shortening develop. In very early cases, physical signs may be so minimal that repeated roentgenologic examinations are required to confirm the diagnosis.

Legg-Perthes' Disease (Coxa Plana)

This condition occurs in children between the ages of 3 and 10. There is flattening of the head of the femur with a broadening of the neck.

Inspection

A limp is characteristic and usually directs attention to the condition. Associated muscle atrophy will be present and can be demonstrated by measurement of the thigh circumference.

Motion

The extremes of mobility are restricted, especially in abduction and rotation. In more advanced cases muscle spasm may limit motion in all directions; the findings then become similar to those seen in tuberculosis, with which the disease is often confused. The differential diagnosis is established by x-ray examination.

Coxa Vara

The angle between the neck and the shaft of the femur is lessened. The condition may be congenital or rachitic in origin. The physical findings may simulate congenital dislocation as the femur is shortened.

Slipping Upper Femoral Epiphysis or Epiphysitis

A weak connection at the epiphyseal plate permits displacement of the head of the femur on the neck. The condition occurs in children between the ages of 10 and 15 during the period of rapid adolescent growth. It frequently affects fat, overweight children. The habitus is often so characteristic that the diagnosis can be made at a glance.

Inspection

There is a distinct limp, and the affected limb is held in external rotation. Pain may be referred to the knee or the hip.

Motion

Internal rotation is markedly restricted, and abduction is reduced. Flexion is likely to be limited and painful.

Septic Arthritis

High fever, toxemia, and pain in the hip call attention to the condition, and on examination there is exquisite pain at the slightest motion of the hip.

Acute Bursitis

Acute bursitis of the hip joint may be confused with arthritis. There is no toxemia, and there may be little or no rise in temperature, but if the bursa communicates with the joint, there may be marked pain on motion. It is more common for motions to be restricted to those which compress the involved bursae. There are many bursae around the joint, but the two principal ones lie posteriorly beneath the gluteal muscle and anteriorly beneath the iliopsoas. Careful palpation around the joint will often indicate that the pain and tenderness are restricted to a particular area as opposed to the diffuse tenderness found in arthritis.

chapter 11

EXAMINATION OF THE BLOOD VESSELS AND LYMPHATICS

Examination of the peripheral blood vessels usually provides accurate assessment of the vascular system. The physical findings often closely reflect the state of the arterial and venous systems that may be delineated further by arteriography or venography. Because many arterial, venous, and lymphatic insufficiency disorders may be diagnosed solely by physical findings, these examinations should be done in an orderly and careful fashion.

I. DISORDERS OF ARTERIES

Cerebrovascular Insufficiency

The location of arterial lesions in the majority of patients with cerebrovascular ischemic syndromes is in the mediastinal or cervical portions of the brachiocephalic outflow arteries. The symptoms are generally manifest as transient neurologic deficits or transient ischemic attacks (TIAs). There may be ipsilateral loss of vision (amaurosis fugax), or contralateral sensory or motor changes involving the extremities. Less discrete signs are those of lightheadedness, vertigo, bilateral visual blurring, or mentation deficits. The symptoms occur as a result of stenotic arteriosclerotic lesions causing diminished cerebral blood flow or ulcerated atheromata causing retinal or cerebral microemboli (Fig. 11–1). Patients with this condition often are candidates for surgical revascularization; therefore, it is important not to overlook the physical findings.

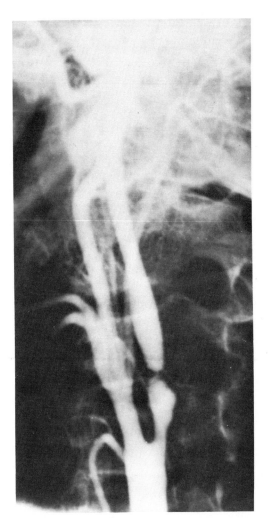

Figure 11–1. Carotid arteriogram showing marked stenosis of the proximal internal carotid artery in a patient with transient cerebral ischemic attacks. A loud bruit was audible by auscultation at the level of the carotid bifurcation in the neck.

Palpation

The subclavian pulse can be felt by digital compression in the neck above the center of the clavicle. The common carotid pulse is best felt by displacing the artery laterally and compressing it against the vertebral column. A totally occluded common carotid artery can be felt as a firm cord with occasionally a transmitted systolic quiver which may be misinterpreted as a pulse. Except for patients with an unusually low carotid bifurcation, the pulse of the internal carotid artery is not palpable in the neck. It was formerly thought that this pulse could be felt from within the oropharynx. The internal and external carotid arteries course together at this level and the pulse in one cannot be differentiated from the other.

Auscultation

Auscultation for bruits detects stenotic arterial lesions and is an essential part of the examination. Cervical bruits may be caused by aortic valvular stenosis. In these cases, they are heard with equal intensity over the carotid and subclavian arteries. Innominate stenosis produces bruits over the right subclavian and right common carotid arteries which diminish in intensity from the level of origin.

A bruit heard only over the subclavian artery above the midclavicle usually arises from stenosis at the origin of the subclavian. Vertebral artery stenosis often produces a faint bruit heard best over the top of the shoulder. Stenosis at the common carotid bifurcation or at the orifice of either of its branches produces a bruit best heard below the angle of the mandible which is not audible low in the neck.

Severe stenosis or total occlusion of the innominate or subclavian artery is generally associated with sufficient collateral blood flow to maintain a weakened pulse in the brachial and radial arteries. When the stenosis is hemodynamically significant the blood pressure in the appropriate extremity will be decreased. *Thus, determination of blood pressure in both arms is essential.*

Lesions which cannot be diagnosed from the physical findings are total occlusion of the internal or external carotid arteries and total occlusion, and often stenosis, of the vertebral arteries. An ulcerated lesion in the proximal internal carotid artery may occasionally exist in the absence of significant stenosis and will be undetectable by physical examination.

The most common pathologic cause of cerebrovascular disease is arteriosclerosis. Only in recent years has it become known that cerebrovascular accidents are more often caused by extracranial rather than intracranial arteriosclerotic lesions. Less commonly, fibromuscular hyperplasia of the cervical or internal carotid arteries is a cause of cerebrovascular insufficiency. This disorder is a common cause of renovascular hypertension. A rare cause of occlusion of the extracranial cerebral arteries is the arteriopathy known as Takayasu's arteritis.

Gastrointestinal Ischemia

Chronic visceral ischemic syndromes are often associated with characteristic clinical findings. The celiac, superior and inferior mesenteric, and internal iliac arteries are the principal sources of blood supply to the stomach and intestines.

Clinical Findings

The main complaint is abdominal pain that occurs about 15 to 30 minutes after eating a meal. This complaint is so characteristic that it may be diagnostic. The pain has also been called abdominal angina. The pain is most often in the epigastrium but may occur anywhere in the abdomen. Weight loss appears in the later stages of the disease as a result of reluctance to eat because of the associated pain. Palpation of the abdomen is generally not contributory but occasionally a thrill from celiac artery stenosis may be palpable in the epigastrium. Auscultation is most important because many of the patients have an audible bruit in the midline between the xiphoid process and umbilicus. This may be a result of narrowing of either or both celiac or superior mesenteric arteries. The pathologic cause in older patients is usually atherosclerosis. In the younger age group, especially in females, visceral insufficiency may be caused by arterial compression from the median arcuate ligament of the diaphragm. An interesting finding of note in these patients is that the bruit becomes noticeably louder with expiration. The diagnosis is confirmed by assessment of the arteriographic and clinical findings. Surgical revascularization is associated with dramatic relief of the preoperative complaints. It is very important that the diagnosis of chronic visceral ischemia be made, promptly because intestinal infarction results from progression of the chronic state.

Renovascular Hypertension

Hypertension may occur as a result of any disorder that causes diminished blood supply to one or both kidneys. Patients may be asymptomatic or display symptoms from their high blood pressure. including headache. irritablility, or emotional depression. Persistent elevation of the diastolic blood pressure is usually the only abnormal physical finding. A bruit may be audible to one or both sides of the midline of the upper abdomen. The bruit may be best heard in the flank or towards the back. The diagnosis is confirmed by arteriographic demonstration of stenosis of the renal artery and elevation of the concentration of renin in the ipsilateral renal vein.

The most common cause of this vascular disorder is arteriosclerosis. The next most common disorder, found frequently in middle-aged females or children, is fibromuscular hyperplasia (Fig. 11–2). These patients, in particular, respond favorably with return to normal blood pressures after surgical revascularization.

Ischemic Disorders Involving the Lower Extremities

Arteriosclerosis is the most common cause of impaired peripheral circulation. If it is recognized early its most serious sequelae, such as gangrene, may be prevented or postponed by proper care and judicious measures, including direct arterial surgery to relieve claudication or

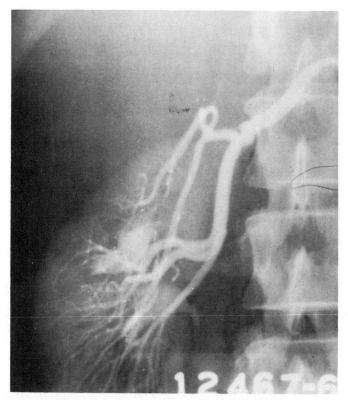

Figure 11–2. Selective right renal arteriogram showing moderate stenosis of the distal main renal artery due to fibromuscular hyperplasia. This patient had renovascular hypertension corrected by reconstructive vascular surgery.

prevent gangrene. Many patients who seek medical advice for other conditions are suffering from moderately advanced peripheral arteriosclerosis; this should be recognized in order to institute appropriate prophylactic measures. Frequently, such patients complain of a painful toe or toenail; ill-advised chiropody or surgery precipitates a sequence of trauma, infection, and gangrene. Thus, a limb is lost that might have been saved if the underlying condition had been correctly appraised.

Ordinarily, the patient will have had symptoms referable to the legs if any of the signs of impaired peripheral circulation are present; intermittent claudication is the most common of these. However, often no complaint is made, and the condition may be difficult to elicit in the history because the patient may have subconsciously limited his activities in order to prevent the onset of pain in the calf.

It is of the greatest importance, therefore, to recognize the manifestations of obliterative arteriosclerosis of the leg in the absence of obvious gangrene or advanced symptoms.

Chronic Segmental Arterial Occlusion

A relatively large group of patients have intermittent claudication as their primary symptom. It may be caused initially by a segmental occlusion of one of the major peripheral arteries.

LERICHE'S SYNDROME (INSIDIOUS THROMBOSIS OF THE LOWER ABDOMINAL AORTA)

This syndrome is found in relatively young men who complain of pain or fatigue in the hips, buttocks, or thighs on walking; they frequently

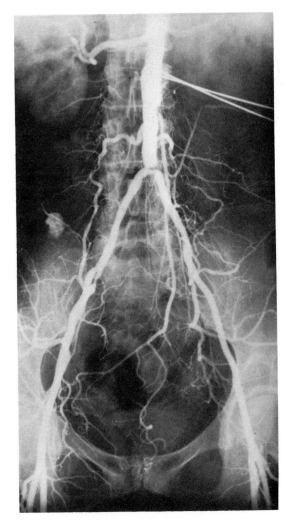

Figure 11–3. Translumbar aortogram of a patient with impotence and bilateral thigh claudication. There is severe stenosis of the terminal abdominal aorta and both common iliac arteries. Both femoral pulses were markedly reduced and bruits were noted at the level of the umbilicus and over each common femoral artery at the groin.

have become sexually impotent. The salient physical findings are pallor, wasting, and a complete absence of arterial pulsations in the lower extremities. In the more advanced stages of the disease, ulceration and gangrene develop. The obstructive process is found predominantly in the lower abdominal aorta (Fig. 11–3).

SEGMENTAL OCCLUSION OF ILIAC OR FEMORAL ARTERIES

This phenomenon may occur in any of the branches of the aorta and distal arteries but it most frequently involves the superficial femoral artery in the adductor canal (Fig. 11–4). Early in the course of the disease there may be no abnormal physical findings except diminished or absent

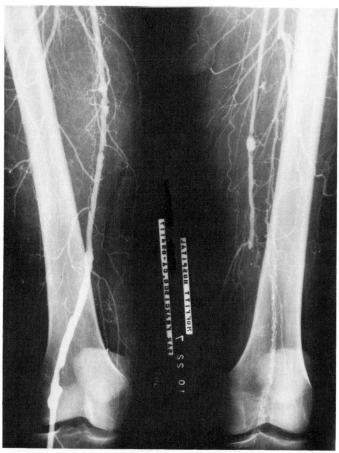

Figure 11–4. Bilateral femoral arteriograms from a patient with claudication of the left leg. There is occlusion of the left superficial femoral artery and irregular atherosclerotic changes of the right superficial femoral artery. On examination the femoral pulses were normal but there were no palpable pedal pulses noted in the left foot.

peripheral pulses. With the passage of time, other signs of obliterative disease of the arteries become apparent. Claudication usually appears early. Recognition of this form of disease, namely, chronic segmental arterial occlusion, is important since it is in this group of patients that direct arterial surgery is of the greatest value.

Determining the Level of an Arterial Occlusion

The precise level of an arterial occlusion should be determined if possible. It is always higher than the area of gangrene or impaired circulation suggests. Variability in the effectiveness of the collateral circulation makes it extremely hazardous to base estimation of the level of the occlusion on the extent of the ischemia. Ischemia of the toes or foot may occur with occlusion below the knee but it is also seen in popliteal and femoral occlusions. Popliteal lesions may lead to the loss of the lower leg. Ischemia extending above the knee indicates an occlusion of the external or common iliac arteries.

The Signs of Obliterative Arteriosclerosis of the Leg Without Infection, Necrosis, or Gangrene

Inspection

There is an atrophic appearance to the leg. The muscle bundles, particularly of the gastrocnemius, appear thin and wasted. The skin is taut and shiny. There is diminished or absent growth of hair. The growth of the nails is retarded in more advanced cases, and the nail plate is thickened and roughened by the presence of eccentrically placed transverse ridges

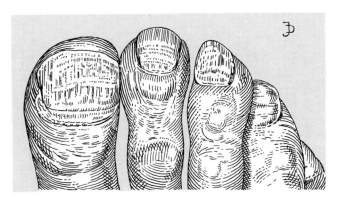

Figure 11–5. Nail changes in obliterative arteriosclerosis. The nails are thickened and roughened by transverse ridges.

(Fig. 11–5). A claw-shaped nail may develop. The toes should be separated, and the interdigital spaces should be carefully inspected for minute ulcerations, which are often the first signs of impending necrosis. The skin may be mottled, but usually its color is normal when the legs are in the horizontal position. The color changes which can be induced by change of position are of such importance that they are described in detail below.

Color Changes in the Skin on Elevation and Dependency

A simple but most valuable test of adequacy of the peripheral arterial circulation is the change in the color of the skin which occurs on elevation and dependency.

The patient should be supine; the legs should be inspected first in the horizontal position. Quite normal pink color may be present. The legs are then elevated to an angle of about 45 degrees and supported in that position by the examiner. Slight blanching and loss of color in the extremities is normal. The skin will quickly lose all color and become dead grayish white if there is significant impairment of the arterial circulation. This may be limited to a toe or may involve the entire foot and lower leg. The legs are then allowed to hang over the edge of the table in the dependent position. A quick pink flush will appear with normal circulation; in the presence of impaired arterial flow a bright red color which slowly changes to a cyanotic hue will develop. This phenomenon is known as dependent rubor. The color changes reflect oxygen saturation and volume flow in the subpapillary venous plexuses of the skin. This is a highly sensitive test. It will indicate an impaired circulation in the presence of seemingly adequate peripheral pulses, color, and warmth.

Palpation

The peripheral pulses may seem normal or may be markedly diminished or absent. The examiner should be certain that the dorsalis pedis is not aberrant if it cannot be felt in the normal location and that the posterior tibial is not unusually prominent. Failure to identify a dorsalis pedis artery pulsation is not in itself a sign of faulty peripheral circulation since it is absent in 10 per cent of normal subjects.

There may be an obvious coolness to the foot or leg when compared with the opposite member or the thigh of the same side. The temperature of the extremities can best be appraised after the part has been exposed to room temperature long enough to come to equilibrium (15 to 30 minutes). The dorsum of the middle phalanx of the flexed finger is the optimum thermotactile surface.

Auscultation

After palpation of the peripheral pulses the examiner should listen over the common femoral arteries for bruits. The presence of an audible bruit connotes stenosis. The loudness of the bruit may be increased after asking the patient to ambulate to the point of claudication. At this point the femoral pulses and especially the peripheral pulses may diminish or disappear. This would indicate a significant degree of proximal stenosis or occlusion.

Venous Filling Time

An added test of adequacy of peripheral blood flow is the determination of the time necessary to fill superficial veins of the foot after emptying. This test is valuable in diabetic patients with "small vessel disease." The feet are elevated until the superficial veins are collapsed, then the legs are allowed to hang over the edge of the table, and the length of time necessary to fill the veins is noted. A prolongation beyond 10 to 15 seconds is evidence of arterial insufficiency. This test is not valid in the presence of varicose veins.

The Signs of Acute Thrombosis

Gangrene or a sudden increase in the signs and symptoms of peripheral arteriosclerosis is usually the result of a thrombotic occlusion of a major vessel. The extent of the change depends upon the site of the occlusion and the adequacy of the collateral circulation. This may be so obvious that an embolus to the extremity is suspected, or so slight that the true nature of the disorder is overlooked.

In general, any sudden impairment of the circulation of the arteriosclerotic extremity suggests a thrombosis. Pain is characteristic but may be so mild as to be described as "numbness." It may be likened to a muscle cramp or it may be agonizing.

Inspection

The color of the leg distal to the occlusion is blue or white. The superficial veins are empty even when the leg is slightly dependent; this is an important point of distinction from venous thrombosis. A bluish, mottled appearance which fails to disappear when the foot is elevated heralds the onset of gangrene. The interdigital spaces are apt to be the intitial site of necrosis, particularly if they are affected by epidermophytosis.

Palpation

The finding of tenderness and no pulsation in the vessel over the site of the thrombosis is a most important observation. The vessel may be identified as a tender pulseless cord in popliteal or femoral occlusions. Tenderness in the calf or in the anterior compartment of the leg indicates posterior or anterior tibial thrombosis, respectively. The corresponding pulse will be absent at the ankle. Occasionally, tenderness will be found at a lower level with absent pulsation at a higher level; this is suggestive of an old occlusion above with a fresh thrombosis below.

The involved area is cold and numb. A well-marked stocking anesthesia develops in severe cases.

Sometimes a superficial or deep venous thrombosis occurs as a complication of an arterial thrombosis. Marked cyanosis and fullness of the superficial veins indicate venous involvement.

The Signs of Acute Embolic Occlusion

It may be impossible to distinguish between an acute arterial thrombosis and an embolic occlusion. The onset of agonizing pain in embolism is instantaneous, while in thrombosis it may take many minutes to reach its maximum. This distinction is so fine that it often cannot be elicited from a patient in severe pain who is obviously threatened with the loss of a limb. On the other hand, as in acute thrombosis, the pain following an embolus may be very mild. The patient may describe the extremity as being "asleep" or "numb."

The nature of the underlying disease is the best guide. The diagnosis of an embolic occlusion is obvious if there is a recognized source of embolism, particularly auricular fibrillation, and the peripheral arteries are normal. A previous history of embolism increases the probability of a recurrent attack. The differential diagnosis may be impossible when there are considerable arteriosclerosis of the peripheral vessels and a source of embolism, such as a recent coronary thrombosis.

In embolism, 99 per cent of the occlusions occur at the site of major divisions of the peripheral arteries. This fact, combined with the evidence provided by the level of the ischemia, the site of disappearance of the palpable pulsation, and the evidence provided by an oscillometer, permits accurate localization for the purposes of surgical exploration (Fig. 11–6).

Ancillary Techniques

Oscillometry is a simple and effective way of determining the level of an arterial occlusion if it is below the iliac vessel. Auscultation over the

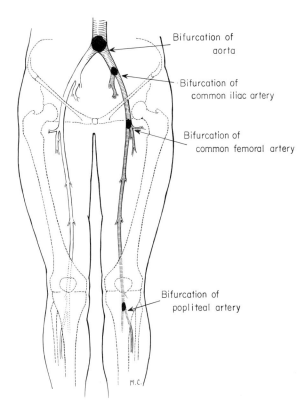

Bifurcation of
aorta

Bifurcation of
common iliac artery

Bifurcation of
common femoral artery

Bifurcation of
popliteal artery

Figure 11–6. Common sites of embolic occlusion.

peripheral arteries while an assistant occludes and releases the femoral artery by pressure is a useful maneuver. A booming arterial sound is heard as the blood re-enters the temporarily occluded vessel. This sound is reproduced each time until the level of the complete occlusion is reached; it then abruptly disappears.

The Doppler flowmeter permits evaluation of arterial and venous flow velocity by sensing and amplifying the frequency shift that occurs when ultrasound is passed through moving blood. This technique is non-invasive and permits localization of arterial and venous obstructive lesions in clinical disorders. Use of this technique has become increasingly widespread; however, its application is limited because of its inability to quantify blood flow adequately.

Thromboangiitis Obliterans (Buerger's Disease)

Defective peripheral circulation may be due to thromboangiitis obliterans. Physical examination usually makes the differential diagnosis between this condition and arteriosclerosis quite easy. Thromboangiitis obliterans occurs predominantly in men below the age of 45; arteriosclerosis is less common before this age. Exceptions occur in both diseases, of course, and occasionally the two conditions are present simultaneously.

The following points are of particular value in differentiation. Superficial phlebitis is common in thromboangiitis and occurs only by coincidence with arteriosclerosis. Pitting edema of the extremity is frequently seen in thromboangiitis and may be the presenting symptom. It is not seen in peripheral arteriosclerosis. Gangrene produces a deep, moist, exquisitely painful ulceration in thromboangiitis, whereas in arteriosclerosis it tends to be superficial, dry, and not very painful.

Raynaud's Syndrome

Raynaud's syndrome is produced by spasm of the digital arterioles. It is characterized by local ischemia of the fingers in response to cold and psychic disturbances. The ischemia of the involved area is manifested by a waxy pallor or severe cyanosis which changes to a compensatory erythema as the attack subsides and the hands are warmed. The syndrome is readily recognized by its obvious relationship to an inciting factor. Although it may first appear unilateral, it is always bilateral when once well established.

The traumatic variety is an occupational disease. It has been de-

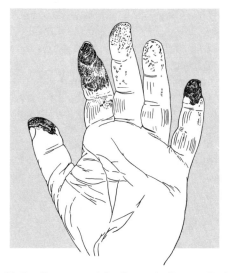

Figure 11–7. Gangrene of the fingers in Raynaud's disease.

scribed in typists, piano players, telephone operators, and individuals who use vibrating machine tools.

The term "Raynaud's disease" is applied to the more severe and progressive form of Raynaud's syndrome. Gangrene of the tips of the digits may ensue as a consequence of repeated severe spasm (Fig. 11–7). The characteristic appearance in advanced cases is manifested by ulceration of the finger tips, tight shiny skin, thickened subcutaneous tissue, and atrophy and shortening of the bones of the fingers.

Allen's test is very useful in delineating small vessel diseases involving the upper extremities. The examiner occludes the brachial artery and washes all arterial blood from the fingers and hand and then releases the brachial artery. Normally, there will occur marked reactive hyperemia within 10 to 15 seconds. In the abnormal situation, there will be pallor for 30 or more seconds and delayed or very delayed return of red color. Digital arterial occlusions may be localized when half or all of a finger remains pale. Further localization may be implemented by finger compression of the radial or ulnar arteries separately.

Scleroderma

In scleroderma the skin becomes hard, tense, shiny, and pigmented. The capillaries of the skin can no longer be visualized. Eventually ankylosis results from fibrotic fixation of the thickened skin to bones and joints.

Erythermalgia (Erythromelalgia; Weir Mitchell's Disease)

The patient complains of severe burning pains in the palms of the hands or soles of the feet. The pain is precipitated by exposure to heat. Even mild warmth, such as placing the extremity beneath the bedclothes, is sufficient to precipitate an attack. Examination reveals marked redness, sometimes with a slightly cyanotic hue, and swelling of the involved extremities. There is a sense of increased heat on palpation. The peripheral pulses are normal and may be full and bounding. A syndrome resembling this may be encountered in diabetes and in polycythemia vera.

Post-traumatic Vasomotor Disorders

Varying degrees of vasomotor instability may result from trauma and subsequent immobilization of a limb. The condition has been confused with Raynaud's disease, thromboangiitis obliterans, and chronic thrombophlebitis.

Pain of an intermittent type, usually accentuated by activity, and blueness, coldness, and swelling are the presenting manifestations. There may be hyperhidrosis and sensitivity to cold. Frequently one symptom is dominant.

Examination discloses edema, atrophy, muscle weakness bordering at times on paralysis, and stiffness of the joints. The skin may be blue or red and shiny. Generally the extremity is colder than its opposite member. The pulses may be diminished or normal. As a rule there is no peripheral nerve injury, and there is no incompetency of the deep veins of the leg. Acute osteoporosis (Sudeck's atrophy) may be demonstrated by x-ray.

The longer the time from injury to the institution of remedial measures, the worse are the symptoms and signs. The history of injury and immobilization, the lack of peripheral nerve injury, the inconstant pain, the variable vasomotor signs, and the acute osteoporosis are important diagnostic points. (See *Causalgia,* Chapter 21, p. 366.)

Aneurysm of a Peripheral Artery

An aneurysm of a peripheral artery manifests itself as a pulsating swelling in the course of the vessel. It has an expansile pulsation so that if the fingers are placed on the swelling in a fanlike manner, they are not only lifted but also separated. A palpable thrill may be present, and on auscultation a systolic bruit may be heard. The patients will not infrequently complain of pain radiating toward the distal portion of the extremity because of pressure on sensory nerves adjacent to the aneurysm. It is important to evaluate the circulatory and nutritional status of the more distal portion of the extremity because this variety of aneurysm not infrequently will thrombose with occlusion of the vessel distal to the aneurysm.

A popliteal aneurysm is a frequent precursor of thrombosis. Early recognition and restorative surgery may prevent loss of the limb.

Traumatic or False Aneurysm

A wound or mycotic infection of the wall of an artery may result in a local rupture with the formation of an organized pulsating hematoma. The sac is formed by the perivascular tissues, not by a weakened bulging arterial wall.

False aneurysm following trauma is distinguished from traumatic arteriovenous fistulae by a systolic pulsation and murmur rather than a continuous one. Branham's sign cannot be elicited (see below).

Rapid enlargement and rupture may occur so that corrective surgery should not be delayed.

Arteriovenous Fistula

An abnormal direct communication between an artery and a vein may be congenital or traumatic. The physical signs in a peripheral location are characteristic and diagnostic. Over the lesion there is a continuous bruit with a systolic accentuation and a continuous palpable thrill. Compression so as to occlude the fistula causes prompt slowing of the pulse (Branham's sign).

The peripheral circulation in the presence of an arteriovenous fistula is usually increased. There may be an increased size in the extremity in congenital lesions or in ones acquired before the completion of epiphyseal growth.

Less commonly there are ischemic signs particularly in the early stages of acquired arteriovenous shunts.

II. DISORDERS OF VEINS

Varicose Veins

The diagnosis of varicose veins is often obvious at a glance. At other times it may be suspected because of increased pigmentation, edema, and enlarged cutaneous veins at the medial side of the ankle. The examiner must seek the answer to the following questions when confronted with the presence or probable presence of varicose veins.

1. ARE THERE DEFINITE VARICOSITIES?
   ARE THE GREATER OR LESSER OR BOTH
   SAPHENOUS SYSTEMS INVOLVED?

Inspect the course of the venous channels carefully. The greater saphenous system is obviously involved if there are dilated veins in the thigh. Similarly, a large venous trunk arising in the popliteal space indicates involvement of the lesser saphenous system. Occasionally the veins may be masked by edema or obesity or are not visible in the thigh although prominent in the leg. The presence and course of the veins can then be accurately determined by the *Schwartz test* (Fig. 11–8). By this means the course of the vein can be traced upward through the thigh or laterally and posteriorly to the popliteal space.

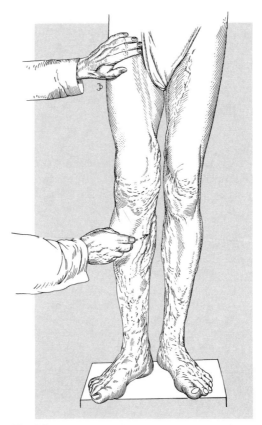

Figure 11–8. The Schwartz test. The flat of the fingers of the left hand is placed over the probable course of the saphenous vein in the thigh. A prominent vein in the leg is gently tapped with the finger of the right hand, as indicated by the arrow. An impulse is transmitted through the column of blood to the palpating finger if there is a direct communication between the vein in the lower leg and the greater saphenous system.

2. IS THERE EVIDENCE OF SUFFICIENT VENOSTASIS TO IMPAIR THE CIRCULATION TO THE LOWER LEG?

The question is answered affirmatively if there is pigmentation of the skin, edema, brawny induration, or actual ulceration in the lower leg. Eczematous changes and epidermophytosis are common accompaniments of peripheral venous congestion.

3. ARE THE VALVES OF THE COMMUNICATING VEINS BETWEEN THE SUPERFICIAL AND DEEP VENOUS SYSTEMS COMPETENT OR INCOMPETENT?

This question is best answered by the *Trendelenburg test*. The veins are emptied of blood by elevation of the leg. The upper thigh is then lightly constricted with a length of gauze bandage or rubber tubing, and the patient is asked to stand up. The entire greater saphenous system will remain collapsed if the valves in the communicating veins are competent (Fig. 11–9). If the tourinquet is not released, the veins will gradually fill from the arterial side, but as soon as the constricting tourniquet is released, blood promptly pours down the incompetent greater saphenous system into the veins of the calf (Fig. 11–9 *B*). Blood will promptly enter the superficial system below the tourniquet if there are incompetent communicating veins below it. The precise site of these perforating veins may be identified by successive reapplication of the tourniquet at lower levels after previous emptying of the leg veins by elevation.

The terminology of the Trendelenburg test is often confused. Trendelenburg wrote:

"Lay the patient flat; lift the leg up vertically; the varices empty. Now compress the saphena magna with the finger. Stand him up quickly. The

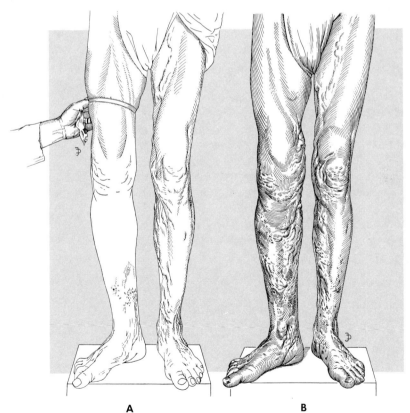

A   **B**

Figure 11–9. The Trendelenburg test. *A,* The veins have been emptied of blood by elevation of the leg, and reflux down the leg when the patient stands up is prevented by the constricting tourniquet. *B,* On release of the tourniquet the veins promptly fill with blood.

varices fill slowly, but not as much as previously. Now let the finger go, and the varices fill very quickly and fully by a column of blood which is seen to shoot downward in the saphena magna."

This is a *positive Trendelenbrug* test. It indicates that the valves in the greater saphenous vein are incompetent. A *negative Trendelenburg* test implies that there is no retrograde filling of the saphenous vein either before or after the compressing finger or tourniquet is removed. A *doubly positive Trendelenburg* test is characterized by rapid filling of the saphenous system through the communicating veins while the greater saphenous vein is compressed, and an additional downward reflux through the saphenous vein after its release. It denotes incompetency òf the valves in both the greater saphenous and the communicating veins.

4. ARE THE DEEP VEINS NORMAL OR IS THERE EVIDENCE OF AN OLD, DEEP THROMBOPHLEBITIS?

The manifestations of thrombophlebitis are discussed in more detail later. *As a general rule it is wise to suspect deep venous incompetence in a patient with varicose veins and brawny edema, ulceration (particularly on the medial aspect of the leg), and stasis changes.* At other times there may be such slight edema of the leg that it may be attributable to the varicosities. In this circumstance one must be most careful to exclude pathology in deep veins.

This is best done by the *comparative tourniquet* test (modified Perthes' test). The patient is allowed to walk about and then the varicose veins are inspected in the standing position. The tourniquet is now applied high in the thigh tightly enough to prevent reflux down the varicose veins. The patient walks vigorously with the tourniquet in place. If the varicosities below the tourniquet shrink, the deep veins are normal. If the varicose veins below the tourniquet become more prominent, the deep veins are incompetent. Gentle compression of the varicosities from ankle to thigh with an elastic bandage is another modification of this test. The patient is then asked to walk vigorously. Circulation of the foot will remain pink and healthy if the deep veins are normal. Cyanosis of the toes will develop rapidly if there is an incompetency of the deep veins.

The comparative tourniquet test demonstrates that the valves in the communicating veins and deep veins are competent.

5. ARE THE VARICOSITIES PRIMARY OR SECONDARY?

Varicose veins are usually primary, but this question must always be answered before attention is directed primarily to the varicosities.

A rapid development of varicosities in the female is frequently seen in pregnancy.

Varicosities may be secondary to a deep thrombophlebitis with incompetence of the main and communicating systems of veins.

Varices in the lateral thigh which extend on to the abdominal wall above the pubis result from deep venous incompetence or occlusion.

6. DO THE VARICES ORIGINATE IN THE SAPHENOUS SYSTEM?

Varices which stream down the medial thigh of a woman from the area of the vulva come from veins in the vulva, vagina, or pelvis. There is usually a history of extensive vulvar varices during pregnancy. Although the varices in the thigh connect with the saphenous system, a conventional operation for primary saphenous varicosities will be followed by recurrence of varicose veins.

Acute Thrombophlebitis

The manifestations of acute thrombophlebitis are sufficiently variable to suggest two supposedly distinct forms. The term "phlebothrombosis" describes those types in which local inflammatory signs in the leg are minimal and in which pulmonary embolism is common. The term "thrombophlebitis" has been applied to those instances in which there are obvious local inflammatory signs and in which pulmonary embolism is somewhat less common. However, since all gradations between these forms are seen and since pulmonary embolism may occur in any of them, most authorities prefer to use the term thrombophlebitis for all of them. Individual cases may be characterized by descriptive terms such as "silent" or "latent" or "acute inflammatory." There appears to be no etiologic difference. In fact, quite often a patient with a marked inflammatory type of thrombophlebitis in one leg will have a silent thrombosis in the opposite leg which is the source of a fatal pulmonary embolism.

Acute Femoroiliac Thrombophlebitis; Phlegmasia Alba Dolens

The onset of the acute inflammatory type of thrombophlebitis is sudden. There is considerable pain which may be excruciating and often localized over the site of the maximal vein involvement. Inspection will disclose swelling of the entire leg. The color of the skin varies. It may be white, pinkish blue or intensely cyanotic. Varying degrees of arterial spasm occur, and in extreme forms acute thrombophlebitis resembles an acute arterial embolism.

Massive Venous Occlusion; Phlegmasia Caerulea Dolens

This relatively rare condition is probably a variant of acute femoro-iliac thrombophlebitis in which the entire venous return of the extremity is occluded. There is a characteristic clinical pattern. Occasionally it may develop in the course of a typical thrombophlebitis, but more often, the onset is sudden, with signs and symptoms developing in a matter of minutes or hours. These consist of an excruciating pain eventually involving the whole limb. The discoloration is characteristic. Within a matter of minutes, the whole extremity takes on a violaceous cyanosis. This is associated with rapidly developing edema. Early in the course, arterial pulsations are present but rapidly diminish and disappear. Circulatory collapse may ensue. The differential diagnosis between an arterial and venous occlusion is difficult.

The prognosis is grave for salvage of the limb because gangrene rapidly ensues unless treatment is instituted promptly. *Intravenous anticoagulation with heparin is indicated. Controversey exists as to the efficacy of venous thrombectomy in this disorder, but if gangrene appears imminent in spite of heparin anticoagulation it should be undertaken.*

The Differential Diagnosis of Acute Thrombophlebitis and Acute Arterial Occlusion

The leg may become dead white, the peripheral pulses may disappear, and the characteristic intractable pain of peripheral ischemia may develop in either. There is more cyanosis in thrombophlebitis than is seen in the dead white, dusky pallor of an arterial occlusion. Sensation in the extremity disappears promptly in an acute arterial occlusion while it usually persists in acute thrombophlebitis. The finding of marked tenderness in the femoral and iliac region is in favor of a diagnosis of thrombophlebitis. Fullness of the superficial veins with the legs slightly dependent is one of the most significant and reliable indications of a venous rather than an arterial occlusion. An arterial occlusion may be excluded if an oscillometer or the ordinary sphygmomanometer placed on the thigh or calf discloses oscillations even though these are diminished. A regional anesthetic block of the lumbar sympathetic chain may help distinguish between the two conditions in doubtful cases. There are instances in which the arterial spasm in thrombophlebitis has been so severe that gangrene has occurred (phlegmasia caerulea dolens).

Pain may be minimal in less acute forms of femoroiliac thrombophlebitis, and the presenting manifestation is that of a white, uniformly swollen, edematous extremity, the so-called milk leg. Palpation will reveal tenderness along Hunter's canal or along the course of the iliac vessels just above the inguinal ligament.

Silent Thrombophlebitis ("Phlebothrombosis")

An obvious thrombophlebitis is not as common as a relatively silent thrombophlebitis or "phlebothrombosis." The following signs should be sought each day in patients with cardiac failure, in postoperative patients, and in all patients in whom a pulmonary infarct has been suspected:

1. A slight irregularity in the pulse rate or temperature.
2. Minimal swelling of the calf of the leg, which may be detected only by careful measurement and comparison of the legs.
3. Minimal pitting edema of the ankle.
4. Slight tenderness to palpation along the course of the deep veins of the calf.

Tenderness in the muscle may be distinguished from *tenderness along the vein* by lateral compression of the muscle bundles which lift the gastrocnemius muscle away from the tibia (Fig. 11–10). The source of the tenderness probably lies within the muscle itself if the pain produced by this maneuver is greater than that produced by compressing the muscle against the posterior aspect of the tibia. Conversely, if pressure deep into the posterior aspect of the calf produces more pain, it is indicative of a deep phlebitis. The degree of pressure necessary to elicit tenderness in deep phlebitis is not great, and the maneuver should be gently performed since rough manipulation may dislodge a clot.

Dorsiflexion of the foot with the leg slightly flexed may produce pain and discomfort in the calf due to slight traction on the involved vein. It may be the only indication of a latent thrombosis. This sign is extremely useful if care is taken to exclude tender, sensitive, shortened heel cords. Women who are accustomed to wearing high heels and who are allowed to walk in slippers or moccasins in the immediate postoperative period frequently develop sensitive heel cords. These may be mistaken for thrombophlebitis on the basis of the dorsiflexion sign alone.

Occasionally no evidence of a deep thrombosis will be found on physical examination; it is only by careful repetition of these maneuvers that the source of suspected pulmonary infarcts or severe pulmonary embolism may be found.

Postphlebitic Syndrome

Incompetence of the deep veins of the leg secondary to a chronic thrombophlebitis produces changes which are quite characteristic in ad-

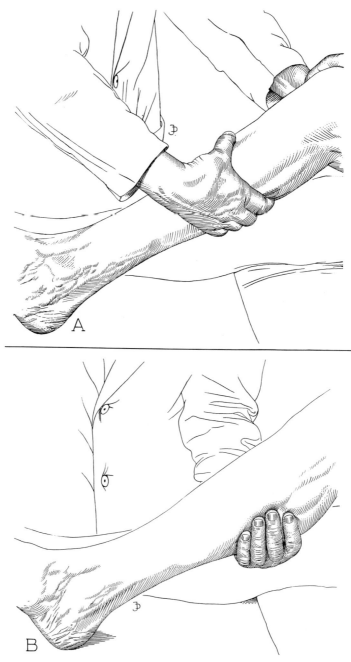

Figure 11–10. *A,* Palpation of the calf for deep tenderness in thrombophlebitis. *B,* Tenderness in the muscle may be distinguished from tenderness in the vein by lateral compression between the thumb and fingers, lifting the gastrocnemius away from the tibia.

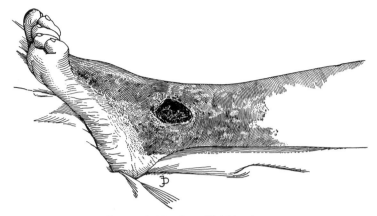

Figure 11–11.   Postphlebitic ulcer.

vanced cases. Ulceration is common (Fig. 11–11); there is a brawny edema of the leg which is most marked at the ankle. Impairment of circulation is manifested by brownish pigmentation, with dry scaly skin and ulceration. There may be associated varicosities or there may be no noticeable superficial veins. Sometimes there is a dusky cyanosis of the lower leg with purplish mottling, but more often, except for pigmentation, the color of the skin does not suggest impaired circulation. Epidermophytosis and eczematous changes in the skin of the leg are usually present.

The only manifestations in less advanced forms may be a moderate tendency to edema, slight cyanosis, and rather prominent varicosities. Here one must be careful to distinguish between the edema attributable to varicosities and that associated with involvement of the deep veins of the leg.

Superficial Thrombophlebitis

Thrombophlebitis may occur in a superficial vein anywhere in the arm or leg, although it is more common in the leg. It is manifested by pain, redness, and induration in the involved segment of vein and in the adjacent skin and subcutaneous tissue. The local reaction around a superficial thrombophlebitis may be so severe that it suggests an acute cellulitis.

Thrombophlebitis in a superficial vein which is already varicose is accompanied by less inflammation. It is also less apt to be associated with a deep thrombophlebitis. The thrombosed vein stands out as a solid cord with a small zone of redness and induration around it. At times there may be no reaction adjacent to the vein, but one will detect a thickened, irregular, tender cord extending along the course of the vein. Fluctuation and abscess formation may occur if secondary infection develops.

Embolism rarely occurs from a superficial thrombophlebitis unless the process is propagating along the upper end of the great saphenous vein. *In this instance sapheno-femoral interruption is indicated to prevent extension of the process into the deep venous system.*

Do not overlook a deep thrombophlebitis associated with a superficial thrombotic process.

Phlebitis Migrans

This is a form of recurring thrombophlebitis. It may be seen in superficial veins on any limb in the body. As one area subsides, a fresh area appears at a higher level or in a different vein. Migrating phlebitis is an early manifestation of thromboangiitis obliterans. It is seen in patients with carcinomatosis, especially from cancer of the pancreas. In such instances the deep as well as the superficial veins may be involved.

Phlebosclerosis

This is probably the end result of small areas of thrombosis. It is most commonly seen as small calcified nodules on an x-ray film of the pelvis and may also be found in the leg as tiny, hard nodules along the course of a superficial vein. The only significant clinical symptoms are the presence of the nodules.

Thrombosis of the Axillary Vein

Straining with the arm elevated may produce an acute thrombosis of the axillary vein. There is marked swelling of the arm and venous congestion about the shoulder. Cyanosis is more pronounced than in thrombosis of the veins of the lower extremity, since there is a less abundant collateral flow. *Although embolism is rare with axillary vein thrombosis recurrences are frequent.*

Effort Thrombosis of the Deep Veins of the Leg

Thrombophlebitis of the deep veins of the leg is so commonly associated with factors which produce stasis in the vein that the term "thrombophlebitis decubiti" has been assigned to it. It is important to recognize, therefore, that this process may occur as a consequence of vigorous athletic activity. It often simulates a muscle strain or partial rupture of the gastrocnemius muscle. The differential diagnosis is of great importance since pulmonary embolism frequently follows effort thrombosis of the deep veins of the leg. The two conditions may be present simultaneously.

Indications of a thrombophlebitis may be detected with careful scrutiny; these include a slight cyanosis in the dependent position, a dilatation of superficial veins, a positive dorsiflexion sign, and tenderness in the calf. Lateral compression of the muscle bundle as compared with anteroposterior compression is particularly helpful. Some hours of observation may be required to distinguish between the two conditions if the patient is seen early after an apparent strain.

III. DISORDERS OF LYMPHATICS

Acute Lymphangitis

There is pain in the affected extremity and usually fever and general malaise.

Examination discloses a fine red line or series of lines extending up the arm or leg. Often this can be felt as a slightly elevated tubular swelling. There may be evident cellulitis and edema around the original focus of infection but very often the portal of entry is hard to find. The interdigital spaces of the feet should be carefully scrutinized because the cracks of chronic epidermophytosis are often the primary site of invasion. There may be remarkably little evidence of local reaction in the presence of a fulminating lymphangitis.

Lymphedema

Several types of chronic lymphedema may be recognized: 1. *Primary:* Congenital and lymphedema praecox. 2. *Secondary:* which is caused by obstruction to the normal lymphatics.

Primary lymphedema. *Congenital lymphedema* is manifest at birth and is often associated with other congenital abnormalities. There may be gross distortion of arms and legs. The underlying cause is a severe hypoplasia or aplasia of the lymphatic system.

There are certain types of hereditary or familial lymphedemas such as "Milroy's disease." An inborn error in the development of lymphatics appears to be associated with these forms of congenital and familial edema. Lymphangiograms usually show atrophy and maldevelopment of the lymphatic channels.

Lymphedema praecox is the classic form of primary lymphedema.

The syndrome characteristically affects a young girl or a woman in her early twenties. It is manifested by the gradual development of a spontaneous edema of one or both extremities. The patient usually relates the edema to some specific episode, such as an operation or an injury, but it is doubtful that there is any direct relationship.

Examination shows a comparatively normal skin with diffuse swelling of the ankle and lower leg. In the later stages the skin loses its hair and may become thickened. Gradually, the entire limb and thigh become swollen and constitute a considerable burden to the patient.

Lymphangiograms may show extensive varicosities of the lymphatics (Fig. 11–12), or marked hypoplasia.

LYMPHATIC COMPLICATIONS. Patients with various abnormalities of lymphatics leading to congenital lymphedema or lymphedema praecox may also have other signs of abnormal lymphatic communications. These may be manifested by chylous ascites, chylothorax, chyluria, or chylous reflux into the lower limb.

Chylous reflux is a rare but particularly interesting variant of lymphedema praecox. There are communications between the lymphatics of the limb and the intestinal tract so that after eating, chyle appears in the subcutaneous lymphatics of the thigh (Fig. 11–13 *A* and *B*). In all cases of dilated incompetent lymphatics, including chylous reflux, operative inter-

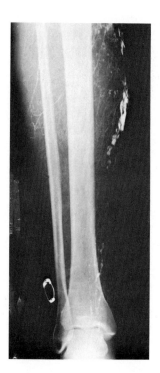

Figure 11–12. A lymphangiogram showing varicosities of the lymphatics in a case of lymphedema praecox.

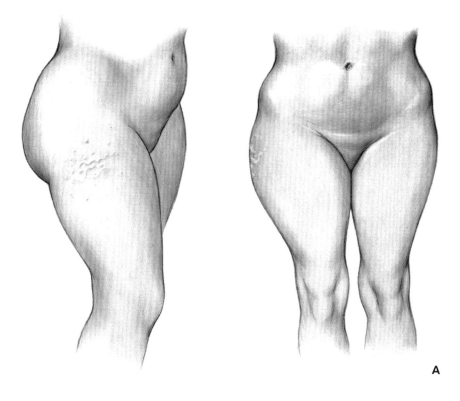

A

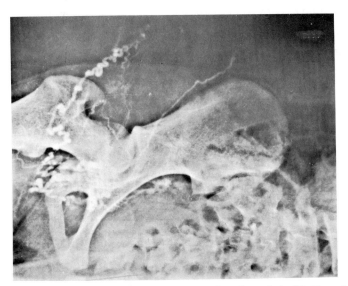

B

Figure 11–13. *A,* A case of chylous reflux. Note the white, chyle-filled lymphatics in the skin of the thigh. *B,* A lymphangiogram in the same case showing extensive dilatation and communications between the thigh and intestinal lymphatics.

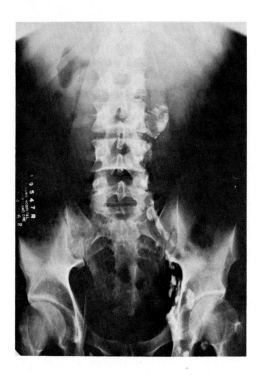

Figure 11–14. Lymphangiogram showing the appearance of lymphoma in retroperitoneal nodes.

vention with division of the lymphatic chains may eliminate or alleviate the edema.

Secondary lymphedema. Lymphedema is encountered in many conditions in which there is a blockage of the normal lymphatics. This occurs following operations on the regional nodes as in radical mastectomy or radical groin dissection. It may follow as a complication of the extension of pelvic cancer into lymphatics. This occurs in advanced cancer of the cervix with or without x-ray therapy.

Lymphangiograms shows signs of obstruction and partial destruction of lymph nodes. Lymphoma produces a characteristic appearance on lymph nodes (Fig. 11–14).

Edema of lymphatic origin is not accompanied by cyanosis, venous enlargement, increased pigmentation, or leathery induration. Edema usually is firm and does not pit well.

Infection may lead to an increased blockage of lymphatics. This is characteristically the case in elephantiasis.

Elephantiasis

This is the end result of extensive lymphatic stasis (Fig. 11–15). It may be a sequel of either the congenital or acquired forms of lymphe-

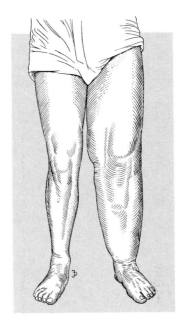

Figure 11–15. Elephantiasis of the left leg.

dema. The edematous extremity is susceptible to recurrent infection and episodes of cellulitis often lead to chronic thickening of the skin. Recurrent attacks of nonsuppurative infection lead to extensive fibrosis of the edematous tissues (Fig. 11–15).

chapter 12 # ULCER AND GANGRENE OF THE EXTREMITIES

The nature of an ulcer or an area of gangrene can be clarified in most instances by physical examination, particularly if the problem is analyzed in an orderly and systematic fashion. The following definitions are pertinent: The term *necrosis* implies the death of tissue; this may be localized or extensive. An *ulcer* is the result of a localized area of necrosis in the skin or mucous membrane. The term *gangrene* is applied to an area of necrosis involving a part of the body such as the finger or leg.

I. THE APPRAISAL OF AN ULCER

In many instances the history renders the etiology of an ulcer obvious, as in a burn or following exposure to x-ray or chemical irritants. At times careful questioning is required to bring out the fact that the patient has been exposed to agents such as carbolic acid, and it must be remembered that radiation ulcers may not develop for years following exposure. Frequently the cause of an ulcer is not evident although the patient may attribute it to inconsequential injuries. In such circumstances the following potential etiologic factors must be considered: circulatory? neoplastic? infectious? neuropathic? radiation? or traumatic?

The physical characteristics of the ulcer provide many clues, particularly its shape, location, the character of the tissues in the base, the edges, the exudate, if any, and the state of the surrounding tissues. Ulcers associated with deficient circulation are, with the exception of those occasioned by Raynaud's disease or Buerger's disease, almost invariably on the lower extremities. Neoplastic ulcerations appear on the exposed surfaces of the body and at sites of chronic irritation. An ulceration in the sinus tracts of chronic osteomyelitis should immediately arouse a suspicion of carcinoma. Malignant melanoma is frequently mistaken for a chronic nonspecific ulceration of the sole of the foot.

A perfectly round ulcer suggests that it is associated with trophic disturbances (Fig. 12–1). *Neuropathic ulcers* commonly appear upon the ball of the foot or the pulp of the fingers. They are usually of very gradual development. Examination will show a loss of sensitivity in the tissues surrounding the ulcer. Peripheral nerve injuries, spina bifida, or diabetic neuritis are common primary causes. An *irregular serpiginous ulcer* is likely to be due to infection. *Tertiary syphilis* is said to produce a punched-out ulcer, whereas deeply overhanging edges in an ulcer suggest *tuberculosis* or a low grade spreading infection often associated with a *microaerophilic hemolytic streptococcus.*

A *decubital ulcer* appears over areas of pressure such as the heel or sacrum in bedridden debilitated patients. In black persons a chronic punched-out ulcer of the leg suggests the possibility of *sickle cell anemia.*

A *varicose ulcer* is found on the inner side of the lower third of the leg along the course of the great saphenous vein. It may be small and clean or large, ragged, and dirty with slough and exudate. The surrounding skin is pigmented and atrophic, indicating the long-standing vascular congestion which has produced the ulceration. Varicose ulcers, even of long standing, are superficial. They do not have punched-out or overhanging edges. Pain is customary and may be exquisite, especially if the lesion is close to the internal malleolus.

The relationship to a large incompetent superficial vein and the absence of signs of an incompetent deep venous system are important diagnostic features (see Chap. 10).

A *postphlebitic ulcer* is more variable in location than a varicose ulcer. It may appear anywhere on the lower third of the leg. The extent

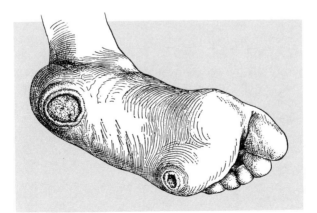

Figure 12–1. Neuropathic ulcers of the foot associated with peripheral nerve injury. (From Homans, J.: Textbook of Surgery. Springfield, Ill., Charles C Thomas, 1945.)

varies from a minute break in the skin to a huge, superficial, weeping sore. Multiple shallow ulcers are common and constitute an important differential point from varicose ulcers, which are always single. Pain is less severe in postphlebitic ulcers. The superficial veins usually are not evident.

Brownish edema and induration spreading far beyond the area of the ulcer are significant diagnostic features. Incompetency of the deep veins of the leg can be demonstrated (see Chap. 11).

Arteriosclerotic ulcerations.   Extensive ischemic ulcerations of the skin of the leg may occur without gangrene of the extremity. Although there is atrophy and wasting of the limb as well as diminished or absent pulses, the adjacent tissues may be warm and so well preserved that it is hard to accept arterial insufficiency as the underlying cause. These ulcers are exquisitely painful.

Two forms occur. Isolated rather deep circular areas of necrosis may result from occlusion of small end arteries, or there may be extensive superficial serpiginous ulceration of the skin of the lateral aspect of the ankle and calf. The foot is often spared. An arteriogram will show obliterative vascular disease.

Confronted with an ulcer the etiology of which is not clear, one should systematically determine the state of the peripheral circulation, both venous and arterial, test the sensation of the tissues in the region of the ulcer, examine microscopically and by bacterial culture the scrapings and exudate from the surface of the ulcer, examine the blood for anemia, test the urine for sugar, perform a Wassermann or Hinton test, and finally, if the etiology remains obscure, perform a biopsy of the lesion. In many instances, of course, the location and character of the ulcer will immediately lead to the performance of a biopsy.

II. GANGRENE

The term *gangrene* implies the death of a part or a region of the body, such as the finger or the foot. Any factor capable of producing necrosis or ulceration may, if sufficiently extensive, result in gangrene. Thus, the topical application of phenol to a wart might produce a local ulcer, whereas immersion of an entire finger in the same solution would produce gangrene. Commonly, however, gangrene occurs as a consequence of deficient blood supply, bacterial infection, or trauma. Frequently, a combination of two or all three of these factors is encountered. The history and physical examination permit an accurate determination of the contributing factors in most cases.

Circulatory Gangrene

Two types of circulatory gangrene occur, dry and wet. In *dry gangrene* the arterial circulation is gradually occluded so that the part in-

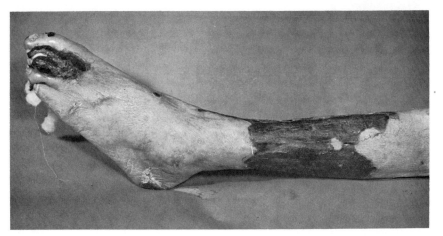

Figure 12–2. Dry gangrene of the foot and leg. A case of progressive arteriosclerosis.

volved becomes anemic first and then slowly mummifies. The end result is a shrunken, withered, black extremity (Fig. 12–2). Unless the surface of the skin is broken, infection is not likely to ensue. The appearance is classic and is the result of slowly progressive arterial obliteration. *Wet gangrene* is the consequence of sudden occlusion of the arterial supply, particularly in a limb in which the circulation has not previously been deficient, as in acute embolism. The area involved becomes mottled and swollen. The skin frequently blisters and constitutes a site of entry for infection (Fig. 12–3). Superimposed infection is common; it may enter through areas of previous epidermophytosis. The characteristics of wet

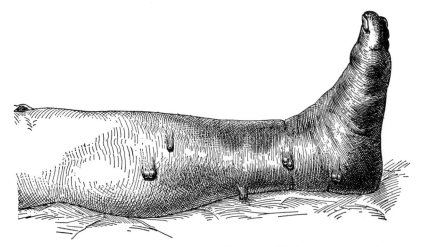

Figure 12–3. Wet gangrene of the leg. This type of lesion may occur after acute embolic occlusion. (From Homans, J.: Textbook of Surgery. Springfield, Ill., Charles C Thomas, 1945.)

gangrene are in part due to infection, since some degree of infection is inevitable. Redness, swelling, and progressive edema ascending from the involved area are indicative of a spreading infection. Crepitation may develop in the necrotic tissues from gas-forming organisms, although these are not primary factors. In diabetic patients circulatory gangrene, whether wet or dry, is apt to be complicated by infection because of the vulnerability of the tissues. Frequently, the septic process becomes the dominant one, producing an area of gangrene and necrosis much greater than would result from impairment of the blood supply alone. Although the process is primarily arteriosclerotic in origin, the term *diabetic gangrene* has been coined to signify the important and often dominant role which infection plays.

Traumatic Gangrene

Traumatic gangrene is the consequence of severe crushing and bruising injuries to an extremity. The term implies that the tissue destruction is caused by direct contusion with local arterial damage rather than by injury to the main vessel to the extremity. Marked arterial spasm or venous occlusion may complicate such injuries. Superimposed infection may lead to loss of the limb, but with proper débridement many limbs which appear hopelessly damaged can be salvaged if infection is prevented. The condition is recognized by the fact that the principal blood supply to the area is intact although in the early stages arterial spasm may render such a conclusion difficult. If major arteries are injured, traumatic gangrene is complicated by ischemic gangrene. Arterial repair or amputation become necessary.

Bacterial Gangrene

This term implies that there is tissue necrosis as a consequence of bacterial action. Although infection is responsible for the course of the disease, there is always some degree of initial ischemic gangrene, which furnishes the necrotic tissue essential for the rapid growth of bacteria.

A common lesion in warfare, bacterial gangrene is so rare in civilian life that its various forms are not always properly distinguished. Failure to do so may lead to the loss of life or the unnecessary sacrifice of a limb.

There are two distinct forms of bacterial gangrene, one associated with the anaerobic clostridial organisms and the other with the streptococcus.

Anaerobic clostridial infections and gangrene. It must be stressed in the first place that the finding of anaerobic spore-bearing organisms including *Clostridium perfringens (Cl. welchii)* in a wound is of no significance unless there are physical signs of bacterial gangrene. The gas-forming organisms may be cultured from many wounds which do not develop gangrene. Secondly, the presence of air in the tissues about a wound, usually manifested by crepitation, is no indication of a clostridial infection. Localized traumatic emphysema around a wound of the chest or neck is fairly common. Lacerated wounds in the region of joints may open and close with motion so as to permit air to enter fascial planes and spread for some little distance around the site of injury. Crepitation alone, therefore, is no cause for alarm, and even if there are signs of local infection in a wound, crepitation does not presuppose the presence of a gas-forming organism.

Infection with the clostridial organisms produces a classic appearance which is seen in several different forms.

DIFFUSE CLOSTRIDIAL MYOSITIS (GAS GANGRENE). This fulminating and very lethal form of bacterial gangrene appears within a few hours or days of injury. It may appear as late as 10 or 12 days following an inadequate débridement or an unrecognized arterial injury, especially if the limb has been encased in a tight-fitting plaster cast.

The onset of gas gangrene is heralded by a sudden change in the condition of the patient. He becomes pale or livid, anxious and restless. There may be severe pain in the limb. The temperature may rise, but often is subnormal. In the early stages the pulse rate and blood pressure may not reflect the gravity of the illness, but later there are tachycardia and hypotension progressing to collapse, with cold cyanotic extremities. The face becomes cyanotic or develops a peculiar bronze tinge due to extensive hemolysis.

The appearance of the involved limb is characteristic. It is tremendously swollen, edematous, and discolored. At first it may be blue or mottled, but later assumes a waxy pale, cadaverous shade. An unmistakable "deadhouse odor" may be detected. This is best appreciated as one approaches the patient's bed or litter. It is often less obvious when one attempts to sniff the wound. A thin serosanguineous discharge frequently is found oozing from the wound. Crepitation of the tissues extending up the entire limb and often onto the trunk is a classic sign of gas in the tissues. However, it may not be detectable and failure to demonstrate it is of no diagnostic significance. An x-ray will demonstrate gas in muscle planes, but such confirmatory evidence is not needed and under no circumstances should therapy be delayed to secure it.

The nature of the initial wound is of great significance. Extensive muscle damage and major arterial injury are fundamental factors. The character of the wound, particularly the compromising of the blood supply, the acute onset of symptoms, the profound toxemia, the extensive swelling of the leg, and rapid progress of the disease make the diagnosis evident, whether or not crepitation is demonstrable in the tissues by palpation. The experienced observer can tell at a glance that the leg is lost. He will know that the patient will be lost too unless an amputation is performed.

EDEMATOUS GANGRENE.   This is a highly fatal variant of gas gangrene produced by *Cl. novyi (oedementiens).* No gas is produced but massive muscle edema occurs without primary vascular injury. The course is fulminant and the only effective therapy is early and extensive débridement.

The diagnosis is often overlooked in its early stages because of the absence of gas and crepitation in the tissues.

LOCALIZED CLOSTRIDIAL MYOSITIS.   This condition must be carefully distinguished from the diffuse variety, since its course and management are entirely different. It should not be designated as "gas gangrene," although it may lead to that state if it is unrecognized and untreated. The late development of diffuse clostridial myositis is usually the result of imprisoning an unrecognized localized myositis in a tightly constricting plaster cast.

Fundamentally the two conditions are quite different. In localized myositis the initial wound is limited in extent, the muscle damage is slight and confined to a few muscles and there is no major arterial injury.

The physical examination reveals the purely local character of the lesion. There may be a thin serosanguineous discharge from the wound. The wound edges are marked by edema, tenderness, and redness bordering on cyanosis. Palpation often reveals crepitation extending for some distance beyond the wound. The systemic reaction varies. At times the patient may not be appreciably disturbed by the infection and at other times there may be tachycardia and high fever, but there is not the profound toxemia of gas gangrene. Most important of all, the physical examination will indicate that the blood supply to the limb is intact. Despite the evident infection and gas in the tissues, the limb distal to the area of infection is warm, and peripheral pulses are normal. The experienced observer sees a viable limb and knows it can be saved by adequate excision of the necrotic, infected muscle bundles. Amputation is never indicated for a localized myositis.

CLOSTRIDIAL CELLULITIS.   Clostridial cellulitis is a spreading anaerobic infection in the subcutaneous tissues. As in other clostridial infections, Welch's bacillus *(Cl. perfringens)* is most commonly encountered. In advanced cases the entire leg becomes edematous, swollen, and pale. The skin may become discolored and necrotic. Crepitation is usually detectable throughout the entire extremity. The extensive swelling of the leg, the edema, the necrosis of the skin, the pallor, and the diffuse crepitation may lead the inexperienced observer to a hasty conclusion that he is dealing with "gas gangrene" in the sense of a diffuse clostridial myositis. Actually the differential diagnosis from clostridial myositis is fairly obvious on physical findings alone.

In contrast to true gas gangrene, clostridial cellulitis is a process which progresses rather slowly. It usually appears 10 days or more after wounding. The initial wounds are not associated with extensive muscle injury although compound fractures are frequently present. The wounds themselves tend to be superficial. Most important of all, there is no major blood vessel injury. Despite the diffuse swelling and rather frightening appearance of the limb, examination will demonstrate that there is excellent circulation to the extremity. The systemic reaction of the patient to clostridial cellulitis may be fairly severe, but it does not approach the profound toxemia of gas gangrene. The patients usually have been chronically ill since they were wounded. A secondary anemia is common, and the general appearance of the patient is one of chronic, fairly severe sepsis rather than one of an acute toxemia.

The diagnosis of clostridial cellulitis is confirmed at operation, which will reveal that the process is limited entirely to the subcutaneous tissue planes. Following an adequate drainage and excision of totally necrotic tissue, prompt recovery will ensue (Fig. 12–4). Amputation is not indicated for this condition.

In all forms of anaerobic infections hyperbaric oxygen therapy is beneficial but it cannot be substituted for early and extensive débridement of the involved tissues. Oxygen inhibits the formation of clostridia lecthinases but has no effect on toxin. It may inhibit bacteremia but has no

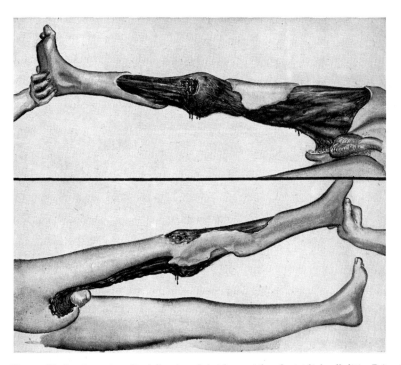

Figure 12–4. An extremity following debridement for clostridial cellulitis. Prior to operation, there was tremendous swelling and edema with diffuse crepitation, but the wounds were superficial and the blood supply to the limb was intact. The end result was similar to an extensive third degree burn.

effect on organisms in necrotic muscle or abscesses. Penicillin in massive doses prevents growth of other organisms and is always indicated.

Streptococcal infections and gangrene. Subcutaneous necrosis and gangrene in association with streptococcal infections have been recognized for many years. The term *necrotizing erysipelas* has been applied to this lesion. The antibiotics have made it exceedingly rare. It may be associated with streptococcal infection secondary to local ulcerations of epidermophytosis. The essential feature of the disease is a spreading cellulitis in the fascial planes rather than in the skin itself. Prostration may be severe. The skin of the involved extremity assumes a dusky hue and eventually blisters and becomes necrotic.

Adequate drainage, particularly of fascial planes, is necessary. The disease is disappearing because of the liberal use of antibiotics in the treatment of wounds and localized infections, especially when the presence of streptococci is suspected.

Mycetoma (Madura foot). This rare fungal lesion should be considered whenever one encounters a painless, slowly progressive destructive lesion of the foot. The disease begins following trauma of mild degree such as stepping on a thorn. Apparently not only the specific fungus, *Madurella mycetomi,* may be involved but the lesion may be induced by other fungi such as a variety of actinomyces.

The lesion begins as a painless swelling with an area of deeper induration beneath it. The course is inexorable with progressive destruction of tissues and bone, swelling of the part, and the appearance of small ulcerations and sinuses. Pain is minimal so that in many instances patients have continued weight-bearing despite partial or complete destruction of the foot.

Surgical excision is curative because the process is a purely local one. Although rare, mycetoma is encountered occasionally in the United States, especially among farm workers who have worked without footwear.

chapter 13 # EXAMINATION OF THE FEMALE EXTERNAL GENITALIA AND PELVIS

I. CONDUCT OF THE EXAMINATION

The pelvic and rectal examination are the final parts of the complete physical examination, for the convenience of the patient, the nurse, and the examiner. A nurse should be in attendance to assist the examiner and act as chaperone. The patient is given an opportunity to empty her bladder and disrobe; she is draped and placed in position on a suitable examining table equipped with stirrups.

Position

The lithotomy position is preferable for pelvic examination (Fig. 13–1 *A*). The Sims or lateral prone position (Fig. 13–1 *B*) is not generally used because it is not as satisfactory for bimanual palpation. It is useful for rectal examination or in the occasional patient who cannot assume the lithotomy position because of disease of the hips or knees. The knee-chest position (Fig. 13–1 *C*) is excellent for complete inspection of the vaginal walls, since the vaginal rugae are smoothed out when air is introduced into the vagina in this position; it is more adaptable for proctosigmoidoscopy in both sexes.

The examiner is seated on a stool facing the patient's perineum with an instrument table within easy reach. This table is equipped with rubber gloves, surgical lubricant, glass slides, aspirating tubes, fixative for cytology smears, long pickup forceps, uterine probes, biopsy forceps, aqueous

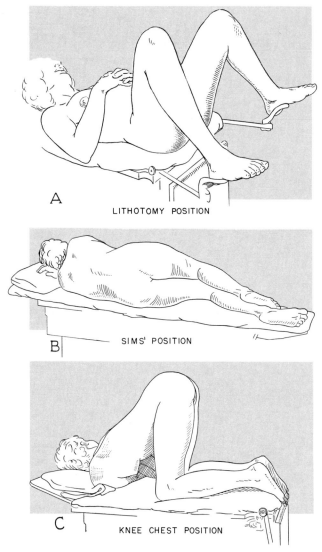

A
LITHOTOMY POSITION

B
SIMS' POSITION

C
KNEE CHEST POSITION

Figure 13–1. Positions for rectal or pelvic examination. The customary drapes have been omitted to show the position of the patient.

iodine solution, culture tubes, cotton swabs, and assorted sizes of vaginal speculums. The perineum is brightly illuminated either by a lamp placed behind the examiner or by one of several types of head lights which are available. An ordinary flashlight provides excellent illumination for the whole procedure, but has the disadvantage of immobilizing one of the examiner's hands. It is important that both the patient and the examiner be comfortable, and that the examination be gently performed. The examiner wears a rubber glove on the hand used for the digital examination (usually the left hand).

Cytology Smear

The cytology smear (Papanicolaou) can be made by aspirating the vaginal contents or obtaining scrapings directly from the cervix (Fig. 13–2). The material obtained should be smeared on a glass slide and the slide immediately placed in the fixative solution.

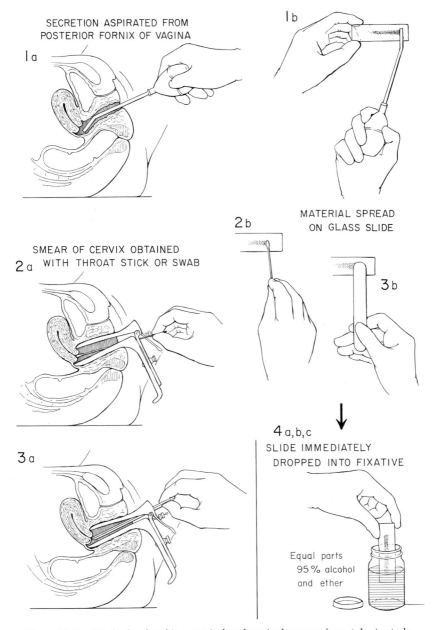

I a SECRETION ASPIRATED FROM POSTERIOR FORNIX OF VAGINA

I b

MATERIAL SPREAD ON GLASS SLIDE

2 b

3 b

2 a SMEAR OF CERVIX OBTAINED WITH THROAT STICK OR SWAB

3 a

4 a,b,c SLIDE IMMEDIATELY DROPPED INTO FIXATIVE

Equal parts 95% alcohol and ether

Figure 13–2. Methods of making cervical and vaginal smears for cytologic study.

Inspection

Inspection of the external genitalia is made, and their configuration and development are noted (Fig. 13–3). Unilateral elongation of the labia minora may be the result of self-manipulation. The skin of the vulva is searched for ulceration, tumor, condylomata, irritation, discoloration, sclerotic whitish areas (leukoplakia), and furunculosis. The perineum and anal region are inspected for scars, sinus openings, and hemorrhoids. In the lithotomy position a pilonidal sinus cannot be seen. The labia are next separated by the thumb and forefinger of the gloved hand, and the vestibule is inspected (Fig. 13–4). The size and shape of the clitoris are noted. The presence or absence of discharge from the urethral orifice and the size, color, and configuration of that orifice are determined. A urethral caruncle appears as a pouting, cherry red, smooth lump at the urinary meatus. The vaginal outlet (introitus) is inspected for discharge which, if present, may be bloody (menstruation, cancer, cervical polyp, cervical erosion, miscarriage, or benign tumor), clear mucoid, whitish, or purulent

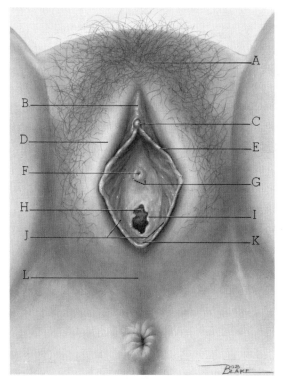

Figure 13–3. The external genitalia. *A,* Mons pubis. *B,* Prepuce. *C,* Clitoris. *D,* Labia majora. *E,* Labia minora. *F,* Urethral meatus. *G,* Skene's ducts. *H,* Vagina. *I,* Hymen. *J,* Bartholin glands. *K,* Posterior fourchette. *L,* Perineal body. (From Sabiston, D.: Textbook of Surgery. Philadelphia, W. B. Saunders Co., 1972.)

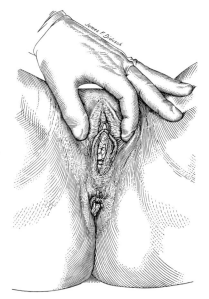

Figure 13–4. Inspection of vaginal vestibule.

(vaginitis, cervicitis, or endometritis). Slight cyanosis or "blueing" of the introitus may be seen in early pregnancy.

The hymen is inspected and may be described as virginal or marital. The virginal hymen has a small, sharp-edged opening which may be relaxed enough to admit one finger, but which usually prevents the introduction of more than the finger tip. In rare instances the hymen is imperforate, and the menstrual blood accumulates in the vagina (hematocolpos).

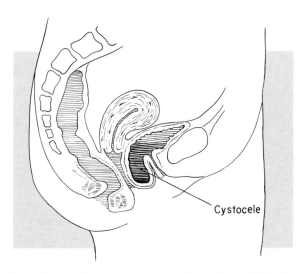

Figure 13–5. Diagram showing a cystocele in sagittal section.

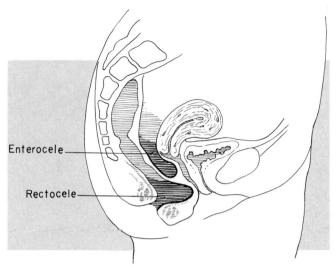

Figure 13–6. Diagram showing a rectocele and enterocele in sagittal section.

Enterocele

Rectocele

Palpation

The digital examination of the introitus and vagina is made next. The strength of the vaginal structures is ascertained by asking the patient to "bear down" to increase intra-abdominal pressure. A cystocele or rectocele will usually become apparent, as will a uterine prolapse (Figs. 13–5 and 13–6). The patient is now asked to cough; this effort may demonstrate

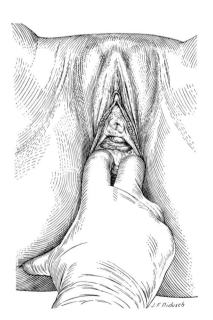

Figure 13–7. Method of testing for perineal relaxation.

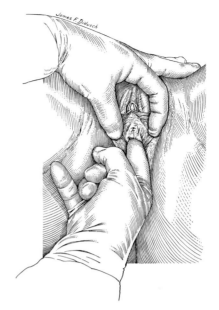

Figure 13–8. Method of expressing exudate from Skene's glands.

urinary incontinence. The strength of the perineum can be further tested by pressure against the levator muscles (Fig. 13–7). Normal Skene's and Bartholin's glands are not palpable, but if diseased, are examined as follows: Skene's glands lie just within the urethral orifice laterally and posteriorly. Compression of the floor and sides of the urethra may "milk out" purulent material (Fig. 13–8); the orifices of the glands are exposed by gently spreading the urinary meatus. The normal Bartholin's gland is not palpable. A Bartholin cyst or an abscess is palpated between the

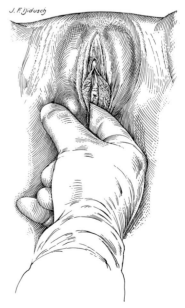

Figure 13–9. Method of palpating a Bartholin's cyst. Note the globular swelling between the finger and thumb.

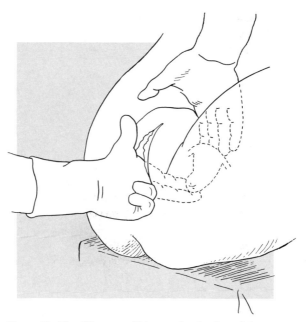

Figure 13–10. Diagram of bimanual palpation of the uterus.

thumb on the vulva and the index finger in the introitus. The finger should be placed just above the levator ani muscle in the posterolateral quadrant. Bartholin's gland may become infected and form a large painful abscess or cyst which gives a globular, swollen appearance to the vulva on the involved side (Fig. 13–9).

Bimanual palpation of the pelvis is next made by introducing the lubricated forefinger and midfinger of the gloved hand into the vagina; in many instances only the forefinger can be inserted. The vaginal walls and cervix are then felt. The position, consistency, mobility, sensitivity, size, contour, and presence or absence of lacerations of the cervix are noted. A softening of the cervix occurs in pregnancy. The normal cervix points toward the posterior vaginal wall, making approximately a 45 degree angle with the vagina.

The body of the uterus is now outlined by pushing the cervix with the corpus uteri upward with the vaginal fingers, while the four fingers of the abdominal hand, palpating suprapubically, feel for the fundus of the uterus (Fig. 13–10). The size, shape, mobility, consistency, sensitivity, and position of the uterus are noted. Normally the uterus is freely movable, firm, and insensitive. If it is soft and symmetrically enlarged, pregnancy is suspected. If the mobility is lessened and it is painful, inflammation and resultant adhesions are suspected. A large movable nodular uterus is characteristic of fibroids (Fig. 13–11), while an enlarged uterus is suggestive of carcinoma of the uterus or pregnancy.

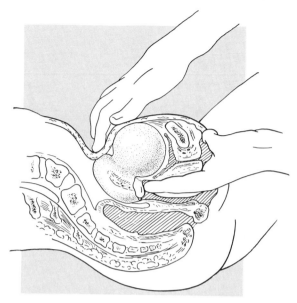

Figure 13–11. Bimanual palpation of a leiomyoma of the uterus. The mass involves the anterior uterine wall and is being felt with the vaginal fingers above the cervix.

Positions of the Uterus

The uterus may be anterior or posterior, and if it is turned back on its horizontal axis it is said to be in retroversion (Fig. 13–12). If the long axis of the uterus in relation to the axis of the vagina is more than a right angle, it is in first-degree retroversion. If the long axis of the uterus corresponds to that of the vagina, it is in second-degree retroversion. Any position posterior to that is called third-degree retroversion. The fundus is best palpated by rectum when the uterus is in third-degree retroversion.

Combined rectovaginal bimanual examination is performed for suspected retroversion or masses in the pouch of Douglas (Fig. 13–13). The middle finger is inserted into the rectum and the index finger into the vagina. The vaginal finger orients the rectal finger, and any posterior mass can be felt since only the rectal wall and thin floor of the cul-de-sac separate the palpating fingers. This combined examination also may be done by inserting the thumb into the vagina and the index finger into the rectum; it is particularly useful for palpation of the rectovaginal septum, the examiner's index finger is in the rectum and the thumb is in the vagina. This is best done with the patient in the standing position. This method forces air, fluid, or intestine into the hernia which can be easily compressed between the fingers, indicating that the lesion is not a rectocele but a hernia in the rectovaginal septum.

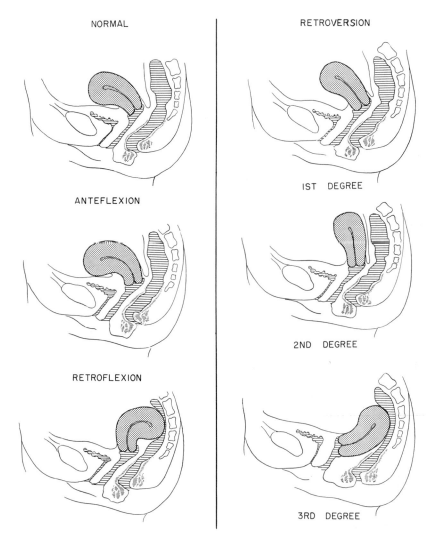

NORMAL

RETROVERSION

IST DEGREE

ANTEFLEXION

2ND DEGREE

RETROFLEXION

3RD DEGREE

Figure 13–12. Diagram of the positions of the uterus in sagittal section.

Palpation of the Adnexa

After the characteristics of the uterus have been determined, the vaginal fingers are slid into one of the fornices, lateral to the cervix. The abdominal hand is now used chiefly to push the adnexa into the pelvis for the vaginal fingers to feel. The ovary is the most sensitive structure in the normal pelvis. It feels like a large almond and is about 4 centimeters long and 2 or 3 centimeters wide. It is firm, solid, and moves freely. If the ovary is located, its size, sensitivity, shape, consistency, mobility, and position are noted. More often than not, normal ovaries cannot be clearly

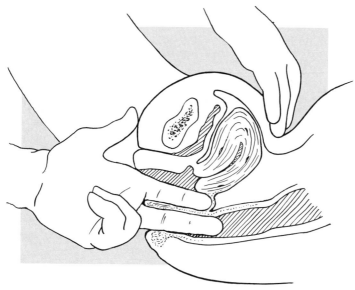

Figure 13–13. Diagram of bimanual rectovaginal examination. This technique provides a more adequate palpation of the pelvic viscera than can be accomplished by the vaginal examination alone.

palpated, but if they are enlarged or a mass is present in the vault, its characteristics and its relation to the uterus, rectum, and pouch of Douglas are noted. Both sides of the pelvis are examined and compared in this fashion. The normal fallopian tubes are not palpable, so that any mass or thicken-

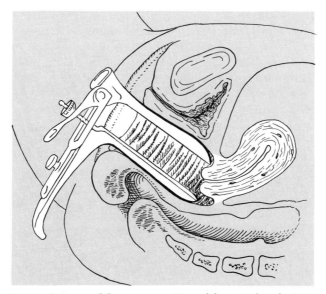

Figure 13–14. Diagram of the proper position of the speculum for inspection of the cervix uteri.

ing in the region of the adnexa is considered evidence of disease until proved otherwise.

The parametrium, which includes the structures immediately lateral to the cervix, is palpated last. It is normally soft, pliable, and insensitive. The chief causes of parametrial induration and thickening are carcinoma of the cervix and puerperal infection.

Speculum examination of the vagina and cervix uteri is now made by introducing a suitably sized, well lubricated, warm bivalve speculum into the vagina. The speculum need not be sterile and can be warmed under tap water. Its blades are closed, and the outer surfaces are lubricated; the instrument is held in the right hand while the left hand separates the labia. The speculum is then introduced into the full length of the vagina, using pressure against the posterior vaginal wall at a 45 degree angle to conform with its normal axis. The blades are then opened and the cervix is exposed (Fig. 13–14).

Inspection of the Vagina

The vagina is inspected for any inflammation or discharge (leukorrhea). The amount, color, and character of the discharge are noted. A smear and culture should be made if indicated. A vaginal discharge which is granular, white, and mucoid is apt to be normal. A frothy, purulent, greenish exudate suggests *Trichomonas vaginalis*. Brownish discharge often originates from the endometrium, while discharge containing unchanged blood is probably from the cervix. A fluid purulent discharge is found in any type of infection of the genital tract. Vaginal fluid normally is acid, while in vaginitis the reaction is usually alkaline. Any discharge which contains blood, except during menstruation, is at once suggestive of carcinoma of the cervix or body of the uterus.

The vagina and cervix are inspected for laceration, polyps, condylomata, ulceration, erosion, senile atresia, tumors, and areas of infection. The size and condition of the cervix are noted, as well as the size of the cervical os. The presence of nabothian glands gives the cervix a nodular appearance. These cysts are a pale, yellowish gray color.

Schiller's test for lesions of the cervix is based on the presence of glycogen in the normal vaginal and cervical mucosa. Pathologic epithelium is often deficient in glycogen or contains none. When a weak aqueous iodine solution (Iodine 2, Pot. Iodide 4, Water q.s. ad 300) is applied to the cervix, the normal epithelium stains a deep mahogany brown while any deficient or diseased area remains unstained. This test is not specific for any type of malignancy, but it is of definite value in selecting suspicious areas for biopsy. Direct smears for cytologic study may be taken from the exposed cervix by scraping the area with a throat stick or other instrument and then making a smear.

II. THE RECTAL EXAMINATION

The rectal examination should now be made by inserting the forefinger into the rectum, after the rubber glove has been changed or washed. A bimanual examination similar to the vaginal examination should be made for confirmation; in children and virgins it is the only way the examination can be done. The tone of the rectal sphincter is noted, as is the presence or absence of hemorrhoids. The presence of masses in the pouch of Douglas should be determined. Confirmation of the strength of the posterior vaginal wall is obtained by pulling gently but firmly with the finger hooked against the anterior rectal wall. A rectocele will become apparent at once. In the physical examination of the pelvis it must be remembered that tumors from elsewhere in the abdomen may metastasize there and that pelvic abscess is a common complication of abdominal sepsis. If there is a question concerning a pelvic mass, it is wise to catheterize the patient to determine whether the mass persists.

III. COMMON GYNECOLOGIC FINDINGS

A summary of the physical findings of some important and common gynecologic conditions follows:

Kraurosis vulvae. A progressive atrophy of the vulva may occur in postmenopausal women. The labia are flat, and the skin is thin and white; it may be reddened or may have a spotted appearance. The vaginal orifice may be stenotic; pruritis is commonly present.

Leukoplakia vulvae. There are milky white, filmy plaques irregularly scattered over the clitoris and labia minora and on the perineum. Kraurosis is often associated with leukoplakia. Pruritis may be extremely severe.

Condylomata acuminata. These so-called venereal warts are not caused by venereal disease. They appear as raised papillary growths with a wide base and may be quite extensive. If the lesions become ulcerated or infected, a darkfield examination may be necessary to rule out syphilis. A *chancre* appears as a firm oval ulcer. Multiple chancres may occur if the site of the original lesions is on the labia where the folds come in contact with each other. *Secondary lesions of syphilis* occur as mucous patches or low broad warts. Gonorrhea does not ordinarily involve the vulva except for Bartholin's and Skene's glands.

Chancroid or soft chancre with bubo (inguinal lymph node involvement) occurs as a granular ulcer but lacks the firmness which is associated with syphilitic chancre. Ducrey's skin test is specific.

Granuloma inguinale (granuloma venereum). Granuloma inguinale initially appears as a small papule which ulcerates, spreads, and may eventually involve the entire vulva and perineum. The disease is almost exclusively limited to Negroes. The finding of the characteristic Donovan bodies in scrapings from the ulcer confirms the diagnosis.

Lymphogranuloma venereum (lymphogranuloma inguinale). Lymphogranuloma venereum starts as a shallow spreading ulcer. The disease is frequently carried by the lymphatics to the rectum and groin. Extensive scarring with dense strictures develops in late stages of the disease. The Frei test is diagnostic.

Carcinoma of the vulva. This occurs chiefly in postmenopausal women. It may originate in an area of leukoplakia. The tumor grows slowly from a small roughened area or papule into a bulky ulcerated lesion.

Melanocarcinomata may arise from pigmented moles of the vulva; they are rapidly progressive tumors.

Chronic cervicitis. There are wide variations in extent and appearance. The universal symptom is leukorrhea. The cervix is often distorted by hypertrophy and old lacerations from childbirth. As a rule, the lacerations are situated laterally; they are visible and palpable. The entire vaginal portion of the cervix may be red and granular. Schiller's test (see p. 278) is an excellent means of determining the extent of the disease. Eversion and erosion of the cervical mucosa are commonly present. Biopsy is the only method by which the presence or absence of carcinoma can be established.

Leukoplakia of the cervix. Leukoplakia of the cervix is usually seen without difficulty as a pearl gray area against the pink cervical mucosa. Schiller's test will intensify the contrast.

Cervical polyp. A cervical polyp is a common cause of intermenstrual bleeding. It is a soft, movable, pedunculated mass which may be attached to the portio vaginalis or to the cervical canal. Polyps which present themselves at the external os may have their origin in the uterine cavity. Malignancy in a cervical polyp is rare.

Carcinoma of the cervix. Carcinoma of the cervix is one of the most common malignant tumors of the female. The clinical features and extent of the disease are so important to prognosis and therapy that they constitute the basis for classification of all cases at the time of the first examination (Fig. 13–15).

The earliest lesion is *carcinoma in situ*. There are no distinguishing clinical features between this early stage and the chronically inflamed or irritated cervix. Early malignancy can only be distinguished from chronic cervicitis or erosions by biopsy. The cytology of a cervical smear (Papanicolaou) is valuable in arousing suspicion of these early lesions.

As the lesion progresses, it may produce a bulky external cauliflower mass which bleeds easily or it may invade deeply into the cervix with little or no superficial spread. Later the entire cervix and vagina become involved.

When the diagnosis of carcinoma of the cervix is made, the extent of its growth must be determined by physical examination. *Speculum exami-*

STAGE 0	CARCINOMA IN SITU – ALSO KNOWN AS PREINVASIVE CARCINOMA AND INTRA-EPITHELIAL CARCINOMA
STAGE I	THE CARCINOMA IS STRICTLY CONFINED TO THE CERVIX UTERI
STAGE II	THE CARCINOMA EXTENDS BEYOND THE CERVIX UTERI BUT HAS NOT REACHED THE PELVIC WALL, OR THE CARCINOMA INVOLVES THE VAGINA BUT NOT THE LOWER THIRD
STAGE III	THE CARCINOMA HAS REACHED THE PELVIC WALL (ON RECTAL EXAMINATION NO "CANCER FREE" SPACE IS FOUND BETWEEN THE TUMOR AND THE PELVIC WALL); OR THE CARCINOMA INVOLVES THE LOWER THIRD OF THE VAGINA
STAGE IV	THE CARCINOMA INVOLVES THE BLADDER OR THE RECTUM, OR BOTH; OR HAS EXTENDED BEYOND THE LIMITS PRE-VIOUSLY DESCRIBED

Figure 13–15. International classification of carcinoma of the cervix uteri.

nation shows whether the tumor has reached the vagina and how deeply the portio vaginalis of the cervix has been invaded. *Bimanual palpation* determines the mobility of the cervix and the relation of the bladder to the tumor. The presence of any thickening of the tissues surrounding the cervix is determined. *Rectal examination* is performed to search for a tumor involving the rectum, the broad ligaments, and the pouch of Douglas. It is also effective in detecting parametrial involvement. Unfortunately, carcinoma of the cervix is quite often more extensive than is evident from palpation.

Normal pregnancy. The pregnant uterus is the most common "abdominal tumor" in the female of childbearing age. The pregnant uterus is symmetrically enlarged and has a doughy, elastic consistency. The cervix may be softened (Hegar's sign). There may be "blueing" of the introitus (Chadwick's sign). Amenorrhea may be a warning sign, but a regular menstrual flow may continue during pregnancy. If the pregnancy is advanced, movements of the fetus and fetal heart sounds may be detected. The fetal bones become opaque to the x-ray at about the fifth month of pregnancy. An Aschheim-Zondek test is indicated in doubtful cases.

Leiomyoma of the uterus (fibroids). These are benign tumors. They occur more frequently in the black than in the white race. The characteristic physical finding is an insensitive enlarged uterus which is hard, nodular and movable (Fig. 13–11). The nodules may be quite small or so big that they fill the pelvis. A large, degenerated, soft myoma may feel like a pregnant uterus or an ovarian cyst. Pedunculated myomas may simulate an ovarian cyst because of their extreme mobility. On the other hand, lesions of the adnexa which have attached themselves to the uterus may feel like solid fibroids.

Carcinoma of the endometrium. This diagnosis can only be made by microscopic examination of the endometrium. In advanced stages of the disease the uterus is enlarged but there are no characteristic physical findings. Daily intermenstrual bleeding and postmenopausal bleeding are important, but they are not necessarily early symptoms of the disease. The cytology smear may be valuable, but a smear which shows no tumor cells does not rule out the disease.

Tumors of the ovary. Attempts at classification of the many types of ovarian tumors and cysts have been the despair of many clinicians. No such attempt is made in this text, but the physical characteristics will be described.

LARGE OVARIAN TUMORS. Large ovarian tumors are usually cysts. The abdomen is large, round, and more prominent in the para-umbilical region than in the flanks. A soft cystic mass may be outlined; it must be differentiated from ascites. Percussion of the abdomen and the "ruler test" (see Chap. 7, Fig. 7–9) are of value. The mass may be palpable upon bimanual pelvic examination, or it may have risen out of the pelvis; it may even have pulled the uterus up so that the cervix cannot be felt. Normal pregnancy, obesity, large fibroids, free fluid, and distended urinary bladder may be confused with large ovarian cysts by physical examination.

SMALL OVARIAN TUMORS. Bimanual pelvic examination discloses a pelvic mass which may or may not be freely movable. A pedunculated fibroid, an intestinal tumor, an ectopic kidney, a parovarian cyst or tubal masses are difficult to eliminate upon physical examination. *Bilateral, firm, freely movable pelvic masses* are likely to be dermoids. *A solid, hard, mobile pelvic tumor* associated with a pleural effusion is apt to be a fibroma. *Bilateral tumors* fixed to the pelvis may be endometrial cysts. If precocious sexual development or sexual rejuvenation beyond the menopause is associated with an ovarian tumor, it may be a *granulosa cell tumor.* If masculinization is associated with an ovarian tumor, it may be an *arrhenoblastoma.* Bilateral solid tumors of the ovaries may occur secondary to carcinoma of the breast, stomach, or intestinal tract *(Kruken-*

berg tumor). Torsion of the pedicle of an ovarian tumor may produce the picture of an acute surgical abdomen. The palpation of an ovarian tumor mass is the characteristic feature in addition to the signs of abdominal tenderness. Examination under anesthesia may be required to outline the pelvic mass.

Ruptured tubal pregnancy. Ruptured tubal pregnancy is featured by amenorrhea or delayed menstruation followed by severe lower abdominal pain and a feeling of weakness, syncope, nausea, and vomiting. The picture may develop acutely or gradually. Pain is usually marked and may be referred to either shoulder. The signs of hemorrhagic shock may be present. The abdomen is diffusely tender and rebound tenderness is present, but spasm may be absent. Pelvic examination may reveal a soft adnexal mass, but more commonly the pelvis is so sensitive that the mass cannot be felt. Immediate laparotomy is imperative as soon as the diagnosis is made. Rarely a ruptured ectopic pregnancy produces signs of collapse without significant abdominal symptoms. The diagnosis should be considered in all instances of collapse in otherwise healthy young women.

Many tubal pregnancies do not present such a typical picture. Vague, mild abdominal pain without menstrual irregularity or signs of pregnancy may be the only symptom. Tenderness in the vault without a distinct mass may suggest inflammation. Anemia may occur from slow bleeding into the peritoneal cavity without signs of acute blood loss.

Culdocentesis will show blood in the peritoneal cavity. Laparoscopy is often required to establish the diagnosis.

Endometriosis. This may be confined to the uterus (internal endometriosis) or may involve the adnexa, bowel, or peritoneum (external endometriosis). The disease is difficult to diagnose, since the symptoms are not entirely distinctive and the findings on palpation are not always typical. The uterus may be enlarged if it is involved, but the main findings are revealed in the adnexa. The ovaries may be fixed and enlarged. Implants may be felt in the pouch of Douglas. The uterus is frequently retroflexed and partially fixed. These findings plus a history of sterility and progressive dysmenorrhea indicate endometriosis. An abdominal or pelvic mass which appears late in the menstrual cycle and subsides after the flow is highly suggestive. Constipation, distention, and crampy abdominal pain late in the cycle suggest endometrial implantation on the pelvic colon or the rectum. Endometrial implants in the umbilicus or vagina have a bluish nodular appearance, but are uncommon.

Adenomyosis (internal endometriosis). Moderate enlargement of the uterus with tenderness to palpation, especially premenstrually, is suggestive of this condition in women between 30 and 50 years of age with irregular menses.

chapter 14 # EXAMINATION OF THE ANUS AND RECTUM

I. CONDUCT OF THE EXAMINATION

The anus and rectum can be examined with the patient in one of several different positions. The indication for and limitations of each position are described.

Positions

The left lateral prone (Sims' position) (see Chap. 13, Fig. 13–1). This position is ideal for inspection of the perianal skin and the pilonidal region and for palpation of the anal canal and lower rectum. It is also suitable for anoscopy and proctosigmoidoscopy. Since the upper rectum and pelvic structures tend to fall away from the examining finger, pelvic masses or high rectal lesions may be overlooked; it also may be difficult to demonstrate a rectal prolapse.

Lithotomy (see Fig. 13–1). The lithotomy position is generally used in a routine physical examination. It is considered the best position in which to palpate the upper rectum, the pouch of Douglas, the pelvis, and the prostate and seminal vesicles. Prolapse of the rectum and protruding internal hemorrhoids are readily demonstrated, while small fistulous tracts, pruritus ani, and pilonidal sinuses are easily overlooked.

Knee-chest (see Fig. 13–1). The knee-chest position has the advantages of the left lateral prone and is the position of choice for sigmoidoscopy, which can be done to high levels without air insufflation. It is awkward and uncomfortable for the patient unless a special table is available.

Standing. This position is frequently employed for examination and massage of the prostate gland. It does not allow satisfactory palpation of the rectum.

Squatting. If there is a history indicative of rectal prolapse, and the lesion cannot be demonstrated, it can often be brought out in this position. Masses lying in the rectosigmoid, sigmoid, or pelvis may be palpable only in this position.

Anatomy

The elements of anorectal anatomy which are essential to an intelligent appraisal of the physical examination are shown in Figures 14–1 and 14–2. The anal canal is a tubular structure, about 3 centimeters in length, which extends from the skin of the buttocks to the mucosa of the rectum. It is lined by stratified squamous epithelium which merges with the skin at its outer end. The junction is identified by the presence of pigmentation and hair in the skin. The inner end of the canal is lined by transitional epithelium which joins with the columnar epithelium of the rectum at the "pectinate line." The presence of teatlike prolongations of the anal epithelium extending upward onto the longitudinal folds of the rectal mucosa gives a serrated or comblike appearance to the anorectal juncture. The teatlike projections of anal epithelium are the *anal papillae,* which

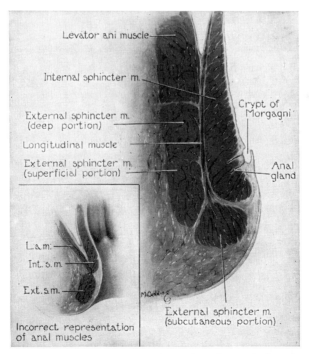

Figure 14–1. Anatomic relationships of the anal canal in sagittal section. Insert illustrates a common misconception. (From Arch. Surg., 57:791–800, December, 1948.)

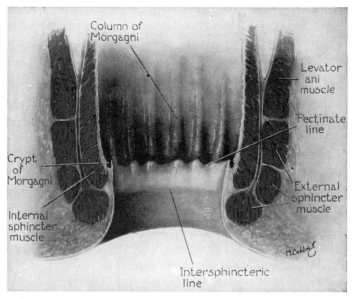

Figure 14–2. Relationship of muscles to anal and rectal mucosa. (From Arch. Surg., 57:791–800, December, 1948.)

are frequently connected by transverse plicae; the anal crypts, or *crypts of Morgagni,* lie behind the plicae.

Hypertrophy of an anal papilla produces a polypoid lesion which is frequently mistaken for an internal hemorrhoid or a rectal polyp. The anal crypts are the site of origin of 95 per cent of all anal fistulae. External hemorrhoids arise distal to the pectinate line and are covered by skin or the squamous epithelium of the anal canal. Internal hemorrhoids arise above the pectinate line and are covered by the moist red columnar epithelium of the rectum (Fig. 14–10).

It is a common mistake to think that the external sphincter lies distal to the internal sphincter. Actually, only a small portion of the external sphincter is distal to the internal sphincter, and the bulk of it embraces the internal sphincter; it is external to it in a lateral rather than a caudal direction (Fig. 14–2). Much of the anal musculature can be identified by palpation, which is a valuable maneuver in tracing the course and direction of a fistulous tract.

A complete examination of the anus and rectum consists of *inspection, palpation, anoscopy,* and *sigmoidoscopy.*

Inspection

The buttocks should be separated. The perianal skin is pigmented and of a coarser texture than the adjacent skin of the buttocks. It is often thrown into irregular shallow folds which radiate outward from the anus to the skin of the buttocks. Normally these folds are easily obliterated when the buttocks are separated; they should be clean and free from detritus or fecal matter. The presence of fecal residue in these folds is indicative of inadequate perianal hygiene or of abnormal thickening of the skin which occurs in the early stages of pruritis ani. Look for the excoriations and abrasions of pruritis ani and the presence of warty excrescences and external hemorrhoidal tabs. The pilonidal area is inspected for dimples, sinuses, or evidence of acute or chronic inflammation. The patient is then asked to strain (as in defecation) and by slight traction on the perianal skin, prolapsing of the rectum or of internal hemorrhoids or polyps may be demonstrated.

Palpation

One should palpate the pilonidal area and the ischiorectal fossae for induration or swellings before examining the anal canal. The presence of an acutely tender fissure is suspected if pain is elicited by gentle pressure against the posterior edge of the anal canal without actually introducing the finger into the canal.

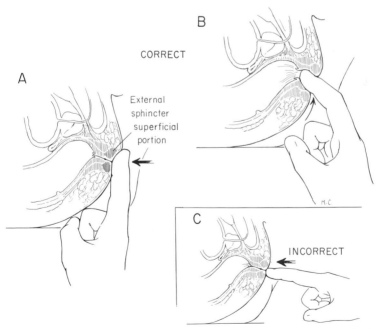

Figure 14–3. *A*, Before introducing the finger into anal canal, the external sphincter should be relaxed by gentle pressure with the palmar surface of the fingertip. *B*, The finger is then inserted into the anal canal. *C*, Incorrect method of anal digital examination.

As the well lubricated finger is introduced into the anal canal, it first meets the normal resistance of the superficial portion of the external sphincter ani. This should be relaxed by gentle pressure with the palmar surface of the finger (Fig. 14–3). Relaxation is aided by asking the patient to strain slightly. If the sphincter does not relax and if further pressure is acutely painful, it indicates the presence of a painful stenosis or acute inflammation of the anal canal. Under these circumstances further attempts at examination will cause unnecessary pain to the patient and will be uninformative to the examiner. It should be postponed until facilities are available to deal properly with the local pathology.

After a little resistance the normal muscle relaxes and the finger can be slipped into the anal canal with a slight rotary motion. The finger should be gently rotated in order to note the smooth lining of the anus before exploring the rectum. The slight depression which marks the boundary between the subcutaneous portion of the external sphincter and the lower edge of the internal sphincter is readily detected. Any palpable irregularities or nodules usually involve the pectinate or anorectal line. The exact nature of these thickenings can best be determined later by anoscopy. One should note the tone of the musculature. In the absence of local lesions marked weakness may be indicative of a neurologic disturbance.

Identification of the anal musculature. The subcutaneous portion of the external sphincter is felt just beneath the skin at the inner aspect of

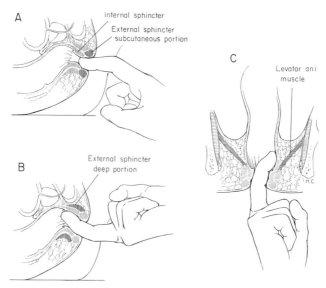

Figure 14–4. Palpation of the anal musculature. *A,* Identification of the subcutaneous external sphincter. *B,* Palpation of the deep external sphincter. *C,* Palpation of the levator ani.

the anal verge. It is a circular or slightly elliptic muscle bundle which can be rolled under the finger throughout the entire circumference of the anal opening (Fig. 14–4 *A*). The intersphincteric line, which is a distinct depression, is located at its upper edge. The lower edge of the internal sphincter is felt above this. When the finger is introduced into the rectum and hooked around the entire sphincter anteriorly, it lies in contact with the anorectal ring, supported only by the deep portion of the external sphincter (Fig. 14–4 *B*). If the finger is kept in contact with this muscle at this exact level and then carried laterally and posteriorly, a distinct thickening will be felt as the levator ani becomes attached to the anal wall. Posteriorly it will be necessary to introduce the finger a little further in order to mark the upper edge of the ring, at which point it will be in contact with the levator ani (Fig. 14–4 *C*).

The finger is then advanced through the sphincter and into direct contact with the wall of the rectum just above the anal canal. It should now be rotated slowly and kept in contact with the rectum while exploring the ampulla systematically in a circular direction. After the entire circumference of the rectum has been palpated, the finger should be advanced and the procedure repeated until all of the rectum within reach of the finger has been explored. Anteriorly the finger comes in contact with the cervix or uterus in the female and the prostate in the male.

The prostate gland and seminal vessels. A careful examination of the prostate gland is an essential part of the rectal examination in the male. One must have a clear conception of the normal surface of the gland in order to recognize abnormalities (Fig. 14–5). The posterior lobes are divided by a *median sulcus* and bounded laterally by the lateral sulci. The junction of the membranous urethra with the prostate may be identified as a soft depression just below the lower end of the median sulcus. Cowper's glands lie on either side of this depression. The seminal vesicles lie just above and to the outer side of the prostatic lobes. Usually these cannot be felt unless they are distended with seminal fluid, in which case one feels a

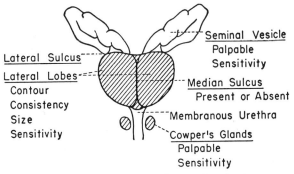

Figure 14–5. A diagram of prostatic palpation.

soft, boggy, nontender, ill-defined swelling above the prostate on each side.

In the routine examination one should (1) identify and palpate the median sulcus; (2) identify and palpate the lateral sulci; (3) feel the surface of each lobe, seeking for nodules or irregularity; (4) test the normal consistency of the gland (it has been compared with that of the slightly flexed biceps muscle); (5) feel for the seminal vesicles; (6) palpate the region of the membranous urethra. The region of Cowper's glands can be felt by palpating between the finger in the rectum and the thumb pressed against the perineum just lateral to the median raphe.

Test for Occult Blood

The examining finger should be inspected for gross evidence of blood or pus after it is withdrawn. A specimen of stool should be smeared on filter paper and tested for occult blood (guaiac test; Fig. 14–6).

Proctosigmoidoscopy

Examination of the rectum and lower sigmoid by means of the sigmoidoscope is an integral part of the rectal examination. Since 75 per cent of all malignant and premalignant lesions of the colon can be seen on sigmoidoscopy (Fig. 14–7), the procedure must never be omitted unless inflammatory or other painful lesions necessitate its postponement. If the physician cannot carry out this procedure, it is his responsibility to make certain it is performed by someone else. The combination of a careful rec-

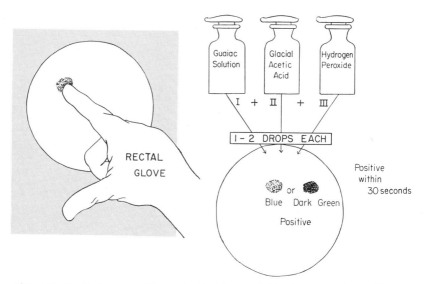

Figure 14–6. Technique of the guaiac test for occult blood in a specimen of feces.

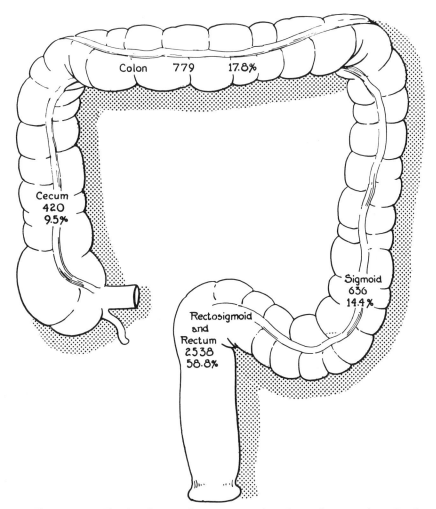

Figure 14–7. The distribution of carcinoma in the colon and rectum. A similar distribution has been demonstrated for benign polyps. About 75 per cent of these lesions are within reach of the sigmoidoscope.

tal examination and a barium enema still leaves a significant area in the lower colon inadequately examined. It should be a rule not to order a barium enema until after proctosigmoidoscopy has been done.

The performance of this examination is simple, but there are certain hazards; it may be painful and dangerous unless gently and skillfully performed. The following precautions must be observed: First, the instrument should never be introduced until a careful rectal examination has indicated that there is no pathologic process, such as a stenosis or tumor, which would prevent satisfactory introduction of the instrument through the sphincter. Second, the instrument should never be advanced blindly, even for short distances. This must always be done under direct vision. Third, severe pain should not be occasioned by the examination; if it is produced, it indicates either inexperience on the part of the examiner or the presence of an inflammatory process, both of which warrant postponement of the examination. Great gentleness is essential. It is rarely necessary to introduce much air during the procedure, and rapid or extensive inflation of the bowel with air is contraindicated. Perforation can occur in the presence of ulcerative diseases. The normal bowel can be seriously damaged by a rough, inept passage of the instrument.

Examination is made by means of a tubular instrument approximately 12 inches in length which is electrically lighted. The patient is prepared for examination by cleansing of the rectum by enema, preferably some hours earlier. Frequently a satisfactory examination may be performed without an enema if the patient's bowel habits are regular and the lower colon has been evacuated earlier in the day. No anesthesia is required for the procedure except in infants and children.

Position. Examination may be performed either in the knee-chest or Sims' position. The inverted position with the use of a special table is ideal (Fig. 14–8). The knee-chest or knee-shoulder position more closely simulates the ideal and in unskilled hands is much more satisfactory than the Sims' position. However, the latter is easy on the patient and usually can be employed satisfactorily in experienced hands.

Manipulation of the instrument. The first step is to introduce the instrument through the anal canal. The patient is asked to strain down gently, and the lubricated tip of the sigmoidoscope is pressed against the sphincter muscle in much the same fashion as is employed in introducing the finger. *The instrument should never be introduced until a rectal exam-*

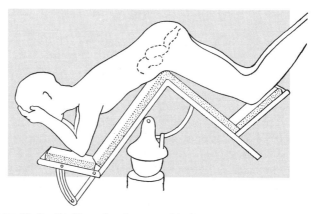

Figure 14–8. Position of patient on table for proctoscopic examination.

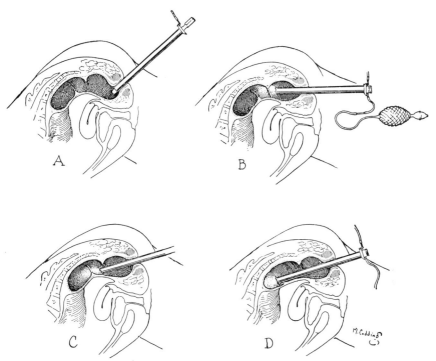

Figure 14–9. Technique of proctosigmoidoscopy. *Step A,* Introducing the instrument. *Step B,* Inspection of the rectal ampulla and inferior valves of Houston. *Step C,* Rotation of the instrument showing the mid valve of Houston. *Step D,* The instrument is about to enter the sigmoid colon.

ination has demonstrated that there is no stenosis of the canal and no obstruction immediately within the rectum. The instrument is pushed with gentle pressure just through the sphincter to avoid the prostate gland in the male and the tip of the cervix in the female (Fig. 14–9). The obturator is then removed, and air is allowed to enter the rectum. Insertion is now continued under direct vision. The instrument may be slowly rotated in order to inspect the rectum and then gradually introduced in an upward and backward direction toward the sacrum. At this point the inferior valve of Houston will be seen (Fig. 14–9) on the left posterior wall of the rectum, and the tip of the sigmoidoscope will be approaching the sacrum. The next step is usually in a more anterior direction to avoid the sacral promontory, and at the same time the middle valve of Houston on the right anterior rectal wall will be visualized (Fig. 14–9). Above this is the superior valve of Houston at about 12.5 centimeters from the anal margin. After passing this point, difficulty may be encountered in introducing the instrument further, since it will be entering the sigmoid colon (Fig. 14–9). Gentle ballooning of the bowel by introducing small amounts of air will show the direction which the colon takes at this point; this is usually to the left, but may be to the right and then to the left, since there is no constant pattern to the course of the sigmoid colon. Usually it can be entered for a short distance, and unless there is sharp angulation or fixation of the lateral sigmoid, one should be able to introduce the instrument to its full length, which is a distance of 25 to 30 centimeters.

When the instrument has reached the highest point to which it can be advanced without discomfort, it should be gradually withdrawn and the mucosal lining again carefully inspected. Since 75 per cent of all polyps and cancers of the colon can be seen with the sigmoidoscope, its routine use is essential in all physical examinations.

Colonoscopy. With the fiberoptic colonoscope, the entire colon may be examined. This examination is particularly useful in establishing the benignity of small polypoid lesions in elderly or poor risk patients, thus avoiding laparotomy in patients with questionable cancer by barium x-ray, and in determining the extent of inflammatory lesions such as granulomatous colitis in areas which appear normal on x-ray. Benign polyps can readily be removed through the colonoscope, but the procedure is hazardous unless performed by an expert.

II. DISORDERS OF THE PROSTATE AND SEMINAL VESICLES

The following disorders of the prostate and seminal vesicles can be recognized on physical examination:

Prostatitis. In *acute prostatitis* the gland is hot, exceedingly tender, and uniformly enlarged. In *chronic prostatitis* the gland is firm and irregularly nodular. The lateral sulci are well preserved. The gland tends to be boggy; it is only slightly tender. Pus may be expressed from the urethra by massage, and the contour and shape of the gland may be altered by massage and firm pressure (contraindicated in the acute stages).

Benign hypertrophy of the prostate. One of the earliest signs of a benign enlargement of the prostate gland is the disappearance of the median sulcus. The enlargement tends to be symmetric. The gland is firm and elastic. It may seem slightly nodular on occasion, but a distinct nodosity is suggestive of malignancy. At times the enlargement may be enormous, it being impossible to get the palpating finger over the surface of the gland.

Carcinoma of the prostate. A loss of the lateral sulci is an early sign in carcinoma. The presence of any firm-to-hard distinct nodule is strongly suggestive of carcinoma. A stony hard irregular enlargement is pathognomonic, but on occasion even the experienced examiner may have difficulty in distinguishing an old chronic prostatitis, with scarring and fibrosis, from carcinoma.

Prostatic calculi. Occasionally, prostatic calculi may be felt just beneath the surface of the gland as tiny, hard, beady nodules.

III. ANORECTAL LESIONS

The following anorectal lesions are easily detected on physical examination:

External hemorrhoidal tabs. These are the end results of previous thromboses of external hemorrhoids. They appear as accentuated fibrotic folds of skin. Usually they cause no symptoms, but may be associated with pruritis ani.

Thrombosed external hemorrhoid. An exquisitely tender, sharply circumscribed, bluish swelling which lies just at the entrance to the anal canal is a thrombosed external hemorrhoid.

Internal hemorrhoids. Internal hemorrhoids which do not prolapse may be difficult to detect except by anoscopic examination. Occasionally, they can be felt as soft folds running upward from the anal canal into the rectum (Fig. 14–10). If prolapse is present, the hemorrhoids can be readily detected by separating the buttocks and asking the patient to strain; the hemorrhoidal mass will appear as a red, moist, elliptical nodule protruding through the canal.

Pruritis ani. The normal radiating skin folds are edematous, swollen, and elongated. The skin is cracked and fissured between the folds; there are often irregular excoriations from scratching. The skin may be completely eroded directly anteriorly and posteriorly, leaving raw, super-

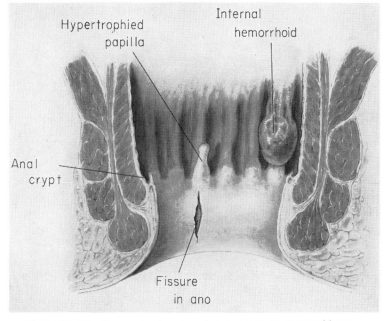

Figure 14–10. Composite drawing of some common anorectal lesions.

ficial fissures. In more chronic cases the skin assumes an irregular pallor. The surface may be moist and lacerated or dry and brittle.

Anal fissure. An anal fissure usually lies directly posterior, and exquisite pain makes examination of the rectum nearly impossible. It should be suspected whenever the external sphincter fails to relax as the patient strains down. Gently separate the buttocks and expose the anal canal; the fissure may then be demonstrated by slight outward traction as a tear in the lining of the anal canal. A chronic fissure is distinguished from an acute fissure partly by the history, but also by the finding of scarring and induration of the tissues. Frequently, a hypertrophied papilla is found just above a fissure (the so-called sentinel pile; Fig. 14–10).

Anal stricture. In anal stricture the finger cannot be introduced into the rectal canal because of the dense fibrous bands which narrow the anal canal. Anal stricture should be distinguished from fibrosis of the subcutaneous portion of the external sphincter.

Fibrosis of the external sphincter ani. Atrophy, contraction and fibrosis of the subcutaneous portion of the external sphincter ani may result in stenosis of the anal canal. The condition commonly is seen in elderly women who have been chronic users of saline cathartics or mineral oil. There is a constricting band at the entrance to the anal canal.

Fistula-in-ano. The external opening of a fistula-in-ano cannot be distinguished from other sinuses or small subcutaneous abscesses in this

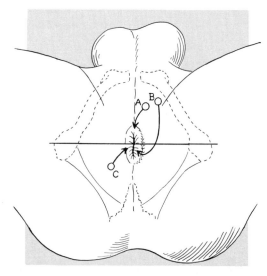

Figure 14–11. A "law" for the location of the internal opening of an anal fistula. An imaginary line bisects the anal canal transversely. *A,* If the external opening is anterior to the line and within an inch of the anal canal, the internal opening will be anterior. *B,* If the external opening is anterior to the line but over an inch away from the anus, the tract will encircle the canal and enter it posteriorly. *C,* If the external opening is posterior to the line, the internal opening will be found to be posterior.

location. The tract should not be probed from the exterior, but careful palpation between the opening and the anus may reveal an indurated cord of tissue extending toward the anal canal. Subsequent anoscopic examination may reveal an internal opening which can be demonstrated with a probe. *Salmon's law* is a convenient guide for locating internal openings in relation to the position of the external opening (Fig. 14–11). An imaginary line is drawn between the ischial tuberosities bisecting the anal canal. If the external opening of a fistula is posterior to this line, the internal opening will be found in a posterior position. If the external opening is anterior to this line and is within an inch of the anal canal, the internal opening will be anterior to the line. However, if the external opening is anterior and an inch or more away from the canal, the fistula will encircle the canal, entering it in a posterior crypt.

Hypertrophied papilla. A hypertrophied papilla can be palpated as a firm polypoid structure lying at the upper end of the anal canal. The diagnosis is unequivocally established by anoscopy, which will show the lesion arising at the pectinate line (Fig. 14–10). Hypertrophied papillae are frequently erroneously described as "thrombosed internal hemorrhoids" or as "polyps." A true rectal polyp arises from the rectal mucosa above the anal canal.

Condylomata acuminata (venereal warts). These cauliflower-like papillomatous lesions develop in a wide area around the anal canal and may extend into it. The lesion is transmitted by a virus, frequently on sexual contact. Anal condylomas in the male often are an indication of homosexuality.

Pilonidal sinus. A pilonidal sinus is a congenital lesion which makes its appearance around the age of 15 to 30. It is more common in males. It may be detected as a mere dimple with a minute opening directly in the midline and well posterior to the anal canal. In some instances no opening is detected, but a small cyst can be seen and palpated. In advanced cases there may be secondary openings to the right or left of the midline, and occasionally the sinus tract may burrow downward and simulate an anal fistula.

Perirectal abscess. A perirectal abscess is evident as a tender swelling adjacent to the anal canal. The usual signs of inflammation are present (Fig. 14–12).

Ischiorectal abscess. The inflammatory process is less obvious in an ischiorectal abscess than in a perirectal abscess. Only a slight swelling is detectable by inspection. Palpation will reveal deep tenderness lateral to the rectum and palpation within the anal canal will reveal a tender mass bulging against the lateral wall. The signs of severe inflammation are present, but fluctuation is very late to appear.

Supra levator abscesses. These may show no evidence of inflammation on external palpation, but internal palpation reveals a tender boggy swelling bulging into the lateral wall of the rectum (Fig. 14–12).

Rectal stricture. The ampulla of the rectum is usually narrowed in

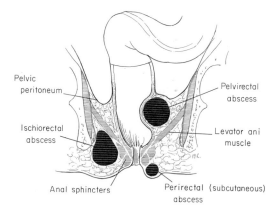

Pelvic peritoneum

Pelvirectal abscess

Ischiorectal abscess

Levator ani muscle

Anal sphincters

Perirectal (subcutaneous) abscess

Figure 14–12. Diagram of the location of rectal abscesses.

inflammatory strictures of the rectum. The palpating finger comes in contact with the entire rectal wall as it approaches the narrowed strictured area. There may be bleeding and tenderness if there are inflammatory changes.

Rectal polyps. Polyps of the rectum may be detected by palpation if they are within the reach of the examining finger. The usual polyp will be felt as a pedunculated, soft nodule attached to the wall of the rectum. At times it is difficult to distinguish from a small amount of adherent fecal material. On sigmoidoscopic inspection two types of polyp may be recognized. The pedunculated polyp has a narrow stalk by which it is attached to the rectal mucosa. Sessile polyps have a broad base so that the attachment of the nodule to the wall of the rectum is often as wide as the polyp. Pedunculated polyps with a distinct stalk are rarely malignant. Sessile polyps may be indistinguishable from cancer except on biopsy.

Prolapse of the rectum. Prolapse of the rectum usually can be demonstrated by having the patient strain as in defecation while the buttocks are separated. Occasionally there is a clear history of prolapse but no abnormality is demonstrable. In such instances the prolapse may be produced only when the patient strains in the sitting position as at stool.

A true prolapse or procidentia should be distinguished from prolapse of the mucosa alone and from sigmoidorectal intussusception. The distinction is easily made on physical examination.

In a mucosal prolapse the lesion is small, more or less symmetric, and tends to have radial mucosal striations (Fig. 14–13 *A*). A true prolapse, because of the presence of a peritoneal sac on the anterior wall, is always assymmetric. The anterior wall is longer than the posterior and the opening is thus rotated somewhat posteriorly (Fig. 14–13 *B*).

In sigmoidorectal intussusception the examining finger can be passed into the rectal ampulla without reduction of the protruding mass (Fig. 14–13 *C*).

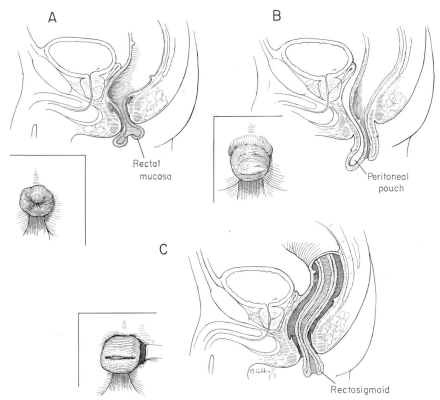

Figure 14–13. *A,* Cross section and appearance of mucosal prolapse. *B,* The appearance and cross section of procidentia of the rectum. Note the greater length and thickness of the anterior wall due to the presence of a pouch of peritoneum. *C,* Sigmoidorectal intussusception. It is obvious that the finger can be passed into the rectum along the protruding mass.

Villous adenoma. A villous adenoma is a soft, compressible, sessile lesion which may reach enormous size, encircling the entire rectum. Microscopically, it is made up of multiple frond-like villi. The surface is often covered with thick, tenacious mucus.

There may be a massive loss of potassium associated with a mucoid diarrhea, resulting in dehydration, weakness, and vascular collapse. There is a high incidence of carcinoma in villous adenomata, often requiring repeated biopsy or total biopsy excision in order to establish the malignant nature of the lesion.

Polypoid carcinoma. The carcinoma may present as a polypoid lesion. Although benign in appearance, it is often highly malignant.

Carcinoma in a polyp. Sometimes carcinoma develops in a polyp, usually at the tip. If there is no invasion of the stalk, metastases are very rare and most surgeons treat the lesion as benign.

Carcinoma of the rectum. Carcinoma of the rectum will be recognized as a hard, irregular lesion arising from the rectal wall and having a central area of ulceration. At times carcinoma may be palpated merely as a huge polypoid lesion without a central core of ulceration. Tenderness or fixation indicates an advanced lesion. It is important to remember that lesions high in the rectum may be palpated only in the lithotomy position. Carcinoma of the rectum is best recognized by means of the sigmoidoscope. It appears as a broad-based fungating or ulcerative lesion. In its early stages it may be indistinguishable from a polyp, especially of the sessile type. Carcinoma may develop in a pedunculated polyp without altering the benign appearance of the lesion. The diagnosis is established by biopsy.

Carcinoma of the rectum is one of the more favorable forms of cancer. Abdominoperineal resection is the accepted form of therapy, but in selected cases, especially in poor risk or elderly patients, electrocoagulation is done preserving the rectum and avoiding colostomy. Preoperative x-ray may be of value in advanced cases of borderline operability.

Malignant tumors of the anal canal and perineum. Epidermoid carcinoma is the commonest anal malignancy but it comprises only 5 per cent of all anal and rectal tumors. Metastases to regional nodes, including the inguinal nodes, is common. Early superficial lesions may be confined to the anal skin. In advanced cases the perirectal tissues and perineum become invaded (Fig. 14–14).

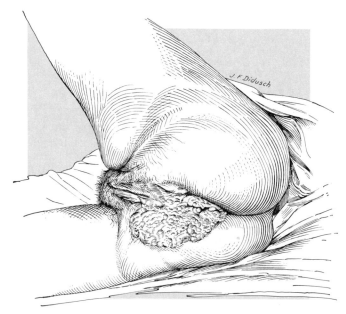

Figure 14–14. Carcinoma of the anus.

Malignant melanomata, Paget's disease, and Bowen's disease (a rare form of intraepidermal cancer) may develop in the anal canal.

Transitional cell cancers arise from embryologic remnants. Growth is rapid, often without symptoms, resulting in large tumors deeply invading the perirectal tissues with a small presenting surface. Metastases are early and rapidly growing.

Early recognition and abdominoperineal resection offers the best chance for permanent control in most cases. Sometimes preoperative x-ray may contribute to operability. Irradiation alone may give significant palliation.

chapter 15   EXAMINATION FOR
THE DETECTION OF
CANCER

Cancer detection can be defined as the diagnosis of cancer before the disease is the cause of signs and symptoms. The diagnosis of cancer at this stage is, in most instances, the most favorable time for successful treatment. Frequently, cancer detection is regarded as an enterprise that can be performed only in large medical centers, or by specialists, but nothing could be further from the truth. It is the practicing physician, whether in his own office or in the hospital clinic, who must do cancer detection. Any physician who is willing to spend the time on a complete physical examination can diagnose a number of important cancers before they are the cause of symptoms. The basic tools required are those adapted for the usual physical examination plus a sharp awareness of the possibility of the presence of cancer in the seemingly well patient. *To forestall a false sense of security on the part of the examiner and the patient alike, the physician must have a realistic idea of what cancers he can and cannot be expected to identify in his examination.*

It is helpful in cancer detection to classify the disease according to its accessibility to the examiner's tools. Thus some cancers are visible, some can be visualized with the aid of instruments, some are palpable, and others are inaccessible except by sophisticated radiologic examination, radioisotopic scanning, or exploratory surgical procedures.

The *visible cancers* (Fig. 15–1*A*) are those arising in the skin, lips, tongue, mouth, vulva, and penis. Cancer of the pharynx, nasopharynx, larynx, vagina, cervix uteri, anus, rectum, and sigmoid colon can be visualized with the aid of simple instruments in the usual office examinations (Fig. 15–1*B*). More specialized endoscopic procedures such as colonoscopy, esophagoscopy, gastroscopy, bronchoscopy, and cystoscopy are performed for specific indications and enable the examiner to visualize lesions of the esophagus, stomach, colon, lung, and urinary tract (Fig. 15–1*C*).

302

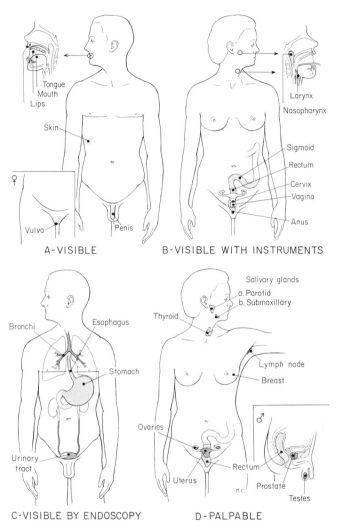

Figure 15–1. *A,* Cancer of the skin and of the buccal cavity can readily be seen on inspection. The examiner should not omit the inspection of the skin of the external genitalia or of the extremities, including the palms of the hands and soles of the feet. *B,* The laryngeal mirror, vaginal speculum, and sigmoidoscope are simple office instruments and enable the examiner to diagnose the frequently overlooked cancers of the throat, cervix uteri, rectum, and sigmoid. *C,* Carcinoma of the bronchus, esophagus, stomach, and urinary tract can be visualized with the aid of endoscopic instruments. However, special skill is required in the use of these instruments; therefore, these examinations are performed only when specifically indicated. *D,* The organs shown in this diagram are easily accessible to the examiner's fingers. Careful palpation of these regions in the search of new growths should never be omitted in either sex.

Many cancers become palpable if their bulk is large, but the malignant tumors which first manifest themselves as palpable masses are those arising in the salivary glands, thyroid, lymph nodes, breasts, rectum, prostate, testicles, and ovaries (Fig. 15–1*D*). Cancers of the liver, esophagus, stomach, pancreas, small intestine, colon, lungs, kidney, brain, and bone are inaccessible (Fig. 15–3*A*) unless their presence is suspected and appropriate examinations are made. Even after the presence of a tumor is suspected and all avenues of investigation are exhausted, exploratory surgical operation is not infrequently the final diagnostic step in patients with inaccessible cancer. The important cancers that, however, can be diagnosed in the office examination can be summarized from the above classification as follows: *About 35 per cent of cancer that occurs in the male is accessible to direct examination (mouth, pharynx, thyroid, skin, prostate, and rectum). In the female almost 65 per cent of cancer is likewise accessible (mouth, pharynx, breast, thyroid, uterus, and rectum). See Figure 15–3 A, B, and C.*

The problem of cancer detection is so inescapably connected with the symptoms of cancer that the following suggestions are included.

First, the alleged cardinal symptoms of various cancers are all too frequently manifestations of well advanced disease.

Second, pain with rare exceptions is not an early symptom of cancer and often is due to a metastasis.

SITE	PREDISPOSING FACTOR
Skin	Excessive exposure to x-rays, sun, arsenic, tar, petroleum products.
Oral Cavity, Pharynx, Larynx, Tongue	Tobacco, syphilis, nutritional deficiency, poor dental hygiene.
Thyroid	Excessive x-ray exposure, iodine deficiency, goitrogenic substances.
Lungs	Cigarettes, exposure to Chromate, metal dust, asbestos, air pollution.
Breast	Nulliparous, previous breast disease, high familial incidence.
Esophagus	Nutritional deficiency, tobacco, alcohol.
Stomach	Pernicious anemia, achlorhydria, high familial incidence, Blood type A.
Liver	Parasites, cirrhosis, nutritional deficiency.
Gallbladder	Gallstones.
Colon-Rectum	Polyps, ulcerative colitis, familial polyposis, high familial incidence.
Cervix uteri	Multiple pregnancies, early age of frequent coitus, uncircumcised partner.
Endometrium	Radiation therapy, endocrine imbalance, obesity, infertility and/or diabetes.
Urinary bladder	Excessive exposure to aniline dyes and related chemicals, exstrophy of the bladder.
Male Genitalia	Uncircumcised, poor hygiene, phimosis, cryptorchidism.

Figure 15–2. Factors that predispose to cancer.

Third, the history must be complete and include a review of factors that may predispose the patient to cancer (Fig. 15–2). The presence of these factors does not mean that cancer is present, or that it will inevitably occur. These factors indicate, rather, the patient who has a higher than average risk of having cancer.

The Examination

The performance of the examination to screen a patient for cancer is essentially that of the elective examination. However, the aspects of the examination especially applicable to cancer detection are outlined below.

1. *History:* Complete.

2. *Head and Neck:* Inspect and palpate the head and neck, tongue, and oral cavity. Don't forget to have the patient remove dentures if present. Use the laryngeal mirror to examine the base of the tongue, pharynx and larynx (see page 24 – Figs. 2–13 and 2–14).

3. *Skin:* Inspect the skin with especial attention to the head and neck, palms of hands, soles of feet, vulva, penis, and scrotum.

4. *Lymph Nodes:* Palpate each regional collection of lymph nodes. If a lymph node is enlarged, search its "watershed" for primary lesion.

5. *Breasts:* Examine the breasts in every patient, male or female. Teach all female patients to examine their own breasts monthly after their regular menstrual period.

6. *Abdomen:* Palpate carefully to determine the size of the liver and search for palpable masses along the course of the entire large bowel and region of each kidney.

7. *Pelvic:* Inspect the vulva for lesions of the skin. Make a cytologic smear on every patient prior to the digital and instrumental examination (see page 269 – Fig. 13–2). Do a bimanual examination of the pelvis and then examine the cervix with a vaginal speculum. Schiller's test is an aid to delineate diseased areas of the cervix for biopsy (see page 278).

8. *Rectal:* Palpate for intrinsic lesions of the rectum and nodules in the prostate. Do a test for occult blood on the finger specimen of feces (see page 290 – Fig. 14–6).

9. *Biopsy:* Any accessible lesions, especially of the cervix uteri, skin, and mouth, should be biopsied. If it is a question of a melanoma, total excision of the lesion, not biopsy, should be done.

10. *Sigmoidoscopy:* Sigmoidoscopy must be performed if there is occult blood in the stool or any change in normal regular bowel habits (see page 293 – Fig. 14–9).

11. *X-ray examination:* A chest film should be made at least once a year on every patient 40 years of age or over. This advice is based upon the alarming increase in the incidence of carcinoma of the lung. Other x-ray examinations, such as barium studies of the gastrointestinal tract, are made as indicated. Mammography or xeromammography is recom-

mended in the female patient in the high-risk group, such as a woman with a strong family history of breast cancer.

12. *Laboratory:* A urinalysis and test for the level of hemoglobin is done; any hematuria or pyuria deserves a more detailed investigation. The cause of anemia must be explained, and it is to be remembered that cancer of the gastrointestinal tract is a frequent cause of secondary anemia.

After the above procedures are completed the physician can be reasonably confident that he has not overlooked any accessible lesion. The interpretation of signs and symptoms and indications for more detailed investigation require good clinical judgment on the part of the examiner; however, there are pitfalls to be avoided.

Pitfalls in Cancer Detection

The chief pitfall to be avoided in cancer detection is the assumption that symptoms or physical findings are caused by benign conditions. Some situations in which cancer is overlooked or mistaken for a benign disease are shown in the lower portion of Figure 15–3 (discussed below). An oral cancer should not be confused with the common "canker sore" since a biopsy will show the true nature of the lesion. In like manner, confusing lesions of the skin can be identified. The physician must assume that any persistent discrete mass in the breast is malignant until it is proved otherwise by biopsy of the lesion and not assume that it is fat necrosis or inflammatory disease. The patient who has the symptoms of gastric or duodenal ulcer should not be treated for such until x-ray and endoscopic examinations of the upper gastrointestinal tract, gastric analysis, and examination of the stool for blood have been performed. To do otherwise will lead to failure to diagnose cancer of the stomach.

It must be recognized that an inguinal hernia, especially of long duration, may become symptomatic from the dynamics of straining to urinate or to defecate. Thus, the presence of carcinoma of the prostate or of the rectum should be considered in these patients as a possible cause of the sudden increase in symptoms of the hernia. Abnormal uterine bleeding should not be treated with hormones or other medications until the diagnosis of cancer of the uterus has been excluded by adequate histologic examination. Hemorrhoids are the most common cause of rectal bleeding but they may mask a coexisting carcinoma of the rectum. Despite the fact that bleeding hemorrhoids are present, the presence of carcinoma of the rectum should be excluded by digital rectal examination, proctosigmoidoscopy, and barium enema. Anemia is a common manifestation of cancer, especially when arising in the gastrointestinal tract. The possibility of cancer should be considered in every patient with anemia.

If, after the examination, no disease is found, the patient should be advised to continue to have a periodic physical examination at a minimal

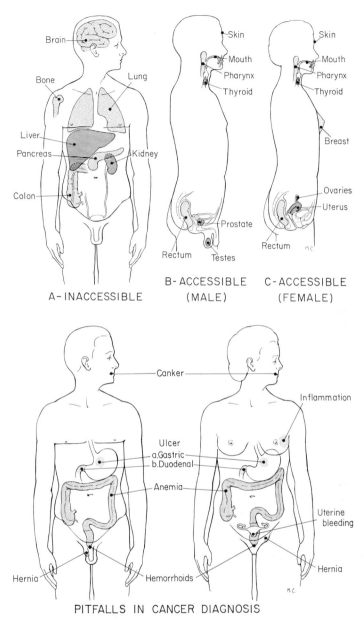

Brain

Bone

Lung

Liver

Pancreas

Kidney

Colon

Skin

Mouth

Pharynx

Thyroid

Prostate

Rectum

Testes

Skin

Mouth

Pharynx

Thyroid

Breast

Ovaries

Uterus

Rectum

B- ACCESSIBLE
(MALE)

C- ACCESSIBLE
(FEMALE)

A- INACCESSIBLE

Canker

Inflammation

Ulcer
a.Gastric
b.Duodenal

Anemia

Uterine
bleeding

Hernia

Hemorrhoids

Hernia

PITFALLS IN CANCER DIAGNOSIS

Figure 15–3. *A,* These anatomic sites are inaccessible to direct examination unless a huge tumor is present. Otherwise, lesions so located are diagnosed when their presence is suspected and endoscopic and x-ray examination is made. At times exploratory surgical procedures are necessary to make the definitive diagnosis. *B,* The lesions shown in this diagram represent about 35 per cent of cancer that occurs in the male. All of these lesions are accessible to inspection or palpation. *C,* The lesions shown in this diagram represent about 65 per cent of cancer that occurs in the female. All of these lesions are accessible to inspection or palpation.

Pitfalls in cancer detection: These supposedly benign lesions may actually be cancerous, or symptoms attributed to them may be caused by cancer. Thus, the examiner must utilize biopsy, sigmoidoscopy, or radiologic examination to determine the true nature of the lesion.

307

interval of one year. A single normal examination is most comforting to the patient at the time, but provides no assurance for the future. It is the repeated periodic careful examination of the well patient that will produce the dividends of better cancer detection.

The Follow-up of the Treated Cancer Patient

The follow-up of patients treated for cancer is important for several reasons, two of which are (1) excellent methods of palliation for recurrent cancer are available and (2) some cancers tend to repeat themselves de novo in contralateral organs or in the remaining segment of the structure originally involved (breast, ovary, colon, skin). Furthermore, a patient who has had one carcinoma may develop a second one. If there is proper communication between physician and patient, a regular schedule of follow-up examinations is not difficult to carry out. The interval between follow-up examinations will vary with the type and stage of the disease when originally diagnosed and treated. In general, for the first year the patient should be seen every few months and at least once a year thereafter.

The follow-up examination.   Above all listen to the patient. New symptoms which the patient may minimize, or vague but persistent complaints may be clues to recurrent disease or a new primary neoplasm.

1. A record of the patient's weight should be kept. The implications of this are obvious.

2. The site of the initial tumor should be examined for signs of local recurrence. This applies especially to tumors of the breast, thyroid, head and neck, skin, and soft tissues.

3. The regional lymphatics are examined for evidence of lymph node metastases.

4. Pelvic and rectal examinations are periodically made and include a Pap smear and test for occult blood in the stool.

5. Sigmoidoscopy and colonoscopy are essential in the follow-up of patients who have had colonic cancer. The hematocrit is done at frequent intervals, since a developing or persistent anemia is an ominous sign. Carcinoembryonic antigen (CEA) may not be as specific for carcinoma of the gastrointestinal tract as originally reported, but it may be very useful in the follow-up of patients with known colonic and possible breast cancer. If the levels have fallen to normal after removal of the neoplasm, and high levels reappear at a later date, the possibility of recurrent disease or undetected metastases exists.

6. Roentgenology and nuclear medicine play an increasingly important role in the follow-up of the patient with cancer. A yearly roentgenogram of the chest is standard, even in the asymptomatic patient. Radiologic skeletal surveys are frequently indicated to detect osseous metastases. The more sophisticated radiologic techniques available—

arteriography, venography, and lymphangiography—are used not only in the diagnosis but also in the follow-up of some malignant tumors. Liver, bone, and brain scanning by radioisotope techniques serves to diagnose primary or metastatic neoplasms and to follow the course of such lesions when extirpation of the primary is not possible. The use of ultrasound, while a different technique, serves much the same purpose. Thus, the progress of a neoplasm that is being treated by radiotherapy or chemotherapy may be followed by these methods as indicated.

Radiologic barium contrast studies of the gastrointestinal tract are still indicated periodically in those patients with treated cancer of the colon or stomach.

The follow-up of the treated cancer patient must not be neglected. Recurrent disease or new primary cancers, if detected early, can be treated aggressively with more optimism than in the past. The discussion above outlines a background for the follow-up examination which the physician can selectively apply to the individual patient.

The Paraneoplastic Syndromes

In any discussion of cancer, some mention of the paraneoplastic syndromes is justified in the hope that it will help the examiner understand and correlate the physical findings in patients suffering from cancer. In fact, the patient may first seek a physician's advice because of the nonmetastatic distant effects of the malignant disease. The term *paraneoplastic syndromes* (Hall and Nathanson) encompasses the diverse distant manifestations of cancer that frequently cause disability or death for reasons other than direct invasion of a vital organ or organs by cancer. In other words, the paraneoplastic syndromes represent distant effects on many organ systems in association with various human neoplasms. Cachexia, anemia without blood loss, and intermittent fevers are common examples. More sharply localized metabolic disorders are seen in pheochromocytomas, islet cell tumors of the pancreas, virilizing tumors of the ovary and adrenal, and carcinoid tumors.

Part Two

THE
EMERGENCY
EXAMINATION

chapter 16   # GENERAL PRINCIPLES IN EXAMINATION OF THE INJURED PATIENT

The approach to the examination of the injured patient is so utterly different from the ordinary physical examination that it requires considerable elaboration. The history may not be obtainable or may be presented in toto by a phrase, such as "auto accident" or "gunshot wound." Although the details of the accident are fully as important in the appraisal of the extent and character of the injury as are the symptoms of any illness, the acquisition of this information is a secondary consideration. The primary consideration is the life of the patient and whether the examination is being performed on a roadside, in a casualty clearing station, or in the emergency ward of a fully equipped hospital, the same general principles apply. In this discussion those general principles which govern the examination of the patient in any situation will be emphasized. The examination cannot be dissociated from management, but the extent to which each is carried out must be governed by the availability of facilities and personnel which permit treatment to be undertaken. The details of first aid and emergency treatment will not be presented.

PROCEDURE

1. PROVIDE AN ADEQUATE AIRWAY

At first glance the patient may appear lifeless. *The number one priority is to provide an adequate airway.* The patient should be turned on his side or face down, head dependent, so that he cannot aspirate blood, mucus, or vomitus. If he is not breathing well the jaw should be pulled forward. Foreign material, food, and vomitus should be cleared from the mouth, and tracheal intubation should be performed. If the patient is cyanotic and his chest is retracting with each respiration, but he does not appear to be getting air, listen to the chest on either side for sounds of aeration. If there are none, it may be that the patient has already aspirated material and has a tracheal obstruction. Under such circumstances endo-tracheal suction is imperative. Rarely, an emergency tracheostomy should be performed.

If the patient is conscious but his respirations are extremely labored, consider the possibility of a sucking wound of the chest, a tension pneumothorax, or a flail chest due to multiple fractures of ribs and ster-num. These complications may have to be dealt with as emergencies before the patient can be transported or further examined. They are dis-cussed in detail in Chapter 18.

2. EMERGENCY RESUSCITATION

On first encounter with the injured patient or at any time during the course of a surgical illness, there may be the need for resuscitation. The possibility of inadequate respiration, inadequate circulation, or failure of either must be uppermost in the mind of the examiner. *Measures for their correction must precede any other treatment or diagnostic maneuver,* for anoxia can cause irreparable damage. A simple plan of action, carefully thought out beforehand, becomes an instinctive action in an emergency. Whether respiratory or circulatory resuscitation should take precedence or whether both are carried out simultaneously depends upon the circum-stances.

Respiratory inadequacy. Respiratory inadequacy may be due to airway obstruction, apnea, or depressed respiration. Absence of cyanosis is an unreliable sign. The diagnosis is made by observation of thoracic movements—whether shallow or of an obstructive nature. Obstructive thoracic movement is indicated by rocking movement, retraction of the supraclavicular fossae, and intercostal spaces. The most common cause is soft tissue obstruction, the jaw having receded and carried the tongue against the posterior wall of the hypopharynx. In the majority of cases this can be corrected by hyperextension of the head and neck, with the chin held upward and the lips apart (Fig. 16–1*A*).

If apnea is present or respiration depressed, mouth-to-mouth or mouth-to-nose breathing is begun with the operator observing the ade-quacy of thoracic movement and compressing the epigastrium to prevent gastric distention (Fig. 16–1*B*). This type of artificial respiration can be effective even if the jaws are tightly clenched. Secretions, vomitus, or foreign bodies can be wiped out of the cheeks, mouth, or pharynx with the fingers, a handkerchief, or gauze. Although it is not recommended to

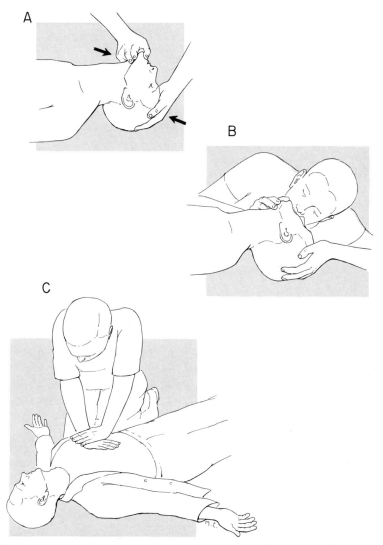

Figure 16–1. Methods of emergency resuscitation. *A,* The jaw is pulled forward to clear the airway. *B,* Mouth-to-mouth or mouth-to-nose respiration. *C,* External manual cardiac systole.

move the injured patient at once, soft tissue obstruction is less apt to occur in the lateral or prone position. Vomitus or secretions can run out of the mouth when the patient is on his side or on his abdomen. On the other hand, mouth-to-mouth breathing is made more difficult in these positions.

Positive pressure breathing applied to the mouth will be ineffective if obstruction exists due to laryngeal or tracheal fracture, vomitus, blood, or foreign body, at or below the glottic level. A direct tracheal airway is best established quickly by intubation. Tracheostomy should not be attempted at the scene of an accident. In a desperate situation, a large bore needle can be introduced into the trachea and will provide a temporary airway until intubation or a formal tracheostomy can be instituted. Removal of foreign bodies and vomitus from below the glottis calls for immediate bronchoscopy and tracheal lavage.

Restoration of adequate respiration will often bring about return of consciousness, improvement of circulation, and reversal of apparent circulatory standstill. *Should there be need for long term artificial respiration, better respiratory exchange can be obtained with an oropharyngeal airway or endotracheal tube, plus intermittent positive pressure carried out with an oxygen face mask, and compression of a reservoir bag, or a mechanical respirator.*

Circulatory standstill. *Circulatory standstill* is diagnosed by the absence of peripheral pulses, blood pressure, and audible heart sounds. *The most immediately effective treatment is utilized—manual closed chest cardiac systole.* While this could conceivably be performed with the patient prone, it is best applied with the patient lying supine on an unyielding surface. The operator straddles the victim and rhythmically compresses the chest 80 times per minute with the heel of the hand over the lower sternum (Fig. 16–1C). The heart is thus compressed between the sternum and spine to mimic cardiac systole. Effective artificial systole is indicated by appearance of a femoral or radial pulse, by disappearance of anoxic pupillary dilatation, and by improvement in skin color.

Manual cardiac systole can be carried out simultaneously with mouth-to-mouth breathing by two operators, or by one person who alternates every fourth compression with inflation of the lungs. Perhaps the only situations in which these measures may not carry the possibility of success are in the presence of a flail chest which cannot recoil after compression, bilateral pneumothorax, or laceration of the heart itself. These conditions may provide the only indications for immediate thoracotomy and direct manual cardiac systole. External manual compression has resulted in fractured ribs and cartilages, laceration of the liver and spleen, and production of fat embolus but these risks must be assumed in an emergency situation. Nevertheless, the most gentle approach consistent with restoration of circulation must be adopted. In the infant and young child mere finger compression may be adequate.

Despite manual systole, circulation may not resume on its own because of continued cardiac asystole or ventricular fibrillation. As soon as possible, therefore, an electrocardiogram should be recorded. If fibrillation is present, external DC shock is applied. Simultaneously, an intravenous line is established and sodium bicarbonate is given to counter metabolic acidosis. Ventricular fibrillation may respond to external electrical countershock, in some instances in combination with injection of procaine amide or quinidine. Correction of blood volume deficit and the use of vasopressor drugs through improvement in the cardiac output and coronary arterial blood flow, along with continued oxygenation, can institute natural systole and revert fibrillation. Persistent asystole calls for cardiac stimulants such as calcium, epinephrine, or norepinephrine or the use of a transverse pacemaker.

In summary, the most important aspects of the emergency treatment of respiratory and circulatory failure are immediate recognition of the problem and instantaneous application of the simplest measures at hand without resort to more complicated methods. Specific treatments have been alluded to, but their application comes later, perhaps after consultation or with the assistance of specialists.

3. CONTROL SERIOUS LOSS OF BLOOD

A. If blood is spurting from a wound of a limb, a tourniquet should be applied proximal to the wound. Such instances are rare.

B. If there is steady oozing of blood from a wound, this can best be controlled by pressure. In the case of an injured limb, elevation of the limb and gentle compression over the wound with any clean cloth will suffice to control bleeding.

4. MAKE A RAPID SURVEY OF THE EXTENT OF THE INJURIES

As soon as possible, but preferably under circumstances which permit therapy to be started, a complete but rapid survey of all potential sites of injury must be carried out. With a little experience it is possible to complete a rapid survey of the body within two minutes. At its completion a reasonably accurate knowledge of the extent of the injuries is obtained. One can be certain that a cerebral injury, a tension pneumothorax, a flail chest or cardiac tamponade—conditions which may contraindicate or affect the extent or type of parenteral fluid therapy to be given—will be recognized. To omit this type of survey of the body and attempt to treat an obvious injury will sooner or later lead to the pitfall of attributing the collapse of an unrecognized chest injury to a fractured femur or to overlooking extensive abdominal injury in the presence of a comparatively mild cerebral contusion. Moreover, information gained at this preliminary examination is exceedingly valuable in the subsequent management of the patient. For example, abdominal spasm and tenderness detected at a later date, when the initial examination showed a soft, nontender abdomen, is sound evidence of a progressing abdominal injury. Although each case must be evaluated on its own merit and no routine warrants blind adherence, the following will serve as a guide.

A. *Inspect and palpate the skull* gently but thoroughly for lacerations or contusions. One particularly looks for fluid or blood issuing from the ears or nose. Note the size of the pupils and the color of the ears and lips. Determine the state of consciousness by response to questions or painful stimuli. Palpate the position of the trachea and feel for crepitation in the tissues of the neck.

B. If there is a *wound of the chest,* be certain that it is not sucking (see Chapter 18). Auscultate the chest sufficiently to determine that there are good breath sounds on both sides; gently compress the thoracic cage to exclude fracture of the ribs. If abnormalities are detected, the chest will require more elaborate examination on completion of the rapid survey.

C. *Palpate the abdomen* for spasm or tenderness.

D. *Gently compress the wings of the ilium* and palpate the symphysis pubis for evidence of a pelvic fracture.

E. *Ask the patient to move his extremities,* or if he is unable to cooperate, gently palpate and move them sufficiently to recognize major fractures.

F. *Separate the legs* and inspect the perineum for ecchymosis, swelling, or extravasation of blood or urine.

G. *Inspect the back and buttocks* for major wounds or hitherto unrecognized points of bleeding. When the patient is turned on his side, a more complete examination of the chest may be done.

H. *Note the color and temperature* of the hands and feet. Feel the pulse, observing its quality as well as its rate. If possible take, or have an assistant take, the blood pressure. Begin at once to record pulse, respiration, and blood pressure on some type of chart, even if it be merely a scrap of paper.

5. SPLINT BROKEN LIMBS AND CONTROL PAIN WITH MEDICATION

The exact sequence of the procedure will vary with the circumstances. Frequently medication must be given and limbs must be splinted before an adequate survey of the extent of injuries can be made.

Do not give medication as a routine. It should be withheld unless there is pain, and it should be given by the intravenous route because in the presence of shock it may not be absorbed from the subcutaneous tissues.

At the conclusion of this examination the following should be accomplished: An adequate airway will have been established, external bleeding will have been controlled, the extent of the injury will have been established, and measures to control pain and immobilize injured limbs will have been taken. Moreover, the examiner will be in a position to interpret abnormalities of respiration or circulation on the basis of pathologic entities rather than by use of the vague term "shock."

In each case a more detailed appraisal of the specific injury will be required. The essential steps are dealt with in the succeeding chapters.

chapter 17

INJURIES OF THE
HEAD AND FACE

Injuries of the head and face are extremely common in civilian life as well as in war. The nature of an injury in this region is often so obvious that it is recognizable at a glance as a "black eye," a "broken jaw," or a lacerated or penetrating wound of the head or face. The principal diagnostic concern is the extent of injury to the brain. This chapter is devoted mainly to a discussion of cerebral injury.

I. CEREBRAL INJURIES

The immediate concern in a patient with actual or potential cerebral injury is to be certain that he has *an adequate airway.* Having done so, investigation should follow the general survey described above. Splinting of major injuries of limbs, control of hemorrhage, and treatment of shock or associated injuries take precedence over the appraisal and management of cerebral injuries except for the establishment and maintenance of an airway. It can be categorically stated that whenever a cerebral injury is so severe that death occurs within a few minutes, despite an adequate airway, no treatment will be of avail.

The primary purpose in the initial appraisal of a head injury is to establish a base line for subsequent observations, to determine the type of injury sustained, and to select those cases in which immediate surgical procedures may be necessary.

Determining the Neurologic Deficit and Establishing a
Base Line for Subsequent Observations

An elaborate neurologic examination is neither necessary nor desirable in patients with severe head injuries. An adequate examination can be performed in a few minutes with a reflex hammer, a pin, and a flashlight or any reasonable substitutes. The most important observations are the *level*

319

of consciousness, the *character of the respirations*, the *state of the pupils*, the *degree of motor activity*, and the *character of the deep tendon reflexes*. Poor prognostic signs during the early period after injury include bilateral, dilated, fixed pupils, extensor rigidity of all extremities, periodic type of breathing, and hyperthermia of 103° to 104° F.

State of consciousness. If the patient is sufficiently awake to answer questions and obey commands, his level of consciousness can be evaluated by the accuracy and speed with which these functions are accomplished. If he does not respond to questions, the usual method of evaluating the state of consciousness is to determine his response to painful stimulation such as supraorbital pressure, pricking with a pin, or pulling hair. Painful stimuli should be repeated in as standard a fashion as possible. Determinations of swallowing, gagging, and eyelid reflex are also of value.

Pupils. The state of the pupils is probably next in importance to the patient's level of consciousness. Their size (large or small), their equality, and their comparative response to strong light and pain should be observed. If both pupils are very small and do not dilate readily with a painful stimulus, the outlook is fairly grave and usually means that the midbrain is damaged, unless the patient is intoxicated or has been medicated. If both pupils are dilated and fixed to strong light in the acute phase of head injury, the prognosis is probably hopeless. This situation is usually accompanied by respiratory irregularity, fever, and decerebrate rigidity.

If the pupils are unequal but both will react, or if one pupil is dilated and fixed and the other is normal in size and activity, evidence is present of local injury involving one oculomotor system more than the other. Unilateral dilation of the pupil, if it appears during a period of observation, usually signifies intracranial bleeding. It may be due solely to severe contusion if present from the moment of injury.

Examination of the eyegrounds may disclose hemorrhages in the optic disks. Usually the appearance of the optic disks is normal. Papilledema will not be found, since it appears after the intracranial pressure has been increased for several days.

Motor and reflex activity. Examination of the extremities for flaccidity or spasticity can be carried out readily no matter what the state of consciousness. The same is true with respect to deep tendon reflexes. The motor and reflex responses of both sides should be compared with each other at each examination, and from one examination to the next. It is sufficient to test the triceps, biceps, radioperiosteal, plantar, knee, and ankle reflexes. Ankle clonus should also be tested (Fig. 17–1). Motor activity can be appraised by having the patient squeeze the examiner's hand or by noting the strength with which he resists passive motion of his extremities. In profound coma the degree of flaccidity may be noted by lifting an extremity and then letting it drop gently.

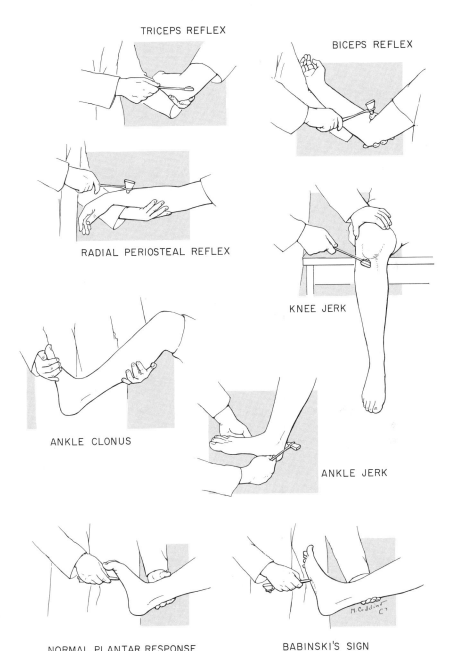

Figure 17-1. Technique of testing for peripheral reflexes.

It is especially significant when a change of motor or reflex activity appears during a period of observation. The development of unilateral pyramidal tract signs some time after injury means localized intracranial hemorrhage until proved otherwise. Extensor rigidity of all four extremities is an ominous sign, especially if present immediately after a head injury and progressive in severity. Complete flaccidity and areflexia in the absence of alcoholism or drug intake also denote severe and probably irreversible central nervous system damage.

Types of Head Injury

Concussion. Any person who has lost consciousness or cannot remember events immediately preceding or following an accident has sustained a cerebral concussion. It may be so slight that the patient appears perfectly well, but he must be kept under observation for a period of several hours because of the potential hazard of intracranial bleeding. Under such circumstances a more complete neurologic examination should be done. A simple but effective means of testing the function of the cranial nerves is shown in Figure 17–2.

Extradural hemorrhage and subdural hemorrhage. The classic sequence of events is a blow on the head, recognized or unrecognized in the midst of other injuries, a brief period of unconsciousness followed by

CRANIAL NERVE	TEST
I—OLFACTORY	SENSE OF SMELL.
II—OPTIC	VISION. OPHTHALMOSCOPIC EXAMINATION.
III—OCULOMOTOR	EXTERNAL OCULAR MOVEMENTS. SIZE, SHAPE, AND REACTION OF PUPILS.
IV—TROCHLEAR	EXTERNAL OCULAR MOVEMENTS.
V—TRIGEMINAL	HAVE PATIENT CLENCH HIS TEETH (ACTION OF MASSETER MUSCLES).
VI—ABDUCENS	EXTERNAL OCULAR MOVEMENTS (LOOK FOR INTERNAL SQUINT).
VII—FACIAL	HAVE PATIENT SHOW HIS TEETH (ACTION OF FACIAL MUSCLES).
VIII—ACOUSTIC	HEARING (TEST BOTH EARS BY RUBBING FINGERS TOGETHER, OR WITH A WATCH).
IX—GLOSSOPHARYNGEAL	TEST POSTERIOR THIRD OF TONGUE WITH A PROBE (SENSORY TO POSTERIOR THIRD OF THE TONGUE).
X—VAGUS	PULSE AND RESPIRATORY RATE AND RHYTHM.
XI—SPINAL ACCESSORY	HAVE PATIENT SHRUG HIS SHOULDERS (ACTION OF TRAPEZIUS MUSCLES).
XII—HYPOGLOSSAL	HAVE PATIENT PROTRUDE HIS TONGUE (MOTOR NERVE OF TONGUE).

Figure 17–2. Rapid tests for gross appraisal of cranial nerve function.

recovery with a period of apparent well-being, and then the onset of confusion, drowsiness, and steadily progressing coma. Characteristically the pulse is slow and full and the respirations are slow and deep. Lateralizing neurologic signs, such as hemiparesis, abnormal reflexes, or asymmetric pupillary dilation, warrant emergency neurosurgical intervention.

The findings are not always so obvious. Any patient who has sustained a head injury and has been shown to have a specific neurologic deficit which remains stable and then progresses after a time should be suspected of having intracranial bleeding.

Diffuse cerebral injury. Extensive, diffuse contusion and laceration of the brain occur in closed head injuries with or without associated skull fractures. The mechanism is sudden deceleration of the head, the brain being snapped against the cranial vault. There is generalized injury to the brain, sometimes with associated massive extradural or subdural bleeding, and usually with subarachnoid bleeding.

Respirations are slow and deep and often stertorous or of a Cheyne-Stokes type. Bleeding from the ear, indicative of a basilar fracture, is common. Spinal fluid may issue from the nose or ears, indicating a dural laceration. Reflexes are diminished to absent. Extensor rigidity is an ominous sign. In general, depth of coma is the best guide to the condition of the patient. A stable neurologic deficit, as determined by carefully repeated examinations, is a reassuring observation. Steadily deepening coma, bilateral dilated fixed pupils, extensor rigidity, and hyperthermia indicate extensive brain damage.

Skull fractures. Simple linear fracture of the skull, associated with cerebral concussion or contusion, may be of little importance and does not in itself alter the management of the patient. Many severe closed head injuries are associated with fractures of the skull, often basilar in location. However, extensive skull fracture may occur without cerebral injury if the deceleration phenomenon is absent. The classic example is the mechanic working under a car with his head on the garage floor. The jack slips, and the car crushes the mechanic's head. The skull may be cracked like an egg shell without serious brain injury. In such types of injury the lack of neurologic deficit should not lead the examiner to overlook an extensive skull fracture. Localized dural injuries may result in delayed but serious extradural or subdural bleeding.

DEPRESSED SKULL FRACTURE. Depressed fracture of the skull occurs from blows on the head with sharp or blunt instruments, weapons, or missiles. Depending on the mechanism of the injury, there may be extensive brain damage or no recognizable neurologic deficit. Although brain damage is frequently minimal, the danger of infection renders surgery imperative in depressed fractures. In all lacerated or contused wounds of the scalp, one should suspect a possible associated depressed fracture, particularly if there are any focal neurologic abnormalities.

Penetrating wounds of the brain. All penetrating wounds of the brain require surgical exploration and débridement as soon as the condition of the patient permits. In many instances the diagnosis is obvious. Brain tissue, shredded dura, clear or blood-tinged cerebrospinal fluid may be seen emerging through a scalp wound, particularly when the patient strains or cries out. High velocity small missiles may produce only minute self-healing wounds of entrance, but extensive intracranial destruction. Intracranial clot formation should be suspected in patients showing evidence of increased intracranial pressure out of proportion to the extent of a visible penetrating wound. Early surgical intervention in such patients may be life-saving. Examination of external wounds in suspected or obvious penetrating craniocerebral injuries should be limited to inspection and to control of severe scalp bleeding by pressure or by ligation or clamping of large arteries. Further wound exploration should be part of definitive neurosurgical treatment.

X-Ray Examination

Every patient with a cerebral injury should be x-rayed. Stereoscopic films are preferable. The time at which x-ray films are made will vary with the type of injury. Considerable judgment must be exercised. Usually little is gained by x-ray examination during the first few hours after a severe head injury, and there may be considerable hazard in unwise manipulation of such a patient. Films are technically difficult to obtain and are unsatisfactory in a restless, overactive, uncooperative patient who may be vomiting or bleeding freely from a wound, or whose respirations are irregular. Such a patient should receive supportive treatment, bleeding from the wound should be controlled, and only after the neurologic deficit has been shown to be stable should the patient be moved to an x-ray table and appropriate films secured. The complications of head injuries which require acute surgical intervention are massive extradural or other localized intracranial hemorrhage. They are recognized not on the basis of x-ray but because of changes in vital signs and neurologic findings. At times, surgical exploration may be necessary without taking time for an x-ray.

The importance of an x-ray examination lies in ruling out certain types of fractures which necessitate special treatment, and in recognizing a fracture in the presence of what seems to be a mild concussion. A depressed fracture or a fracture extending into the paranasal sinuses, the mastoid, or the petrous portion of the temporal bone, indicating that the injury is, in fact, a compound one, can often be recognized by means of x-ray studies. The ultimate management of the patient rests upon such data, although his emergency care is not affected by it. Finally, an x-ray is often required for medicolegal reasons. It is a good rule, therefore, to secure x-ray films of the skull as soon after a cerebral injury as is consistent with the general condition of the patient.

II. FRACTURE OF THE FACIAL BONES

A detailed discussion of all the fractures which may affect the facial bones is not within the scope of this volume. Two very common injuries which are frequently overlooked despite obvious physical signs require mention, however.

Fracture of the Nose

Some fractures of the nose are obvious because of extensive depression or deviation of the nasal contour. More often, however, one finds swelling, edema, and discoloration without obvious distortion. The presence of a fracture may be readily demonstrated by careful palpation and by intranasal inspection. The contour of the nose is best examined from above and behind the patient. If the patient is seated in a chair and the examiner stands behind and looks down on the face, an asymmetry may be detected from this vantage that is not recognized on inspection from in front of the patient. Careful bimanual palpation, placing the fingers of both hands simultaneously along the bridge of the nose, will usually indicate a deviation or depression. If doubt exists, inspection through the nostril will demonstrate deviation or buckling of the nasal septum if any significant break in the contour of the nasal bone or the nasal cartilage has occurred.

Depressed Fracture of the Zygoma

This common injury results from a blow on the cheek. It is frequently overlooked because of the lack of external deformity. The depression of the zygoma is masked by edema and swelling over it. Edema and swelling over the zygoma associated with subconjunctival hemorrhage and a rim of anesthesia just below the eye due to injury of the second division of the fifth cranial nerve make the diagnosis evident. Inspection and palpation of the zygoma is performed from behind the patient as described in fracture of the nose. If the examiner compares the contour of the zygomatic arches simultaneously on the two sides, the depression at the fracture site can be felt.

chapter 18   # INJURIES OF THE THORACIC WALL, HEART, AND LUNGS

The general principles of examination of the injured patient described in Chapter 16 apply. The nature of the injury and the patient's complaints may render an injury to the chest obvious, or in the presence of multiple injuries as from shell fragments, a mangled limb or a head injury may draw attention away from a small but potentially lethal injury to the chest. In every seriously injured, shocked patient one must automatically consider the possibilities of tension pneumothorax, mediastinal emphysema, cardiac tamponade, or an open sucking wound. There may or may not be evidence of injury to the thoracic wall.

I. INJURIES OF THE THORACIC WALL

Fractured Rib

This very common injury of the chest wall occurs from a blow, contusion, or crush. It is a frequent complication of penetrating wounds. It may or may not be associated with intrathoracic damage. Uncomplicated, simple fracture of the rib or ribs occurs usually from a blow or a fall on the chest. The physical findings are definite.

Inspection

The patient should be stripped to the waist. Painful, restricted respiration with limitation of motion of the affected side is generally obvious. If the patient is asked to take a deep breath, he will experience sharp pain at the site of injury. One should carefully inspect the skin over the entire chest wall for signs of an external wound regardless of the type of injury sustained.

326

Palpation

The presence or absence of the crepitant sensation of air in the subcutaneous tissues in the region of the pain should first be determined by very gentle palpation without compressing the chest wall. Then each rib should be compressed separately by gentle pressure with the tips of the fingers. Exquisite pain will be elicited when the injured rib or ribs are compressed.

Percussion and Auscultation

The patient with a fractured rib may have an intrathoracic injury, so the chest must be carefully percussed and auscultated. The position of the trachea and the heart should be determined to exclude a mediastinal shift and to establish a base line for comparison if signs of intrathoracic injury subsequently appear. The manifestations of pneumothorax, pleural effusion, and traumatic emphysema are discussed elsewhere. Usually no evidence of intrathoracic injury is found in simple rib fractures.

Identification of the Injured Rib

The second rib may be palpated anteriorly as the highest rib the upper edge of which can be clearly felt beneath the clavicle. This may be

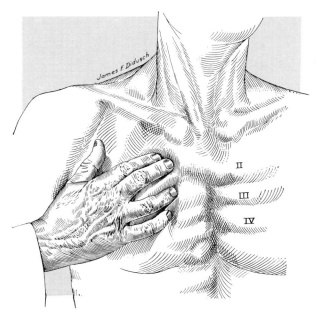

Figure 18–1. Identification of the second rib. The second rib is the highest rib the upper edge of which is clearly palpable anteriorly. This can be confirmed by palpation of a transverse ridge on the sternum which lies directly opposite the second rib.

confirmed by running a finger downward over the sternum from the suprasternal notch until a slight transverse ridge can be identified (angle of Louis). The finger lies directly on the second rib when it is moved laterally from this point (Fig. 18–1). Posteriorly the twelfth rib may be recognized in thin individuals, and each rib then may be identified by palpation from this point upward. Unfortunately, the twelfth rib frequently cannot be felt. Identification of the seventh rib as the one upon which the lower angle of the scapula rests is notoriously unreliable.

The Sign of Compression

In doubtful cases the chest should be compressed by the hands of the examiner placed anteriorly and posteriorly so as to gently spring the thoracic cage on the affected side (Fig. 18–2). This maneuver is particularly helpful in obese or heavily muscled individuals in whom precise palpation of the ribs is difficult. It is not necessary to employ it if the diagnosis of a fractured rib is evident. It should be used to exclude a fractured rib when the signs are equivocal. Lateral compression should also be tried if anterior-posterior compression is painless. The compression test should be omitted if there are signs of a pleural effusion or other evidence of intrathoracic injury.

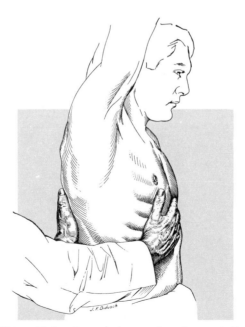

Figure 18–2. Compression test for a fractured rib.

Costochondral Separation

Occasionally, the break in the continuity of an injured rib occurs at the junction of the rib with the costal cartilage; here the physical findings are less marked and x-rays are negative. This injury may occur from coughing or sneezing and may be quite distressing to the patient. Pain on breathing is less striking, but careful identification and palpation of the rib will usually elicit pain localized to the damaged joint.

Fracture of the Sternum

This injury is the result of considerable violence. It is often associated with contusions of the heart.

Inspection

There is pain on breathing; respirations are rapid and shallow. The patient holds his head and neck forward and rigid. There may be deformity at the junction of the manubrium and gladiolus. Usually no deformity is present unless there are extensive fractures of the ribs, in which case there will be a flail chest. In most cases of simple fracture, disability is not great but ecchymosis over the fracture site is common.

Palpation

This should be gentle, as pain will be elicited at the fracture site.

Auscultation

Cardiac arrhythmias or murmurs may be detected on auscultation, since this injury is frequently associated with cardiac contusions. The lung may be injured, with changes in profusion and ventilation of the traumatized segments. The ability of the patient to clear mucus and fluid from the tracheobronchial tree is significantly reduced.

Traumatic Flail Chest

Crushing injuries of the sternum or ribs may result in complete separation of a portion of the chest wall so that it becomes excessively mobile. With each respiration the mobile fragment is sucked inward. The normal expansion of the pleural space is prevented and effective respiratory exchange severely limited.

The diagnosis may be obvious, but very often soft tissue swelling and the restricted expansion of the chest wall obscure the deformity and the paradoxical motion. Initially the patient may be able to compensate for the reduction in respiratory reserve. He may appear so well that corrective measures are not taken until secretions accumulate, pulmonary compliance falls, and severe anoxia, hypercapnea, and collapse occur.

Traumatic flail chest is a surgical emergency requiring immediate treatment. In an emergency, temporary stabilization of the chest wall is helpful, but endotracheal intubation and positive pressure ventilation are the generally accepted methods of restoring respiratory exchange. In addition to assisted respiration, the chest wall can be stabilized by towel-clip traction, or definite stabilization may be accomplished by surgical pinning of the separated fragments.

Flail chest with multiple other injuries is likely to terminate in the respiratory distress syndrome, especially if treatment is delayed.

Associated injury to the lung is so likely that insertion of chest tubes with sealed underwater drainage is usually required.

Wounds of the Chest

If the physical signs associated with wounds of the chest are to be properly interpreted, one must be familiar with certain classifications and definitions (Fig. 18–3).

Nonpenetrating wounds of the chest wall present the physical features of any soft tissue wound. In contrast to contusions or crushing injuries of the chest, they are not associated with damage to the heart or lungs. On the other hand, *penetrating wounds of the chest (closed)*, even

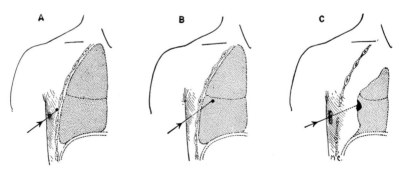

Figure 18–3. A classification of wounds of the chest. *A,* Nonpenetrating wound of the chest. The pleural or pericardial cavities are not entered by the wounding agent. *B,* Penetrating wound of the chest closed. The missile has transversed the pleural space and lung but the opening in the chest wall has sealed. *C,* An open wound of the chest. The wounding agent is so large that it tears an opening in the thoracic cage and leaves a free communication between the pleural space and the outside.

when very small, are associated with some degree of pleural, cardiac, pericardial, or pulmonary damage. The most common of these is simple hemothorax. The physical signs of visceral damage associated with wounds of the chest will be discussed in detail later.

The physical findings associated with an *open wound* are striking. The patient is in great distress, with obvious signs of asphyxiation. Inspiration is labored and expiration is forced. There is marked cyanosis unless there has been an associated loss of blood which produces so severe an anemia that cyanosis cannot be produced. The pulse is rapid and thready and the blood pressure is low. As the air rushes in and out of the wound, an audible sucking sound is created. Inspection of the wound will reveal frothy serum and blood issuing from it with each expiration. These signs will be of lesser degree if the wound is small. There may be crepitation about the wound, which indicates that air is being forced into the soft tissues.

An open sucking wound should be closed by strapping a sterile or clean dressing over it; if the patient experiences marked relief, the diagnosis is confirmed. The closure of a large sucking wound is an emergency procedure which must be carried out as soon as it is recognized. In desperate cases, one should not hesitate to close the wound with anything available, such as a clean cloth pressed over the opening with one's hand. After the sucking wound is closed, a tension pneumothorax may occur because of associated injury to the lung, so that catheter drainage of the pleural space is essential after surgical closure of the defect.

II. INTRATHORACIC INJURIES

A number of intrathoracic lesions occur as complications of crushing injuries, fractured ribs with injury to the underlying pleura or lung, and penetrating wounds of the chest. The basic physical manifestations are essentially the same regardless of cause, and prompt recognition by means of the physical examination may be life-saving.

Hemothorax

Substantial amounts of air and fluid may fill the pleural spaces before the physical signs are obvious. Consequently, in most cases of suspected major thoracic injury, catheters should be introduced into the pleural space or spaces anteriorly with closed drainage.

The extent of the bleeding depends upon the injury. Exsanguinating hemorrhage follows injuries of the main pulmonary artery or internal mammary or intercostal arteries. Venous bleeding leads to a hemothorax with comparatively little circulatory impairment. The signs of hemothorax are those of a pleural effusion. Dullness to flatness on percussion and diminished breath sounds will be found at the base posteriorly on the involved side if the patient is examined in the upright position. There may be a shift in the trachea or mediastinum to the opposite side, and, if the hemorrhage is extensive, the percussion note may be flat over the spines of the lower thoracic vertebrae.

The signs of respiratory impairment will depend initially on the amount of blood in the pleural space. Later, as the hemoglobin breaks down, the initial effusion is often augmented by an additional transudation of fluid greatly exceeding the original volume of hemorrhage. Respiratory embarrassment may suddenly become acute.

Bleeding from a laceration of the parenchyma of the lung is not likely to be excessive, but there is an associated pneumothorax. In such cases hyperresonance, tympany and absent breath sounds will be found above the area of dullness. In the presence of a hemopneumothorax the signs of the pneumothorax tend to be dominant, and rather large collections of blood may produce very few physical signs.

Pneumothorax

The manifestations of a pneumothorax vary with its extent. Small amounts of air in the pleural space are easily missed on physical examination, but if large amounts are present and if the pneumothorax is of sufficient extent to affect the well-being of the patient, the diagnosis can readily be established. When both fluid and air are present, the physical signs are predominantly those of a pneumothorax.

Inspection

There is diminished to absent motion of the chest wall on the affected side. Respirations are increased, dyspnea may be present, and the patient may complain of pain in the chest. The pain of associated lesions, such as a fractured femur, may obscure the symptoms of a pneumothorax. If the patient is in collapse from a tension pneumothorax, particularly with associated blood loss, his complaints may not direct attention to the pneumothorax. Dyspnea and a pallid cyanosis are good clues to the diagnosis but frequently blood loss from other injuries leads to severe pallor rather than cyanosis.

Percussion

The percussion note is distinctly hyperresonant and tympanitic. This may be masked by a pleural effusion posteriorly and dependently. Percussion may indicate a shift in the position of the heart and mediastinum.

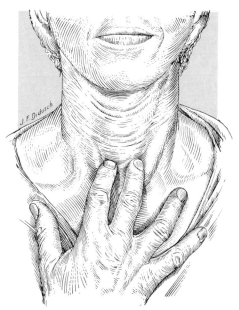

Figure 18–4. Palpation of the trachea, an important maneuver in the appraisal of a pneumothorax.

Palpation

Tactile fremitus is absent. Palpation of the trachea will indicate a shift toward the normal side (Fig. 18–4).

The Coin Test

A coin is pressed against the anterior chest wall and tapped with another coin. While the posterior chest wall is auscultated, a characteristic metallic sound will be heard if there is air in the pleural cavity.

If fluid and air are present and the patient shifts his position suddenly, splashing sounds, the so-called "succussion splash," may be heard. No attempt should be made to elicit this sound by shaking or jarring the patient.

Open Pneumothorax

An open pneumothorax is an invariable consequence of an open wound of the chest wall. The manifestations of the pneumothorax are dominated by the presence of mediastinal flutter and the sucking wound, and there is no reason to demonstrate its presence by physical examination. Attention should be directed at once to closure of the open wound.

Tension Pneumothorax

An untreated tension pneumothorax can be fatal because there is a progressive aspiration and trapping of air in the pleural space from a wound of the lung. More air is drawn into the pleural space from the injured lung with each inspiration; this increases the collapse of that lung, drives the mediastinum further toward the uninvolved side, and reduces the function of the good lung (Fig. 18–5). Tension pneumothorax is apt to develop when an open sucking wound of the chest is closed by packing or strapping. It is commonly seen following penetrating wounds of the chest and is often associated with varying degrees of traumatic emphysema. It may be spontaneous.

Inspection

There is marked dyspnea bordering on suffocation. Cyanosis is a pronounced feature unless there has been an extensive loss of blood. Col-

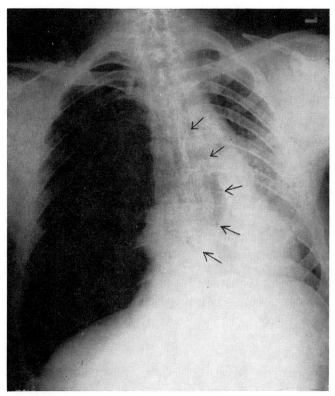

Figure 18–5. An x-ray of the chest showing the extreme mediastinal shift which may occur in a tension pneumothorax.

lapse, with a thready pulse and marked hypotension, results from cardiac embarrassment and the prevention of an adequate venous return to the heart. It is vital not to confuse the circulatory collapse associated with a tension pneumothorax with that seen in hemorrhage or shock. Cyanosis and dyspnea are the best clues which can be noted on inspection.

Palpation

The trachea will be shifted toward the opposite side, as is the apex impulse of the heart (Fig. 18–5).

Percussion

When there is marked tension from pressure of air within the thoracic cage, the percussion note is generally tympanitic, but may be dull due to lack of vibration of the chest wall. Absence of hyperresonance and tympany *does not exclude* a pneumothorax.

Percussion of the mediastinum will provide confirmatory evidence of the shift which has already been noted by palpation of the trachea.

Auscultation

Breath sounds are generally absent; if heard, they will be muffled, hollow, and amphoric. The "coin test" will be positive, but it is not necessary to elicit it.

Aspiration

Aspiration of the trapped air must be done as an emergency procedure. Since it is life-saving, it will be briefly described. The patient should be in the supine position. A one and one-half inch needle with syringe attached should be introduced into the second interspace anteriorly on the involved side. Aspiration should be gently applied to the syringe as the needle is introduced. Sufficient air should be removed to bring about relief of symptoms. As soon as possible, a tube thoracostomy should be performed, because recurrence of the tension pneumothorax is very likely after expansion of the lung.

Under strict sterile conditions, a small incision is made in the second or third intercostal interspace. As the incision is deepened, a finger is introduced into the pleural space to be sure that it has been properly entered; a chest tube is inserted. The tube is placed on suction and later attached to an underwater seal.

Subcutaneous Emphysema and Mediastinal Emphysema

Whenever the lung is injured, air may escape from it with each inspiration and produce tension pneumothorax or traumatic emphysema or both. In traumatic emphysema the air is forced into tissue planes around the wound from which it may spread subcutaneously for variable distances. The physical signs are those of local swelling, edema, and crepitation. Compression injuries involving rib fracture are the most common cause of traumatic emphysema. The violent compression closes the glottis, fractures the ribs, stabs the lung with a rib fragment, and during the instant of tremendous intrathoracic pressure, air is injected along the tissue planes around the ribs into the parietes. As the violent compression passes, the ribs and chest wall spring back and intrathoracic dynamics return to normal. Thus air may be "injected" into the chest wall from the lung without causing a pneumothorax.

The most common cause of mediastinal emphysema is broncheolar or alveolar rupture in the lung without rupture of the visceral pleura. This rupture site then leaks air into the peribronchial planes during inspiration and cannot return it to the airways during expiration. This ball-valve effect may send large amounts of air out the superior aperture of the mediastinum into the subcutaneous tissues over the body. It may then spread with great rapidity, producing fantastic swelling of the neck, face, chest wall, abdominal wall, and scrotum (Fig. 18–6). There is little respi-

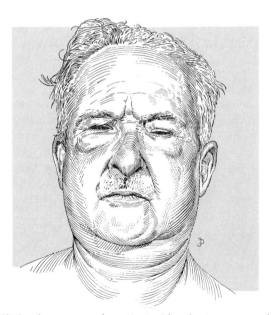

Figure 18–6.   Appearance of a patient with subcutaneous emphysema.

ratory distress, although the appearance of the patient is frightening and dramatic. One should suspect a tension pneumothorax or progressive mediastinal emphysema if dyspnea and cyanosis are present.

Mediastinal emphysema may develop sufficient tension to produce embarrassment to the heart and great veins. In such cases the air is not escaping freely from the mediastinum into the subcutaneous tissues but is accumulating in the mediastinum under pressure. There should be considerably less evidence of generalized emphysema. Auscultation over the base of the heart may reveal a crackling sound synchronous with the heartbeat, the so-called "mediastinal crunch." This sign is strongly suggestive of early mediastinal emphysema. Later on, crepitus may be elicited in the suprasternal notch as the air dissects upward. Percussion should reveal hyperresonance over the sternum. A combination of these physical findings associated with circulatory failure not explained by other causes may be an indication for cervical mediastinotomy. At times, simple aspiration of air from the supraclavicular area suffices to reduce the compression.

Cardiac Tamponade

Oozing of blood from the heart into the pericardial space may occur when the heart is injured either by penetrating wounds or by compression injuries of the chest. This accumulation of blood within the pericardium produces a progressive compression of the heart and obstruction of the great veins. Cardiac filling is impossible and death follows since the heart receives too little blood to maintain an effective output. The recognition of the condition is vital, since aspiration of the pericardium is life-saving. In many wounds of the heart, death results from cardiac tamponade rather than from exsanguinating hemorrhage.

Inspection

Inspection will reveal dyspnea, respiratory embarrassment, and a pallid cyanosis. The high venous pressure is manifested by distention of the neck veins.

Percussion

There may be a widening of the mediastinal dullness, but this is not a reliable sign. Serious tamponade may result from rapid effusions which do not appreciably enlarge the area of cardiac dullness and do not produce significant enlargement of the cardiac shadow on an x-ray film.

Auscultation

The heart sounds are rapid and faint; the blood pressure is low, and there is a diminished pulse pressure. The systolic pressure falls, and the diastolic level rises. Pulsus paradoxicus is present and is best detected with the sphygmomanometer. The systolic pressure falls with each inspiration. This is demonstrated by maintaining the cuff pressure at the level at which systolic sounds are first heard. With each inspiratory effort the sounds will disappear.

These findings in the presence of a crushing injury or penetrating wound of the chest are sufficient to establish the diagnosis.

Fluoroscopy

If readily available, this should be done, as it will demonstrate diminished cardiac pulsation.

Pericardiocentesis

Pericardiocentesis provides conclusive evidence of hemopericardium. Since this procedure may be life-saving, it is described in some detail. The costoxiphoid angle on the left is generally used; a No. 18, 3-inch needle is directed upward at an angle of 45 degrees to the abdomen and midline. If possible, the central venous pressure should be monitored and an electrocardiograph lead attached to the needle. A marked change in the electrocardiograph appears on contact with the heart by the needle. If an electrocardiographic lead is not available, contact with the heart produces a grating sensation, calling for immediate withdrawal of the needle. In most instances the needle is advanced slowly with gentle tension maintained on the syringe. If blood is present, it will be encountered at once.

Intrathoracic Injury without Visible Damage to the Chest Wall

It is not generally realized that severe intrathoracic damage frequently occurs from blows, contusions, or crushes which produce no evidence of injury to the chest wall. These may take the form of any of the lesions described above or may fall into one of several special categories characteristic of crushing injuries.

TRAUMATIC ASPHYXIA

This rare but traumatic syndrome follows violent compression of the thorax. It is probably due to the reflux of blood with a sudden increase in pressure in the great veins of the thorax. There is intense purplish to black cyanosis of the face, neck, and upper chest. The tissues of the face are particularly edematous, and there are extensive subconjunctival hemorrhages. There may be diffuse petechial hemorrhages over the face and upper chest. There is comparatively little impairment of cardiac and pulmonary function in many instances, although the appearance of the patient is frightening. In other cases the injury may be associated with underlying pulmonary damage which is manifested by dyspnea and hemoptysis. Immediate transient loss of consciousness is common. Transient episodes of delirium or other mental aberrations occurring as late as 4 to 14 days after the accident have been ascribed to cerebral hemorrhage and edema.

CONTUSION OF THE LUNG

Extensive pulmonary damage may occur without the slightest evidence of damage to the chest wall. In such cases inspection reveals marked dyspnea, and the patient coughs up frothy or bloodstained sputum. Percussion of the chest shows varying degrees of dullness in proportion to the amount of pulmonary damage. Breath sounds are diminished, and there are usually crepitant to quite coarse bubbling rales. The findings are essentially those of a localized bronchial pneumonia. Differential diagnosis is made possible since the physical findings are present immediately following an injury, and this is much too soon for an inflammatory lesion to have developed. Very careful physical examination of the lungs should be performed in order to exclude unsuspected pulmonary damage whenever a history of crushing injury to the chest is obtained.

TRAUMATIC WET LUNG

The lung may be contused by direct impact or by rapid deceleration injuries. The initial response of the lung to contusion is a marked increase in secretions often associated with an inability to clear the fluid from the bronchi. Pulmonary edema, severe bronchorrhea, and bronchospasm follow.

Inspection

The patient produces copious amounts of frothy white or bloodstained sputum. He is cyanotic and dyspneic.

Palpation

There may be splinting of the injured side. Coarse tracheal and bronchial rhonchi may be perceptible to the hand.

Auscultation

Moist rales of all grades are interspersed with expiratory sibilant and sonorous sounds.

Tracheobronchial aspiration, intubation, and assisted respiration are required. The condition is often associated with other injuries of the chest wall.

CONTUSION OF THE HEART AND PERICARDIUM

Syncopal attacks, cardiac irregularities, bizarre murmurs, and death may ensue from contusions of the chest wall. One should not be misled by the fact that there is no sign of an external injury. The injury may result in extensive valvular damage or rupture of the heart. In other cases, careful auscultation will be necessary to reveal faint cardiac murmurs or friction rubs. Arrhythmias may develop. The findings may be identical with those seen following coronary occlusion. Recognition of such injuries is vital because occasionally the patient's general condition may not be seriously impaired at the time of the first examination, but his management should be similar to that following a coronary occlusion.

Traumatic Rupture of the Thoracic Aorta

Patients subjected to sudden deceleration injuries of the anterior chest wall or clavicle with fractures of the sternum should always be suspected of having a possible traumatic rupture of the thoracic aorta. With complete rupture most patients die before reaching the hospital, but in approximately 20 per cent of cases an acute false aneurysm is formed, the majority of which then rupture within the next few days or weeks. Rarely, the aneurysm becomes stabilized and is discovered as a mediastinal mass on routine x-rays taken many months or years later.

Except for the pain of the associated sternal or clavicular injuries, there may be no specific symptoms. Sometimes with a rapidly expanding false aneurysm there may be increasing chest pain, shortness of breath, difficulty in swallowing, and hemoptysis.

In all suspected cases an emergency chest x-ray should be done, and, if a wide mediastinum and a vaguely outlined aortic knob are present, an emergency aortogram should be performed. Acute medical emergency measures involve the use of hypotensive agents to reduce the blood pressure. Left heart bypass or a temporary external shunt is necessary to permit safe cross clamping of the aorta and operative repair, following which the prognosis is excellent.

chapter 19   # ABDOMINAL INJURIES

An abdominal injury involving rupture of a viscus or hemorrhage from a major vessel is one of the most challenging of surgical problems. It is the most lethal of all injuries which do not cause instant death, since the mortality rate in untreated or badly treated cases approaches 100 per cent. Yet prompt recognition, an accurate estimate of the extent and nature of the injury, and early operation will salvage the vast majority of such patients.

I. PENETRATING WOUNDS

Practically all penetrating wounds of the abdomen, excepting shotgun wounds, and very carefully selected stab wounds, require surgical exploration. There is more to the problem, however, than noting a wound of entrance, treating shock, and carrying out an exploratory laparotomy. The same principles which govern the triage of abdominal wounds of warfare must be applied in the appraisal of the individual patient with a penetrating abdominal injury.

Factors which directly affect the interpretation of the physical findings are:
1. The time which has elapsed since the injury.
2. The nature of the wounding agent.
3. The position of the patient when hit.
4. The therapy or medication which has been given since the injury.

The Time Factor

The time lag is one of the most important single factors in assessing the gravity of an abdominal wound. Under eight hours the prognosis is directly related to the character and multiplicity of the injuries. After eight hours, however, even in simple wounds of the small bowel, the mortality

341

rate rises rapidly. The interpretation of hypotension or shock depends to a considerable extent on the time lag. Profound collapse within a few hours of injury indicates persistent bleeding or massive peritoneal contamination. Persistent hypotension not responding to resuscitation 12 hours or more after wounding is more likely to be due to infection and peritonitis.

The Wounding Agent

Bullet wounds and stab wounds are the least damaging. Severe collapse shortly after a stab wound or bullet wound is probably due to hemorrhage. *High-velocity shells* are the most serious as they produce an expansion and subsequent contraction of the abdominal cavity which damages the viscera far beyond the direct path of the missile. It is as if an explosion occurred within the peritoneal cavity. The wounding of the viscera greatly exceeds that which might be expected from the appearance, size, and location of the wounds of entrance and exit. A direct hit in the epigastrium or midabdomen from a shotgun at short range is lethal. Rarely, a shotgun wound may tear away part of the abdomen and allow surgical salvage. At long ranges, recovery may ensue. The many small, diffusely scattered, penetrating wounds of the bowel cannot be dealt with surgically, but the small size of the wounds frequently allows them to seal spontaneously. Thus the problem is that of the conservative management of peritonitis.

At intermediate ranges, the surgeon must use his own judgment. Exploration is the wiser course in doubtful situations.

The Position of the Patient When Hit

The exact position of the patient when hit is of importance in estimating the probable course of a missile, especially if there is no wound of exit (Fig. 19–1). Reconstruction of the mechanics of injury, particularly in wounds of the thighs or buttocks, will often indicate the probability of an abdominal wound when it might not otherwise have been expected. The likelihood of an associated chest wound may become immediately apparent if the position of the patient at the time of injury is considered. Frequently the exact position of the patient cannot be determined, but at operation the surgeon must always anticipate far more damage than might be predicted from the location of the wounds of entrance and exit or the position of the retained missile.

Previous Treatment and Medication

The amount of emergency fluid replacement or morphine which has been given must be taken into consideration in assaying the physical state

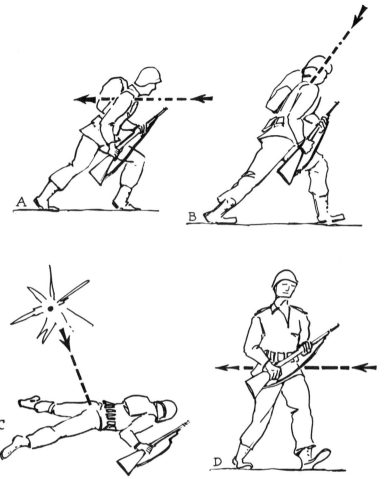

Figure 19–1. Effect of position and trajectory on the probable course of a penetrating missile. *A,* Shoulder wound; abdominal wound excluded. *B,* Shoulder wound; thoracic and abdominal injury probable. *C,* Buttock wound; abdominal wound probable; *D,* Buttock wound; abdominal wound excluded.

of a wounded person. Persistent hypotension after large amounts of blood have been given, particularly if the time lag is considerable, suggests extensive peritoneal soiling and sepsis.

Abdominal wounds are often painful. If morphine is given subcutaneously when the patient is in shock, it may not be absorbed. Because of continued pain, additional morphine may be given. After resuscitation, all the morphine is absorbed, with resulting overdosage. The slow breathing, coma, and pinpoint pupils are readily identified but may be mistaken for a head injury if the circumstances are not appreciated.

To avoid overdosage, morphine should be given by the intravenous route in small repeated doses as required to control pain.

The Physical Examination

In cases of profound shock, replacement therapy must be instituted as the physical examination is being performed. The insertion of major intravenous lines for infusion and for monitoring central venous pressure takes precedence over the physical examination. The pulse, respiration, and blood pressure must be noted and recorded at frequent intervals. The patient should be completely stripped. A rapid physical examination of the "survey type" is done with particular attention being given to the location, size, and appearance of all wounds. Reconstruction of the mechanics of wounding and the appearance of the wound edges usually leave no doubt as to which is the wound of entrance or exit, if there be one. However, high-velocity missiles may produce explosive shattering exit wounds and such small and insignificant wounds of entrance that these can easily be overlooked. A careful scrutiny of the buttocks, perineum, and anal canal is of the utmost importance. In cases of multiple wounds the patient is often unaware of the location of many of the wounds, particularly of the small wounds of entrance.

The appearance of the wound may give immediate information as to the character of the visceral injury, since blood, bile, or intestinal contents may be oozing from it or bowel may have prolapsed into it. Undigested food particles in the wound indicate a gastric perforation. The character of the wound will govern, to a considerable extent, the need for more detailed examination of the abdomen. Obviously, in the presence of an open abdominal wound with partial prolapse of bowel, a lengthy examination of the abdomen is not indicated. In small wounds of entrance, a more detailed examination is required. In cases of penetrating wounds of the back, thighs, or buttocks with potential but not definite abdominal damage, a very careful assay of the abdominal findings is necessary, much as in a patient with a questionable acute appendicitis. Inspection, auscultation, palpation and percussion, all directed toward finding minimal evidence of peritoneal irritation, must be performed. A rectal examination is essential. A skillfully performed proctosigmoidoscopy, using little or no air insufflation, is a most important means of assaying the extent of rectal or colonic injury associated with wounds of the buttocks.

Severe abdominal pain and rigidity with hypotension may result from wounds of the spinal cord alone. Consequently, in all suspected abdominal injuries one must be certain that the patient can move his legs and that there is no peripheral neurologic deficit.

Physical Signs of Penetrating Abdominal Injury

Hemorrhage, peritoneal irritation, and shock of varying degree accompany all abdominal wounds. All gradations and combinations occur, but in a general way three components may be described.

HEMORRHAGE

Hemorrhage may be rapidly exsanguinating, especially in wounds involving the aorta or cava. The patient may appear lifeless and unresponsive, with no obtainable pulse or blood pressure. "Coma with shock" means cerebral ischemia, not cerebral injury. Cardiac massage, massive rapid infusion of fluid, and an immediate operation is often life-saving. Massive but more slowly progressive hemorrhage is often seen in wounds of the liver or spleen. The clinical picture is one of progressive shock with tachycardia, hypotension, sweating, anxiety, thirst, and air hunger. The abdominal findings may not be alarming. Deep tenderness and a sense of fullness may be the only signs. Peristalsis may be quiet or active. Progressive swelling of the abdomen will be evident on repeated observation.

In less severe hemorrhage the findings are indefinite. The pulse rate is of less value than are its quality and fullness. A comparatively normal blood pressure may be maintained but with a narrowing pulse pressure. The trend of the pulse and the blood pressure is of more importance than the actual value. In slow but steady bleeding, the circulation may remain comparatively stable; the physical findings in the abdomen become more significant. Progressive abdominal tenderness, the development of spasm, and signs of shifting dullness within the abdomen may be better indications of continued bleeding than are the levels of the pulse and blood pressure. Progressive swelling of the abdomen as measured by a string tied around it is a very important finding.

PERITONITIS

A penetrating wound involving a major viscus, such as the stomach or colon, may produce the characteristic picture of acute peritonitis, such as is seen in free perforation of gastric or duodenal ulcer. The classic features of acute perforation may be lacking if there are multiple injuries, if medication has been given, or if there has been a significant time lag between injury and hospital admission.

Unless there is associated bleeding, shock is usually slower to appear than with hemorrhage. Severe hypotension shortly after wounding always suggests bleeding. In the late stages after eight or more hours, cyanosis, anxious facies, rapid respiration, and persistent hypotension are indicative of rapidly progressive abdominal sepsis.

SHOCK

Most penetrating wounds of the abdomen result in a combination of hemorrhage and peritonitis. The indication for operation is the presence of the penetrating wound, and operation must be undertaken as soon as possible, consistent with adequate resuscitation. As noted above, however, in massive exsanguinating bleeding, resuscitation and operation take place simultaneously.

On the other hand, when for some reason or another there has been a substantial delay between wounding and admission for definitive care, it is evident that exsanguination is not the problem since the patient would have long since expired. The clinical picture is now one of advanced peritonitis combined with varying degrees of blood loss. Infection from massive contamination of the peritoneal cavity, or a spreading peritonitis or retroperitoneal cellulitis, may produce a state of almost total loss of vasomotor tone. This is septic shock in an advanced stage with circulatory and high-output respiratory failure. Response to fluid replacement is poor and must be combined with continuous monitoring of central venous pressure, blood pressure, and urinary output. As in the respiratory distress syndrome, measurements of arterial Po_2, Pco_2, and pH are critical in the total evaluation of the patient.

Prompt operation with relief of abdominal distention, removal of massive amounts of blood and bowel contents from the peritoneal cavity, control of bleeding, and closure of intestinal wounds are as critical to resuscitation as is control of bleeding in an aortic wound.

Failure of the blood pressure to respond to transfusion is a clinical syndrome, not a specific physiologic state. From a practical point of view, the most important causes are exsanguinating hemorrhage which is not being adequately replaced and septic shock. If the time lag is minimal, the former is clearly responsible and immediate operation is necessary. If the time lag is long, the latter is more likely. Rarely, an explosive wound of the colon in which the peritoneal cavity is literally drenched with liquid feces will produce a state of septic shock immediately.

In septic shock, if blood loss has not been great, the initial pattern may be one of "hyperdynamic shock." The extremities are warm and dry. There is marked hypotension, oliguria, and hyperventilation. Central venous pressure will be high and arterial pH low, with a respiratory alkalosis.

If there has been significant blood loss or marked loss of fluid from damaged or necrotic bowel, or if extensive peritonitis is present, the picture is essentially that of hypovolemic shock with a low blood pressure, lowered central venous pressure, low urinary output, and cold cyanotic facies and extremities.

In this situation, every effort must be made to correct fluid losses and provide respiratory and circulatory support, but operation is essential to resuscitation.

An "irreversible state" in the late hours after abdominal wounding is principally a matter of progressive infection. Blood loss may be a contributing factor, but continued or recurrent bleeding is uncommon. Clostridial infections, retroperitoneal cellulitis spreading from a wound of the rectum, and advanced peritonitis are the clinical states most frequently encountered. The situation may be beyond control, but here again the physical findings are of the greatest importance. Drainage of accessible infection and débridement of necrotic gangrenous tissue, when combined with massive antibiotic therapy, may tide the patient over what has seemed a hopeless situation.

Forty-eight hours or more after wounding and frequently after definitive treatment has been accomplished, malnutrition of extraordinarily rapid onset, electrolyte and fluid imbalance, and renal failure become dominant factors in the management of the patient. Careful monitoring of all biochemical parameters, combined with judicious use of hyperalimentation, has vastly improved care. Here again, however, persistent infection may be a crucial factor. Careful daily repeated examinations searching for signs of residual abscesses in the wound, in the peritoneal cavity, in the retroperitoneal spaces, or beneath the diaphragm are of vital importance. No amount of antibiotic or replacement therapy is a substitute for adequate drainage of residual abscesses.

The exciting feature of all abdominal wounds is that despite their enormous gravity, if the man recovers, he is a whole man.

II. NONPENETRATING ABDOMINAL INJURIES

The liver, the spleen, the intestines, the stomach, and even the pancreas may be ruptured by blows which leave no mark or bruise on the abdominal wall (Fig. 19–2). If the abdomen is relaxed and the spine flexed, the abdominal viscera may be directly bruised or may be crushed between the wounding agent and the vertebral column or posterior parietes.

The physical signs depend largely upon the organ injured and the extent of bleeding or peritoneal contamination. Shortly after the injury the abdomen may appear quite normal. A full-blown perforation syndrome is rare in nonpenetrating abdominal wounds, since the usual points of injury to the bowel are posterior and somewhat protected from the abdominal wall by the omentum. Lacerations of the small intestine occur at fixed points, namely, the duodenojejunal flexures and the junction of the terminal ileum and cecum. Although the colon may be ruptured, it is more apt to suffer extensive mesenteric tears with impairment of blood supply. Progressive gangrene and necrosis then result in a peritonitis which takes some little time to develop. Hemorrhage may be so massive and exsanguinating that the patient dies almost immediately, or it may be so slowly progressive that it is difficult to recognize.

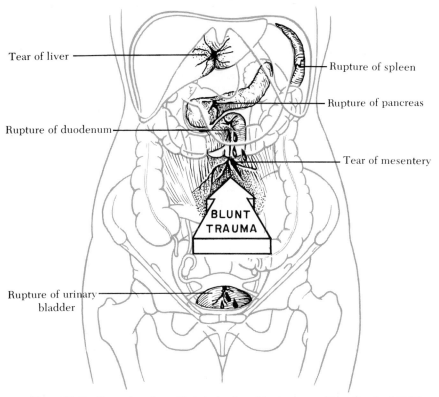

Tear of liver

Rupture of spleen

Rupture of pancreas

Rupture of duodenum

Tear of mesentery

BLUNT
TRAUMA

Rupture of urinary
bladder

Figure 19–2. Examples of specific injuries from blunt trauma. (From Botsford, T. W., and Wilson, R. E.: The Acute Abdomen. Vol. X in Major Problems in Clinical Surgery. Philadelphia, W. B. Saunders Co., 1969.)

In every case frequently repeated examinations of the abdomen are essential. Progression of the abdominal signs is of more importance than the findings on a single examination. If doubt exists, abdominal paracentesis with peritoneal lavage is essential to early diagnosis of intra-abdominal hemorrhage.

Rupture of the Liver

Contusion or rupture of the liver may be caused by a blow over, or severe compression of, the lower portion of the thoracic cage or the upper abdomen. The mechanism of the injury may suggest the probability of hepatic injury. The physical manifestations are dependent upon the extent of the injury.

Massive rupture of the liver results in exsanguinating hemorrhage. In less severe injuries, the signs are those of intraperitoneal hemorrhage, namely, abdominal pain, tenderness, swelling with hypotension, and diminished urinary output. Initially, the signs may be minimal but later sudden hypotension and collapse occur. In massive rupture the initial picture may be one of collapse and coma with cerebral ischemia. Emergency operation with cannulation of the vena cava and control of bleeding now permits salvage of many formerly lethal cases.

A central rupture of the liver may occur without intraperitoneal bleeding but with hemorrhage into the bile ducts and bleeding into the upper gastrointestinal tract (hemobilia). The bleeding may not occur for some hours or days. Gastrointestinal bleeding, days, weeks, or even months after blunt abdominal injury, may be due to a central rupture of the liver.

Rupture of the Extrahepatic Biliary Tract

Blunt trauma in the region of the gallbladder which is sufficient to produce a laceration usually involves the liver. Isolated injury of the common bile duct, however, occurs as a distinct entity.

Direct blunt trauma over the upper abdomen may shear the common duct at the point where it enters the pancreas. If the injury involves the common duct alone, shock and hemorrhage do not occur. The patient, in fact, may complain of very little pain. Bile leaks steadily into the peritoneal cavity, producing biliary ascites for which the patient may not seek medical attention for many hours or days. Uninfected bile is comparatively innocuous. The condition should be suspected when a patient presents with ascites some time after suffering a severe blow on the abdomen which did not appear to produce any serious injury.

Rupture of the Spleen

Rupture of the spleen is a fairly common injury. It may follow severe contusions or blows on the flank or it may be precipitated by very mild trauma. Two forms are generally recognized: immediate and delayed rupture.

In *immediate rupture* there is a history of a blow on the flank or left lower thoracic cage followed by severe abdominal pain, pain in the left shoulder, dyspnea, and shock. The physical findings are those of an acute peritoneal irritation in the left upper abdomen. There are spasm and tenderness of the musculature, plus the signs of progressive intra-abdominal bleeding. Diaphragmatic irritation is manifested by an increased respiratory rate, pain on breathing, and pain in the left shoulder. An interesting and important sign, if positive, is the elicitation of pain by pressure in the neck over the course of the phrenic nerve on the left side. Pressure should be made just under the sternomastoid a little above its clavicular attachment.

The clinical picture is not always so definite. Minor lacerations of the spleen may lead to slowly progressive intraperitoneal bleeding with much less evidence of diaphragmatic and peritoneal irritation. One may be hard pressed to ascertain that there is an intra-abdominal injury with bleeding. Abdominal paracentesis and arteriography are required in doubtful cases.

Delayed rupture of the spleen. A comparatively mild blow in the flank may produce a subcapsular rupture of the spleen with so few symptoms that the patient does not seek medical advice. Several days or more later, rupture occurs with shock, intraperitoneal hemorrhage, and evidence of peritoneal irritation.

On occasion these patients enter the hospital with what appears to be a huge, tender, left upper abdominal tumor and a secondary anemia. Unless the story of an injury is obtained, one may easily mistake the condition for a retroperitoneal tumor. Percussion will indicate that the mass lies anterior to the colon. An x-ray may be helpful inasmuch as it will show the abdominal mass lying above and anterior to the colon rather than behind it as would be the case in a retroperitoneal tumor. Arteriography has proved helpful in doubtful cases of acute as well as delayed rupture of the spleen.

Spontaneous rupture of the spleen. Large diseased spleens, the seat of malaria, leukemia, or infectious mononucleosis, may rupture spontaneously. Very mild trauma may be a factor.

Rupture of the Small Intestine

The small intestine may be ruptured by having a gas-filled loop of bowel compressed against the vertebral column or posterior parietes in such a manner that air is trapped in it under pressure and the lumen of the bowel is burst. Since the small intestine is freely movable and ordinarily does not contain much gas, this is a rare occurrence. More commonly the small intestine is torn at its point of fixation at the duodenojejunal flexure or at the terminal ileum. The duodenum, because of its fixed position, may easily be ruptured. Since these areas are posterior, the leakage of bowel contents does not immediately contaminate the free peritoneal cavity, and the signs of peritonitis may develop rather slowly. Spasm and abdominal rigidity are late signs. It may be difficult to establish a diagnosis of peritonitis until it is fully developed.

Rupture of the Duodenum

The duodenum is frequently injured in major blunt trauma involving the pancreas. Isolated injury of the duodenum is also common; it is usually due to a shearing force which tears the duodenum retroperitoneally so that there is no free leakage of duodenal contents into the peritoneal cavity. Retroperitoneal bleeding may be extensive.

An intramural hematoma of the duodenum may be found in partial rupture. Less commonly, the duodenum is injured without signs which are sufficient to require laparotomy. Progression of the duodenal hematoma produces obstructive symptoms involving the duodenum and common bile duct. The lesion may be suspected of being a tumor unless its relationship with trauma is established. Rarely, spontaneous hematomas of the duodenum occur, particularly in patients receiving anticoagulants.

Rupture of the Pancreas

The pancreas, duodenum, and bile duct may all be crushed in severe blunt trauma. The clinical picture is one of rapidly progressive shock from combined hemorrhage and peritoneal contamination. On the other hand, the body of the pancreas may be completely divided as it crosses the vertebral column as a result of isolated blunt trauma without injury of any other organ. Because of the retroperitoneal position of the pancreas, the initial findings may be so minimal that major abdominal injury is not suspected. Over a matter of hours the clinical picture consistent with acute pancreatitis (deep-seated abdominal pain, steadily progressive peritoneal signs, and shock) develops. Operation with pancreatic resection is life-saving.

Rupture of the Large Intestine

The large intestine is more apt to be devitalized by huge mesenteric rents and tears than to be ruptured. Necrosis and gangrene with eventual perforation of the bowel occur. When first seen, however, although the patient may be in considerable pain, the signs of peritonitis are lacking. The clinical picture is not unlike that seen in mesenteric vascular occlusion. Repeated examinations of the abdomen are necessary to ascertain that there is a progressing intra-abdominal lesion.

chapter 20

INJURIES OF THE KIDNEY, BLADDER, AND URETHRA; FRACTURED PELVIS

I. INJURIES OF THE KIDNEY

Penetrating wounds of the kidney as the principal injury are very rare. Wounds of the kidney are usually associated with injury to other viscera, and the presenting problem is that of a penetrating abdominal wound. On the other hand, contusion or rupture of the kidney from a blow on the flank or a fall is a fairly common injury despite the protected position of the organ.

The cardinal symptoms of renal injury are pain in the flank and hematuria. In mild ruptures pain may be minimal, and the principal evidence of renal damage is blood in the urine. In severe ruptures hematuria may not occur because of rupture of the ureter or occlusion of the renal pelvis or ureter by clotted blood. Physical signs relate to hemorrhage and extravasation of urine into the renal fossa and the flank on the affected side. Initial loss of blood may be serious, but exsanguinating hemorrhage is rare. The local signs consist of muscle spasm, tenderness, and fullness in the flank on the affected side. A mass may be palpable. The fullness in the flank is often better appreciated by inspection than by palpation, particularly in the thin subject. Ecchymosis may develop in the flank, and there may be nonshifting dullness to percussion lateral to the rectus muscle. Psoas spasm with flexion of the thigh on the affected side may occur from retroperitoneal extravasation of blood or urine overlying the psoas muscle.

The differential diagnosis between an injury to the spleen or liver and a renal injury is often extremely difficult. As a rule the physical signs of renal injury are primarily in the flank. Hematuria, ecchymosis and fullness in the flank, tenderness in the flank and costovertebral angles, psoas spasm, and nonshifting dullness point to a renal injury. Progressive abdominal spasm, particularly involving the rectus muscle on the opposite side, shifting dullness, diminished peristalsis, and evidence of continued intraperitoneal bleeding are indicative of hepatic or splenic injuries. Rapidly progressive shock is indicative of intra-abdominal rather than renal injury. There are instances in which a differential diagnosis is impossible, and at operation it may be found that an injury of the spleen or liver, depending upon the side involved, has occurred concomitantly with a renal injury.

In obvious uncomplicated renal injury an intravenous pyelogram provides definitive information as to the extent of the injury and the state of the uninvolved kidney. It is useless, however, to attempt intravenous pyelography in the presence of shock and hypotension. Even in the presence of multiple injuries, intravenous pyelography is valuable in demonstrating or excluding renal injury. Blunt trauma and crushing injuries frequently cause extensive retroperitoneal bleeding which, if stable, may be best left undisturbed at laparotomy. Under these circumstances, it is essential to know that there is no renal or ureteral injury.

II. INJURIES OF THE BLADDER AND URETHRA

Injuries to the bladder and intrapelvic portion of the urethra occur chiefly as complications of fracture of the pelvis. Injury of the bulbous urethra usually is occasioned by a fall astride, with contusion or penetration of the perineum. The possibility of damage to the lower urinary tract must be considered in all fractures of the pelvis and in all perineal wounds and contusions.

Much can be established by determining when the patient last voided. If the bladder was emptied shortly before the accident, an intraperitoneal rupture is extremely unlikely, and serious injuries to the membranous urethra or neck of the bladder may be expected only if there is considerable fragmentation of the pelvic bones. *If the patient voided clear urine* since the accident, serious injury to the lower urinary tract can be excluded. *If the patient has not voided* for some time prior to the accident or if the bladder was known to be full at the time of the accident, and the patient is unable to void, the probability of injury to the lower urinary tract is very high. The passage of a little bloody urine or the presence of blood at the urethral meatus makes such an injury certain.

Catheterization should not be done until the physical findings have been carefully appraised. If it can be clearly determined that there is no injury to the membranous urethra or neck of the bladder, catheterization should be done, as it is a valuable means of assaying the presence of an intraperitoneal rupture of the bladder. If the physical findings point to injury of the bladder neck or membranous urethra, catheterization should be postponed and carried out only by those who will be responsible for the surgical management of the lesion. Untold damage may be done by persistent inept and futile efforts to pass a catheter in the face of major injuries to the extraperitoneal portion of the bladder or intrapelvic portion of the urethra. A cystourethrogram is an essential diagnostic step in all suspected injuries of the lower urinary tract.

Intraperitoneal Rupture of the Bladder

This occurs only if the bladder was full at the time of injury. The diagnosis of rupture of the bladder should always be considered in an alcoholic who has had a "bad fall" and presents with mild abdominal tenderness. The physical findings are those of a mild peritonitis. Urine is not a necrotizing fluid and its presence in the peritoneal cavity, although it eventually leads to infection and peritonitis, does not produce striking physical findings. Deep tenderness and slight muscle spasm may be the only signs initially. A rectal examination may disclose more tenderness than the abdominal examination. It will also demonstrate that the prostate is normal in position and that there is no edema, tenderness, or fullness surrounding the membranous urethra (Fig. 20–1 A). In the female, the entire floor of the bladder and urethra are readily palpated, and major injury is easily excluded.

Having determined that the urethra and bladder neck are not damaged, catheterization should be done to confirm the presence of a bladder rupture by the finding of a small amount of bloody urine.

Rupture of the Bladder Neck or Membranous Urethra

This results in an extravasation of blood and urine into the retroperitoneal tissues surrounding the bladder and extending on to the deeper portions of the anterior abdominal wall. There is no peritoneal or immediate scrotal or perineal extravasation. The extravasated urine surrounds the extraperitoneal portion of the bladder and is often difficult to distinguish from a large, round, tender, full bladder (Fig. 20–1 B). There is a tendency, however, for the palpable mass to be broad, to extend more laterally, and to be less symmetric than a full bladder. Gentle compression will elicit tenderness and usually does not evoke a desire on the part of the patient to void.

The rectal examination provides information of crucial importance since it will distinguish between rupture of the bladder neck and rupture of the membranous urethra (Fig. 20–1 C). If the prostate is normal in position and can be clearly palpated and identified, the rupture has occurred above it in the bladder neck. If the prostate cannot be felt and its presence is replaced by a boggy, tender mass, the rupture has occurred in

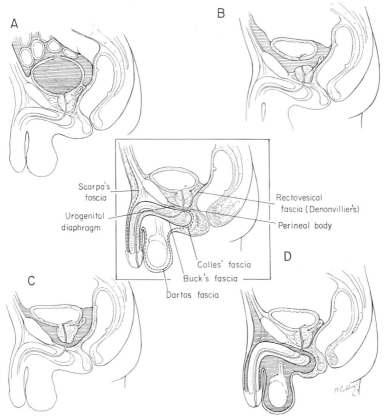

Figure 20–1. Extravasation of urine in injuries of the bladder and urethra. *A,* Intraperitoneal rupture of the bladder. *B,* Rupture of the bladder neck above the prostate gland. There is an extraperitoneal extravasation around the bladder and into the space of Retzius. The prostate remains in its normal position. *C,* Complete rupture of the membranous urethra. The extravasation occurs in the same planes but the prostate cannot be felt. It is replaced by a boggy mass of extravasated urine and blood. *D,* Rupture of the bulbous urethra. The extravasated urine extends into the perineum and scrotum and underneath the superficial fascia of the lower abdominal wall. Center insert shows the fascial layers of the perineum.

the membranous urethra. If both layers of the urogenital diaphragm are torn, as may occur in very extensive injuries, urine and blood may extravasate into the perineum, the periprostatic spaces, and up into the prevesical space.

Perineal extravasation, a mass replacing the prostate, or deep tenderness and fullness around the neck of the bladder are indications for surgical intervention. The importance of a thorough x-ray study of the lower urinary tract by urethrograms and cystograms is emphasized.

Rupture of the Bulbous Urethra

The bulbous urethra is injured by blows or wounds on the perineum. Such an injury commonly occurs when individuals fall astride. The extravasated urine lies anterior to the triangular ligament and extends into the perineum and scrotum, and under the superficial portions of the abdominal wall (Fig. 20–1 *D*). The nature of the injury, the prompt appearance of ecchymosis, edema and fullness in the perineum, and the superficial character of the extravasation on the anterior abdominal wall should point clearly to an injury to the bulbous rather than the membranous urethra. Here again catheterization should not be done until facilities for properly dealing with the urethral injuries are available. The patient should be urged not to void, since the passage of urine will only increase the extent of the extravasation.

III. FRACTURED PELVIS

The extent of a pelvic fracture should be appraised by gentle compression and distraction of the wings of the ilium and by palpation of the symphysis and the pubic rami. An x-ray will be necessary to determine the full extent of the bony injury and to determine whether or not there has been extensive fragmentation.

If a fractured pelvis is suspected, care must be taken not to compress or distract the wings of the ilium during turning, lifting, or transportation of the patient. An accurate evaluation of the extent of injury to the lower urinary tract as described above is of the utmost importance.

Fractures with displacement of the pelvic ring result from severe trauma. There is always associated vascular injury with massive retroperitoneal bleeding. The lower urinary tract may be involved but often is spared. Profound shock with pelvic fractures is diagnostic of massive vascular injuries. Arteriograms may be of great value in identifying an arterial bleeding site. There is always extensive venous bleeding.

chapter 21   # INJURIES OF THE SPINE AND EXTREMITIES

I. INJURIES OF THE SPINE

Fractures and fracture dislocations of the spine result from considerable violence or a fall from a height. Fractures in the cervical region often follow diving accidents and are likely to be accompanied by injury to the cord.

Examination should disturb the patient as little as possible. If a fracture or a fracture dislocation of any portion of the vertebral column is suspected, attention must be directed to the prevention of injury to the spinal cord. The patient should not be moved in the slightest way without protecting and preserving the normal position of the vertebral column. The most serious injuries occur in the cervical spine, and this region must be well protected because of its mobility. Whenever the patient is moved, gentle traction on the head along the axis of the spine should be made by an assistant. Under no circumstances should the patient be allowed to flex the neck voluntarily (as in trying to drink a glass of water). Whether the patient is carried in the prone or supine position will depend largely upon the circumstances and the method of transportation available. It is *a primary consideration* to move the patient as little as possible, turn him as little as possible, and not bring about any rotation, flexion, or extension of the spine during these maneuvers.

Detailed examination of the extent of the injury is an integral part of the arrangement for definitive treatment of the patient; it should be carefully carried out only by those responsible for such treatment. However, a fairly accurate estimate of the location and extent of cord injury can be readily obtained without disturbing the patient.

Test for cord injury. *Ask the patient to move his toes and legs.* If he can do so, major cord damage has not occurred. If the legs are

357

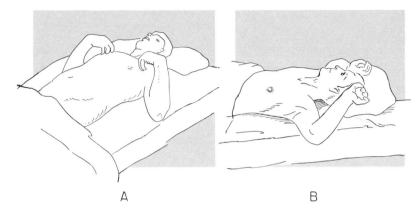

Figure 21–1. Position assumed by the patient in injuries of the cervical cord. *A,* Injury at the level of the seventh cervical vertebra. *B,* Injury at the level of the sixth cervical vertebra.

paralyzed and the patient is able to move his hands readily, the lesion must lie below the cervical region. If there is impairment of arm function, the position assumed by the patient is often diagnostic (Fig. 21–1). In lesions at the level of the seventh cervical vertebra, the elbows are flexed with the half-closed hands resting on the anterior chest wall. In lesions of the sixth cervical vertebra the arms are abducted, the elbows flexed, and the forearms pronated. If a lesion above the sixth cervical vertebra is not immediately fatal from phrenic nerve paralysis, there will be complete flaccidity of the arms. Loss of sensation to pinprick will confirm the impression of a major cord injury at any level.

If there is no evidence of cord injury, but a fracture of the spine is suspected, the examination of the back must be performed very gently. Transportation should be carefully carried out, and x-rays of the spine made to determine the location and extent of the damage.

II. INJURIES OF THE PERIPHERAL NERVES

Injury to the main peripheral nerve trunks is frequently encountered among military casualties, particularly where artillery, grenades, land mines, and bombs delivered from aircraft are in use. In this type of warfare complex wounds of the extremities involving both soft tissues and the long bones are common. In civilian practice injuries to peripheral nerves are less common. They are the result of certain types of closed and compound fractures incident to industrial and vehicular accidents and from lacerations of the extremities.

Determination of the existence and location of a peripheral nerve injury is based on an accurate knowledge of (1) the anatomic course of the major nerve trunks from their segmental roots of origin to their peripheral termination, (2) the individual muscles which receive their motor supply from each nerve, and (3) the skin areas innervated by each peripheral nerve, as distinct from the spinal cord segments (dermatomes). *The examiner should not hesitate to consult textbooks of neuroanatomy to be certain of these relationships at the time an examination is being carried out.*

In peripheral nerve damage it is the axons of lower motor neurons which are injured; the paralysis is therefore flaccid, and atrophy of all muscles supplied distal to the level of injury eventually ensues. In addition to paralysis, atrophy, and sensory loss, certain autonomic changes become apparent in the denervated area. The skin becomes thin and smooth, pale or mottled in appearance; there is absence of sweating, and the associated finger- or toenails become distorted and brittle. It is important to remember, however, that in the acute phase of injury, positive findings may be limited entirely to loss of voluntary muscle power and loss of perception of sensory stimuli (i.e., pinprick).

Certain limitations in the examination of traumatized extremities must be emphasized. If a hand or foot is swollen, shiny, and discolored from dependent, post-traumatic, or inflammatory reaction or from a tight bandage or cast, voluntary function of the distal muscle of the part will be impaired, and sensory evaluation equivocal. If there are extensive soft-tissue wounds or fractures, movements of adjacent muscle groups will be painful and therefore restricted. Actual laceration of muscles or tendons themselves must be carefully differentiated from damage to the nerve supply of these muscles. Patients quickly learn how to compensate for paralyzed muscles by substitution of supplementary muscular activity. Therefore, wherever possible, isolated muscle or muscle group tests should be employed rather than complex purposeful movements.

In civilian life the types of peripheral nerve injury most commonly seen are: the *radial nerve* injury associated with compression of the upper arm or fractures of the shaft of the humerus; the *ulnar nerve* injury associated with fractures about the elbow; the *common peroneal nerve* injury associated with fractures, soft-tissue wounds, or pressure about the knee; the *sciatic nerve* injury associated with dislocations and fractures of the hip joint and misplaced intramuscular injections; the *median* and *ulnar nerve* injuries associated with lacerated wounds about the wrist; and the *brachial plexus* injury associated with stretch injuries from birth trauma and severe traction on the upper extremity. No attempt will be made to describe the findings present in injury of all peripheral nerves at various levels, since this is beyond the scope of this section. Only the major nerves will be considered, i.e., the median, ulnar, and radial nerves in the upper extremity, the brachial plexus, and the common peroneal, posterior tibial, femoral, and sciatic nerves in the lower extremity. Their examination will now be outlined in brief.

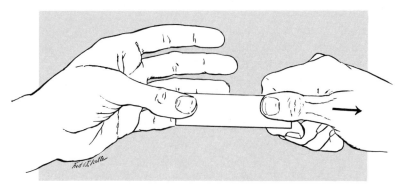

Figure 21–2. Opposition of the thumb and little finger. The thumb is drawn over the palm mainly by the opponens pollicis, which is supplied by the median nerve. Opposition of the little finger depends on palmar elevation of the fifth metacarpal (ulnar action) as well as the action of the opponens muscles. (Haymaker and Woodhall, Peripheral Nerve Injuries.)

MEDIAN NERVE

If the median nerve is injured at the wrist, there is paralysis of the opponens pollicis, the abductor pollicis brevis, and the outer head of the flexor pollicis brevis. The patient cannot flex the first metacarpal at the wrist in order to oppose the volar surface of the thumb to the volar surface

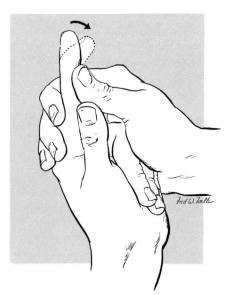

Figure 21–3. Test for median nerve palsy. In complete interruption of the nerve about the elbow or upper arm, flexion of the distal phalanx of the index finger is absent. (Haymaker and Woodhall, Peripheral Nerve Injuries.)

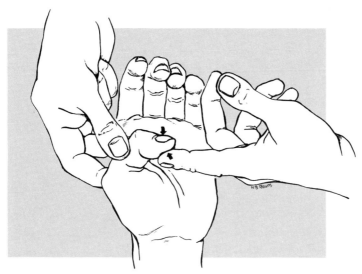

Figure 21–4. Test for median nerve palsy. In complete interruption of the nerve about the elbow or upper arm, the patient will not be able to flex the distal phalanx of the thumb. (Haymaker and Woodhall, Peripheral Nerve Injuries.)

of the hand at the base of the little and ring fingers. The motion may be tested by asking the patient to hold a slip of paper between the thumb and the base of the little finger. An intact ulnar nerve is required, since the maneuver is a combined one involving palmar elevation of the fifth metacarpal (Fig. 21–2). There is anesthesia of the radial portion of the palm and of the volar surface of the first three digits. The autonomous area of complete sensory loss always present in median nerve injury is the volar surface of the distal phalanx of the index finger.

If the median nerve is injured about the elbow or in the upper arm, there are, in addition to the above, paralysis of the flexors of the wrist, except the flexor carpi ulnaris, and paralysis of all the long flexors of the first three digits. The patient cannot flex the distal phalanx of the index finger (Fig. 21–3) or the distal phalanx of the thumb, since these always depend solely on median innervation (Fig. 21–4). The grasp becomes inadequate, and the hand is quickly flattened on its radial aspect.

ULNAR NERVE

If the ulnar nerve is injured at the wrist, there is paralysis of all the interossei, the third and fourth lumbricales, the adductor pollicis, and the inner head of the flexor pollicis brevis. The patient cannot adduct or abduct the fingers if they are held against a flat surface (Fig. 21–5). The proximal phalanx of the thumb cannot be pulled to the proximal phalanx and metacarpophalangeal joint of the index finger held in the plane of the

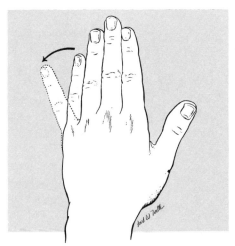

Figure 21–5. Test for ulnar nerve palsy. In complete interruption of the ulnar nerve the power to abduct the little finger is abolished. (Haymaker and Woodhall, Peripheral Nerve Injuries.)

other fingers. There is anesthesia of the ulnar portion of the palm and the volar surface of the fifth digit and ulnar half of the fourth digit. The autonomous area of complete sensory loss, always present in ulnar nerve injury, is the volar surface of the distal phalanx of the little finger. The hand becomes flattened on its ulnar aspect, and atrophy appears quickly.

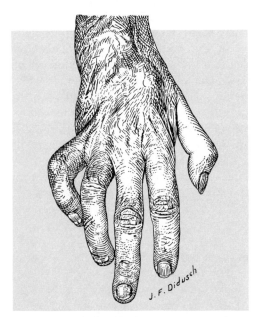

Figure 21–6. Ulnar clawhand. Note the hyperextension at the metacarpophalangeal joints of the fourth and fifth fingers with flexion of the distal joints. Trophic changes are limited to the field of the ulnar nerve.

If the ulnar nerve is injured about the elbow or in the upper arm, there is, in addition to the above, paralysis of the flexor carpi ulnaris and the flexor digitorum profundus to the fourth and fifth fingers. This results in the so-called clawhand deformity (Fig. 21–6), in which the fourth and fifth fingers are held in hyperextension at the metacarpophalangeal joint with flexion of the proximal and distal interphalangeal joints. The patient can grasp with the first three, but not with the fourth and fifth digits. Sensory loss now extends also to the dorsum of the ulnar aspect of the hand.

RADIAL NERVE

When the radial nerve is injured in the upper arm, there is paralysis of the supinator, brachioradialis, extensor carpi radialis and ulnaris, and long extensors of the thumb and fingers. "Wristdrop" is produced by the patient's inability to extend the wrist against gravity (Fig. 21–7). He cannot extend the distal or proximal phalanx of the thumb, and the first metacarpal cannot be abducted in the plane of the palm. He cannot extend the proximal phalanx of the fingers on the metacarpals. He can, however, extend the interphalangeal joints, since this is a function of the interossei and lumbricales (median and ulnar nerves). There is anesthesia on the radial aspect of the dorsum of the hand and forearm. The autonomous area of complete sensory loss always present in radial nerve injury is a small triangular area in the dorsum of the web space between the thumb and index finger.

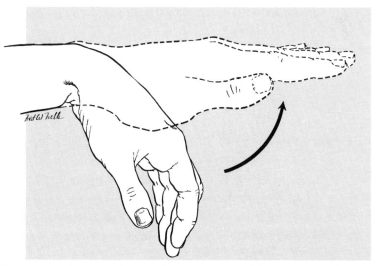

Figure 21–7. Wristdrop. In complete interruption of the radial nerve the patient is unable to dorsiflex the hand at the wrist. (Haymaker and Woodhall, Peripheral Nerve Injuries.)

BRACHIAL PLEXUS

The most common type of brachial plexus injury is the upper arm or so-called Erb's type of palsy due to injury to the fifth and sixth cervical roots or upper trunk of the plexus. These nerves are compressed or stretched as they pass over the scalene tubercle. Here the shoulder is held in adduction and internal rotation, the elbow in extension, the forearm in pronation, and the wrist in flexion. The paralyzed muscles include the deltoid, supraspinatus and infraspinatus, biceps, brachialis, brachioradialis, and sometimes, to a lesser extent, the triceps and long extensors of the wrist and fingers. The biceps and radioperiosteal reflexes are absent. Sensory loss usually involves the volar surface of the hand principally, with some extension to the ulnar aspect of the dorsal surface.

If the major portion of the brachial plexus is involved in a severe traction injury, there is flaccid paralysis of the entire arm. It hangs limply from the shoulder as a dead weight and is areflexic and anesthetic below the middle of the upper arm.

COMMON PERONEAL NERVE

If the common peroneal nerve is injured at any point from the sciatic notch to the neck of the fibula, there is paralysis of the tibialis anterior, the peroneous longus and brevis, and the long extensors of the foot and toes. The patient cannot dorsiflex his foot at the ankle (Fig. 21–8), and he cannot dorsiflex his toes against gravity (Fig. 21–9). A "footdrop" results. He cannot evert his foot against resistance, and he continually stubs his toe when attempting to walk. There is anesthesia on the lateral aspect of the dorsum of the foot and ankle extending one-third to one-half way up the lateral aspect of the lower leg.

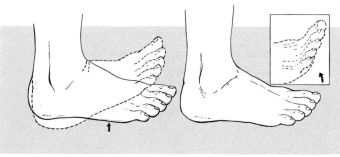

Fig. 21–8   Fig. 21–9

Figure 21–8. Test for common peroneal nerve palsy. In interruption of the common peroneal nerve the patient is unable to dorsiflex the foot at the ankle. (Haymaker and Woodhall, Peripheral Nerve Injuries.)

Figure 21–9. Test for common peroneal nerve palsy. In interruption of the nerve the patient is unable to elevate or dorsiflex the toes. (Haymaker and Woodhall, Peripheral Nerve Injuries.)

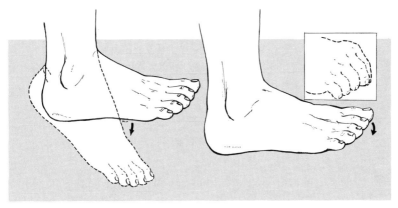

Fig. 21–10   Fig. 21–11

Figure 21–10. Test for posterior tibial nerve palsy. In interruption of the posterior tibial nerve plantar flexion at the ankle is impossible. (Haymaker and Woodhall, Peripheral Nerve Injuries.)
Figure 21–11. Test for posterior tibial nerve palsy. In interruption of the posterior tibial nerve plantar flexion of the toes cannot be performed. (Haymaker and Woodhall, Peripheral Nerve Injuries.)

POSTERIOR TIBIAL NERVE

If the posterior tibial nerve is injured at any point from the sciatic notch to the lower margin of the popliteal space, there is paralysis of the gastrocnemius group of muscles, the tibialis posterior, and the long flexors of the foot and toes. The patient cannot plantar-flex the foot at the ankle (Fig. 21–10). He has no "take-off" on walking and cannot stand on tiptoe. The ankle jerk is absent. He cannot invert the foot against resistance, and he cannot flex the toes (Fig. 21–11). There is anesthesia on the sole of the foot and the volar surface of the toes.

If the posterior tibial nerve is injured below the level of the upper third of the lower leg, all of the muscular branches of the nerve are usually spared, and the only abnormality noted may be the sensory loss on the sole of the foot.

FEMORAL NERVE

This nerve is rarely injured. It may be damaged in penetrating wounds of the groin. There is paralysis of the quadriceps muscle. The patient cannot extend the knee or set his patella (Fig. 21–12). The knee jerk is absent. There is sensory loss over the anteromedial aspect of the lower half of the thigh and a strip extending down the medial aspect of the lower leg almost to the ankle.

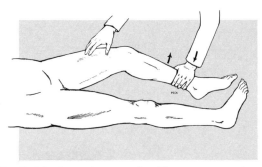

Figure 21–12. Test for femoral nerve palsy. The presence or absence of quadriceps contraction (femoral innervation) is determined by palpation as the patient attempts to extend the leg. (Haymaker and Woodhall, Peripheral Nerve Injuries.)

SCIATIC NERVE

When the sciatic nerve has been divided, the leg becomes useless. Flexion at the knee is greatly weakened, and all ankle and foot movements are abolished. Extension at the knee is unaffected by sciatic nerve injury. Sensibility is lost, except in the area supplied by the saphenous nerve. If the tibial and peroneal components of the sciatic nerve are injured and the nerve to the hamstring is intact, flexion of the knee is preserved; otherwise, the muscle weakness and sensory deficit are the same as in a combined injury of those two nerves.

Causalgia

Partial or sometimes complete division of a peripheral nerve may be followed by an extraordinary type of spontaneous burning pain. Pain may be experienced immediately after injury or it may not develop for several days or longer. The characteristics of the pain are of more diagnostic significance than the physical examination. It is constant and has an intense, predominately burning character. It is exacerbated by moving, touching, tapping, jarring, or emotional stimuli such as fright, excitement, or even hunger. The effect of cold or warmth is variable.

The physical examination will show evidence of a peripheral nerve injury which is almost always incomplete. The sciatic and median nerves are most frequently involved, and the pain is usually experienced in the hand or foot. The skin is often glossy and shiny. It may be red, dry, and scaly. In most instances the affected part is warmer than normal, but it may be cooler. Rarely vascular tone in the limb may seem normal. Prompt relief of the pain by procaine anesthesia of the related autonomic (sympathetic) pathways is an important diagnostic sign.

The severe constant burning pain in the presence of a peripheral nerve injury, the exacerbation of the pain by certain stimuli, and the prompt relief or amelioration of the pain by sympathetic block are the important diagnostic criteria of this condition which distinguish it from post-traumatic vasomotor disorders, trench foot with cold sensitivity, and minor or atypical causalgic states. Sympathectomy is curative.

III. INJURIES OF JOINTS

Injuries in the Region of the Shoulder

Trauma to the shoulder girdle is a common occurrence in athletic events and everyday life. When such injury has taken place, the patient should be examined with both shoulders exposed. Inspection and comparison of one side with the other from in front of and from behind the patient are necessary. *Flattening* of the shoulder may be due to dislocation of the joint or to atrophy of the deltoid muscle. The attitude of the patient and the way the arm and shoulder are held may be a clue to the type of injury.

A fracture, if present, may be suspected on palpation. The shoulder joint is palpated for swelling and tenderness. The sternoclavicular joint and acromioclavicular joint should be identified. The clavicle is palpated by passing the fingers along its subcutaneous surface. If no fracture is demonstrated, the patient is then requested to put the shoulder joint through the normal ranges of motion.

Dislocation of the acromioclavicular joint results in separation of the outer end of the clavicle so that it is elevated while the shoulder drops. This is an unmistakable sign of the injury.

Anterior (subcoracoid) dislocation of the shoulder is the common type of shoulder dislocation. The patient assumes a characteristic position. The acromion stands out above the flattened outer surface of the shoulder; the axillary fold is lowered, and the elbow is held away from the body. Fractures of the surgical neck of the humerus present a somewhat similar appearance, except that the point of the shoulder is rounded. Recurrent dislocations of the shoulder are usually of the subcoracoid type. *Posterior dislocation of the shoulder* is a rare injury. The arm is held in adduction; the shoulder is flattened, and the coracoid process is prominent.

A *coexisting fracture with dislocation* can only be excluded by x-ray examination.

Rupture of the supraspinatus tendon is characterized by the patient's inability to initiate abduction of the arm. The deltoid strongly contracts, but the patient has to shrug or elevate the entire shoulder girdle to initiate the motion. After the arm reaches the horizontal plane, the deltoid can complete the movement.

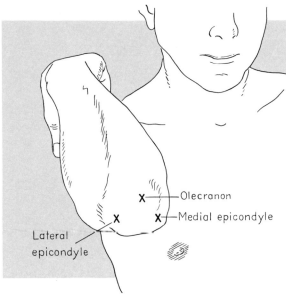

Olecranon

Medial epicondyle

Lateral epicondyle

Figure 21–13. Normal landmarks of the elbow. A triangle is formed by the tip of the olecranon and the medial and lateral epicondyles. When the elbow is extended these points should be in a straight line.

Injuries of the Elbow Joint

The normal anatomic landmarks of the elbow are shown in Figure 21–13. These landmarks may be distorted either by dislocation or fracture.

Posterior dislocation of both bones is caused by hyperextension at the elbow. The deformity is considerable. The olecranon makes a distinct posterior prominence above which is a deep gap. The tip of the olecranon lies in a position behind and above the epicondyles. A fracture through or just above the condyles does not alter the relationship of the epicondyles and the olecranon.

Dislocation of the head of the radius may be associated with fractures, especially of the upper third of the ulna. The forearm is held partially flexed and pronated, and the radial head is prominent anteriorly and is palpable. The posterior interosseous branch of the radial nerve may be injured, resulting in weakness or palsy of the extensor muscles of the hand.

Injuries to the Wrist and Hand

Trauma to this region is so intimately connected with fractures that a brief description of the common fractures will be given.

Colles' fracture.   Colles' fracture is a transverse, usually comminuted fracture through the cancellous lower end of the radius in which the lower fragment is displaced backward to the radial side and rotated in supination. Thus the typical *silver fork* deformity results. The radial styloid process normally is distal to the ulnar styloid, but in this fracture the radial styloid may be proximal to or level with the ulnar styloid.

Smith's fracture.   Smith's fracture (Colles' fracture reversed) results in a deformity just the reverse of Colles' fracture, since the break is transverse or directed from the ventral surface upward and backward. The distal fragment is displaced upward and forward.

Fracture of the carpal scaphoid.   This fracture is often mistaken for a sprained wrist. There may be edema of the "anatomic snuffbox" and tenderness upon the floor of this triangle just distal to the styloid process of the radius. Forced radial deviation of the hand, or a thrust upon the index metacarpal, when aligned with the radius, elicits pain. The diagnosis of sprained wrist is made by exclusion. An x-ray examination is essential.

Dislocation of the semilunar bone.   This results in pain due to pressure of the dislocated bone upon the median nerve. There are an anterior prominence and a pronounced posterior depression below the lower edge of the radius. The wrist cannot be extended.

Fractures of the metacarpal shafts.   Such fractures are commonly caused by blows upon the knuckles. There results posterior swelling due to the dorsal bending of the bone by the action of the interossei. The knuckle is below the line of its fellows owing to shortening of the shaft. The most common metacarpal fracture is that of the fifth metacarpal at its distal end. The second most common is Bennett's fracture of the proximal end of the metacarpal of the thumb.

Dislocation of the thumb.   Dislocation of the thumb at the metacarpophalangeal joint is the most common dislocation at this level. The little finger is next in frequency, and the other fingers are rarely dislocated. Dislocation of the thumb presents deformity due to dorsal displacement of the base of the phalanx over the head of the first metacarpal. The thumb appears shortened and swollen, with a marked dorsal prominence.

Injuries of the Hip Joint

Dislocations of the hip.   Dislocations may be posterior or anterior, but the former is the more common. *Posterior dislocation* is caused by a force applied to the leg when the thigh is flexed, adducted, and internally rotated. The force may be directly against the knee, such as in automobile accidents, and the patella may be fractured. The attitude of the limb is characteristic. The thigh is adducted and internally rotated. The knee is turned inward, and the foot is inverted so the heel may rest upon the other foot. Active motion is absent; the leg is shortened, adducted, and internally rotated.

Anterior dislocation is caused by violent abduction of the hip. The leg is externally rotated; the knee is flexed, and the foot is everted. The attitude of the leg is the reverse of that with posterior dislocation.

Fractures of the neck of the femur. If the fracture is not impacted, there is a characteristic appearance. The foot is everted; the thigh is slightly abducted, and the knee is slightly flexed. The patient does not complain of much pain unless the leg is moved. The leg is shortened. If the fracture is impacted, there is little if any eversion of the foot and no significant shortening is found. The patient may be able to walk with an impacted fracture, so that if the diagnosis is suspected, an x-ray examination should be made before the patient is allowed to bear weight.

Injuries of the Knee Joint

Injuries of the knee joint are very common, especially in athletes. If the patient is seen immediately after the injury, a detailed manipulative examination is impossible. Anteroposterior and lateral x-ray films should be made. If no major fracture is found, a compression bandage should be applied to minimize swelling. Twenty-four hours may be required for enough localization of pain and tenderness to permit a diagnostic manipulative examination. When the injury is of some duration, the manipulative examination need not be deferred.

The knee is examined with the patient supine; both legs are completely exposed and relaxed. Each step of the examination is first performed on the normal knee in order to obtain a standard for comparison.

Inspection

The legs are lifted by the heels, and the knees inspected for swelling, redness, and deformity. The natural hollows on each side of the patella are abolished with effusion into the knee joint. Apparent swelling of the knee may be due to atrophy of the quadriceps muscle. The degree of extension is noted at this time (Fig. 21–14 *A*).

Palpation

The region of the knee is palpated for localized tenderness and masses. The popliteal space is best palpated with the patient prone and with the knee flexed in the same manner as in palpation of the popliteal artery.

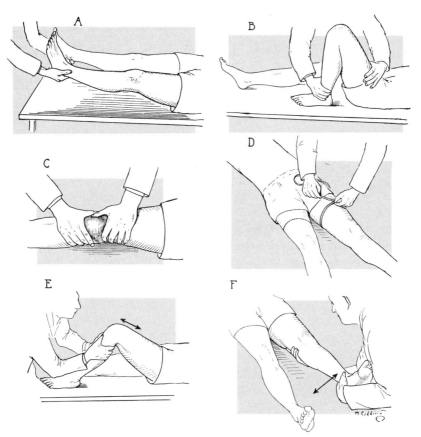

Figure 21–14. Technique of examination of the injured knee. *A,* Inspection and determination of extension. *B,* Determination of passive flexion. This follows a comparison of active flexion with the uninjured leg. *C,* Palpation for fluid. Pressure on the suprapatellar pouch drives small quantities of fluid downward. The right index finger is shown about to compress the anterolateral aspect of the joint, producing a fluid wave palpable by the thumbs and left hand. *D,* Determination of muscle atrophy. The circumference of the thighs is measured at the same level. *E,* Determination of cruciate ligament laxity. The knee is flexed at 90 degrees. The examiner's forearm presses firmly against the lower tibia while both hands grasp the leg just below the knee and manipulate it in the sagittal plane. *F,* Determination of collateral ligament laxity. One of the examiner's hands rests on the table and firmly grasps the femoral condyles. The other grasps the ankle and manipulates the extended knee in the coronal plane. (T. B. Quigley, Surg., Gynec. & Obst., 87:569–575, November, 1948. By permission of Surgery, Gynecology and Obstetrics.)

Flexion

Active flexion of the knees is noted and compared. The normal and then the affected knee are passively flexed (Fig. 21–14 *B*). Flexion is not carried beyond the point of pain.

The method of detecting fluid in the knee joint is shown in Figure 21–14 *C*. Pressure on the suprapatellar pouch forces small quantities of fluid downward. The right forefinger is shown about to compress the anterolateral aspect of the joint to produce a fluid wave palpable by the thumbs and left hand. If the joint capsule has ruptured and there is diffuse hemorrhage, there is a doughy sensation to palpation over the front of the swollen knee. The swelling has no distinct boundaries and does not transmit a fluid wave.

Muscle atrophy. The circumference of the thighs is measured at the same level bilaterally (Fig. 21–14 *D*).

Test for cruciate ligament laxity is shown in Figure 21–14 *E*. The knee is flexed at 90 degrees. The examiner's forearm is pressed firmly against the lower tibia while both hands grasp the leg just below the knee and manipulate the knee in the sagittal plane. The normal knee is stable with this maneuver.

Test for collateral ligament laxity is shown in Figure 21–14 *F*. The examiner rests one hand on the table and firmly grasps the femoral condyles. The other hand grasps the ankle and manipulates the knee in the coronal plane. The normal knee is stable with this maneuver.

Sprains. Any of the ligaments of the knee may be partly or completely ruptured by trauma.

The *medial collateral ligament* is commonly injured by a force tending to bend the knee inward. Pain and swelling may be marked. The diagnosis is established by the presence of tenderness along the course of the ligament, and pain is produced when the ligament is stretched. In severe grades there is laxity of the ligament.

Rupture of the cruciate ligaments is much less common and is produced by a force which violently hyperextends and twists the knee. This injury is suspected when there is abnormal mobility in the anteroposterior direction. Back and forth motion of the tibia on the femur with the leg extended indicates rupture of the anterior cruciate ligament (it is normally tightened by extension). Posterior slipping of the tibia with the knee flexed points to the rare accident of rupture of the posterior cruciate ligament.

Meniscus injuries. Extension of the knee associated with a twisting force is apt to disrupt the semilunar cartilages. The internal cartilage is more likely to be injured than the external. The former may be associated with tears of the internal collateral ligament. Pain is immediate, and the patient frequently has a sensation that something has "given way" in the knee. If the cartilage is displaced, the knee may be locked in flexion. There is usually localized tenderness along the palpable anterior edge of the articular surface of the tibia. This is best searched for with the knee flexed.

Identification of the location of the injured cartilages is made as follows: The patient is prone; the foot is grasped and the knee flexed until the heel almost reaches the buttock. The foot is rotated outward to its extreme limit, and the knee joint is steadily extended. If a "click" is felt during the maneuver, it indicates that the posterior horn of the medial meniscus is torn. The same test is modified for the lateral meniscus by rotating the foot inward to its full extent. Replacement of the cartilage may occur, and the joint effusion may subside. "Locking" and joint effusion may recur with trauma.

Osteochondritis dissecans must be differentiated from meniscus injuries. X-ray films may show a defect or area of diminished density on the articular surface of the femoral condyle. Joint pain is not as severe, and characteristically there is intermittent locking and unlocking of the knee joint with little or no trauma or reaction.

Contusion of the knee results in a painful swollen joint. Fluid is demonstrated in the joint, and ligament injuries are ruled out by manipulative examination.

Injuries of the Patella

The patella is examined while the patient lies at rest. With the quadriceps muscle completely relaxed, the patella can be grasped between the thumb and fingers. Slight lateral mobility is normally present, and excessive mobility of the patella suggests the possibility of recurrent dislocation.

Transverse fracture of the patella is obvious on palpation, provided the fragments are widely separated. If the separation of the fragments is slight, the crevice between them is sought by passing the thumbnail from above downwards over the anterior surface of the patella. A *stellate fracture* of the patella may show only local tenderness and swelling. A "mushy" sensation to palpation is only present in severe comminution of the bone. The knee joint may be distended from hemorrhage, and if the joint capsule is ruptured, as it frequently is, there is a doughy sensation to palpation over the front of the knee which has no distinct boundaries and does not transmit a fluid wave. Fracture of the patella frequently accompanies posterior dislocation of the hip.

Injuries of the Ankle

The bony landmarks of the ankle are the two malleoli, which normally can be easily seen and palpated. Swelling from injury, edema due to heart disease, or stasis from venous or lymphatic disease may obliterate the normal contour of the ankle. In excessively obese individuals there may be fat deposits around the ankle which obscure the landmarks.

Sprained ankle. Sprain of the ankle is usually an adduction injury; that is, the foot is rolled inward under the weight of the body. The external

lateral ligament is thus put under great stress and is more or less completely torn. The tip of the external malleolus may be avulsed (a sprain
fracture). The initial pain of a sprain is severe, and weight-bearing is painful and may be impossible. Puffy swelling over the injured area rapidly
occurs, and there may or may not be ecchymosis. Tenderness is diffuse
and not well localized, but as a rule, by careful palpation the extent of the
damage to the ligaments can be accurately appraised. One-finger palpation over the lateral aspect of the foot and ankle will elicit exquisite tenderness if the lateral collateral ligament has been torn. Pressure anteriorly
between the tibia and fibula will demonstrate tenderness if the tibiofibula
ligament is damaged. In the less common inversion sprain, tenderness
may be found over the medial collateral ligament.

Major fractures can be excluded by precise palpation of the bony
landmarks and by gently springing the tibia and fibula above the ankle. An
x-ray examination is required to demonstrate a minor fracture, in which
there very often may be less pain and swelling than in a severe sprain.

Fracture of the ankle. The ankle may be fractured by a force acting
in eversion, abduction, adduction, or backward displacement. The exact
diagnosis of the fracture can be made only by x-ray examination. If an accurate description of the accident is obtained, the history will aid, since
adduction injuries are more likely to be sprains. Deformity of the foot and
ankle may give a clue to the type of fracture. Swelling may be extensive,
but a bad sprain may produce as much as, or more than, a fracture. Tenderness is more localized in a fracture than in a sprain.

IV. GENERAL PRINCIPLES OF EXAMINATION FOR FRACTURE OF AN EXTREMITY

Fractures are common and intriguing problems in both civil and military practice. Their importance is obvious. However, it is manifestly impossible in a book of this size to describe the characteristics of individual
fractures. Hence, this section will be limited to a discussion of the general
principles of examination of the patient with a fracture.

The classic physical signs common to all fractures are *local tenderness, loss or impairment of function, deformity, abnormal mobility,*
and *crepitus.* In addition, the signs of injury to joints, soft tissue, blood
vessels and nerves may be present. The state of the peripheral nerves and
the blood vessels in an injured extremity must be known to the attending
doctor every moment the patient is under his care.

The examiner rapidly appraises the general condition of the patient
("survey examination") and notes how the injured extremity is held or
protected. The diagnosis may be suspected by inspection alone, as in injuries about the shoulder, wrist, ankle, or hip. *Loss of function* is apparent in

the manner the patient moves or protects the injured region. The pulses distal to the injury are checked. The nerve function is determined by having the patient move the joint or joints distal to the injury.

Deformity is determined by inspection of the injured extremity and comparison with its opposite member. It is an important sign, but soft-tissue swelling from edema or hemorrhage may be misleading. Gentle palpation of the region may disclose whether the deformity is skeletal or soft-tissue, but if doubt exists, a distinction between fracture and sprain can be made only by an x-ray examination.

Shortening of an injured limb is a valuable sign. The measurement of the normal comparable extremity is compared with the measurement of the injured limb. The radial and ulnar styloids are excellent landmarks for comparison at the wrist. The legs are measured from the anterior superior iliac spine to the internal malleolus on the same side.

Local tenderness or pain on pressure is determined unless the subjective pain the patient has is obvious. The bone may be gently tapped, twisted, or sprung to elicit pain, as in suspected subperiosteal fractures when the diagnosis is not clear. However, it is barbaric to elicit this sign in the presence of an obvious fracture.

Abnormal mobility may be elicited by active or passive motion of the involved bone. Its chief significance lies in the fact that it is absent in incomplete or impacted fractures, so its absence does not rule out the possibility of fracture. If present, the demonstration of the sign is painful and will increase the local soft tissue injury, and while it is a classic sign of fracture, it must be rarely sought.

Crepitus (the harsh grating sound heard or the grating sensation transmitted to the examining fingers when the broken ends of the bone move upon each other) is produced as the examiner moves the bone with his hands, one above and one below the suspected site of fracture. This, again, is a classic sign of fracture, but it is rarely necessary.

chapter 22   # THERMAL INJURIES: BURNS AND FROSTBITE

The emergency examination and initial care of a burn patient, the results of which often determine the entire subsequent course of this injury, should be familiar to every competent physician. Because the burn patient may have sustained other injuries in addition to his burn, the general principles in examination of the injured patient described on page 313 are applicable. In addition, there are specific indications of primary importance.

BURNS

The Emergency Examination

At the initial contact, the following points can be settled in a matter of a minute or two.

1. IS THERE A RESPIRATORY PROBLEM?

This must be assumed in any burn sustained in a closed space and in all burns of the face, head, and neck.

Respiratory injury is established by obvious burns of the nasal hair, reddening of the posterior pharynx or by hoarseness, crowing, coughing, or rapid respiration. If respiratory difficulty is threatened, then endotracheal intubation, not a tracheostomy, should be skillfully done. The endotracheal tube can be used for suction, for ventilation, for the oxygen tolerance test, and for other steps as indicated.

376

2. HOW SEVERE IS THE BURN?

Only three points need to be considered in the emergency situation: the location, a rough estimate of the extent of the burn, and the age of the patient. There is no need to consider depth or exact extent of the burn at this point. The following indicate a serious burn:

(a) All burns of the face, hands, or feet; (b) all burns over 10 per cent of the body area; (c) all burns of more than 2 per cent of the body area in aged patients. Under any of these circumstances, hospitalization and definitive examination are indicated.

First Aid

This should be limited to endotracheal intubation when indicated, relief of pain (a small dose of morphine intravenously), and protection of the burned area by a clean sheet or cloth. No local applications should be made to the burn.

Chemical burns require copious washing with water as soon as possible. Sometimes the exquisite pain of superficial second degree burns can be eased by wrapping the burned area in a clean towel moistened with cold water.

In general, the less done to the burned area the better.

THE DEFINITIVE EXAMINATION

In all burns of over 15 per cent of the body area, the definitive examination must be combined with immediate therapy.

1. Appraise the state of the respiratory tract, checking for evidence of a nasopharyngeal burn and noting signs of respiratory injury as described above. If these are present, arrangements should be started to humidify the atmosphere and the probability of endotracheal intubation being needed must be considered.

2. Record the rate of the pulse and respiration and take blood pressure if possible. Weigh the patient. All data should be recorded on a work sheet.

3. Draw blood for laboratory studies and start infusion of saline or colloids if available. The intravenous lines should be placed ideally via the subclavian or jugular route. The indwelling intravenous line should *not* be inserted in a lower extremity because of the high incidence of pulmonary embolism from this source.

4. The most severe burns are often remarkably painless, but a small dose of morphine intravenously will relieve discomfort, restlessness, and anxiety. Second degree burns frequently require more sedation. The more sedation required, the more important it is that it be administered intravenously rather than subcutaneously.

5. In burns of 25 per cent or more of the body area, a catheter should

be inserted in the urinary bladder, as the hourly flow of urine is one of the best guides to the adequacy of fluid replacement. Most burns of less than 25 per cent extent can be handled adequately without catheterization on the basis of vital signs, changes in the hematocrit, and the voiding of urine. There should be no hesitation about resorting to catheterization if there is doubt about the course of the injury. However, infection of the urinary tract, especially in children, has become such a serious complication of burns that "routine catheterization" in the less extensive burns should be avoided.

6. A detailed examination of the extent and depth of the burn is now in order. The examiner and all attendants should be masked and strict aseptic precautions be observed. All clothing must be cut away and the patient placed on sterile sheets. Accurate diagrams of the extent of the burn must be drawn and estimates of depth are made.

Mapping the Burn

The depth of the burn is apt to be underestimated, even by the expert. Any extensive flame burn or scald may be assumed to be mainly full thickness or "third degree." Flash and sunburn may be extensive but usually not full thickness.

When first seen, full thickness burns may present any or all of several appearances. Any of the following should be considered indicative of a deep third degree burn:

1. Black or dark brown leathery char that looks like burned parchment.

2. Deep white cadaveric.

3. Deep pink with thrombosed vessels which do not blanch on pressure.

4. Broken blisters with thin roseate pink beneath.

5. Seemingly transparent with an oily appearance and a network of thrombosed blood vessels visible in the corium.

Some of these changes are illustrated in the color plate.

A third degree burn is anesthetic to pinprick but this is not an unequivocal sign, because certain second degree burns which proceed to third degree in a few days may retain sensation. Occasionally a deep second degree burn which does not progress to third degree may be anesthetic. Anesthesia is, therefore, a useful, but not an absolute sign.

Blister formation is characteristic of a second degree burn but may be present occasionally in some third degree burns.

The final extent of the burn is estimated on the basis of one of the accepted tables or the rule of nines (Fig. 22–1).

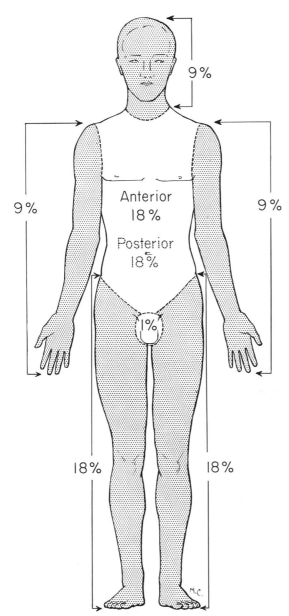

Figure 22–1. Rule of Nines. A rapid method of estimating the extent of body surface burned. The body is divided into areas representing 9 per cent of the body surface or multiples of 9 per cent.

TABLE 22–1. TYPES OF COLD INJURY

Cold Injury	Exposure	Temperature (°F.)
Frostbite	Minutes to 16 hr.	−80 to +20
Trench foot	2 hr. to 14 days	+20 to +50
Immersion foot	12 hr. to 7 days	+25 to +60

FROSTBITE

Frostbite, except in rare instances, is restricted to the extremities of the body or to exposed areas such as the chin, cheeks, nose, and ears. The severity of the injury is directly related to the intensity of the initial exposure and the length of time (see Table 22–1) before adequate circulation can be restored.

The type and duration of contact are the two most important factors in determining the extent of frostbite injury; for example, touching cold wood is not nearly as dangerous as coming in direct contact with cold metal. This is particularly true if one's hands are wet or even damp, because metal is an excellent thermal conductor. Air itself is a very poor thermal conductor. Cold air alone is not nearly as dangerous as a combination of wind and cold; hence, the chilling effect of +20 F. combined with a 45 mph. wind is identical to that of −40 F. temperature with no wind (Table 22–2).

The susceptibility to injury is influenced by training and geographic background. During the Korean War, black soldiers had a six times greater incidence of frostbite than white soldiers, and Southern whites experienced an almost two times greater incidence than Northern whites. In addition, general physical condition influences susceptibility; for example, injured soldiers were much more susceptible to frostbite no matter what their initial injury was.

TABLE 22–2. WIND CHILL FACTORS (EQUIVALENT TEMPERATURES PRODUCED WITH CERTAIN COMBINATIONS OF WIND AND AIR TEMPERATURE)

Wind (m.p.h.)	Equivalent Temperatures (°F.) at		
	+30	0	−30
10	+16	−22	−58
20	+3	−40	−81
40	−4	−54	−101

Pathophysiology

Local. Two types of reaction occur when tissue comes in contact with cold. First, the superficial tissue at the sight of contact actually freezes to a depth dependent on the degree of cold and the duration of contact. With this freezing, ice crystals grow between cells, and if the source of cold is not removed, these crystals continue to grow, dehydrating and severely damaging the adjacent cells. Intense freezing causes crystals to form within the cells, damaging the cells immediately. Second, arteriolar vasoconstriction occurs in the tissue adjacent to the frozen layer, rapidly reducing the blood flow in this zone. With the arteriolar constriction, shunts occur which allow blood to bypass the affected capillary bed, and if the source of cold is not removed, the whole area begins to freeze.

General. There are two general responses to contact with cold, both of which are designed to maintain the body's core temperature. One is shivering, a somatomotor response, which can produce as much as a fivefold increase in metabolism with only a moderate extra load to the heart. The other is peripheral vasoconstriction, an autonomic response mediated through the hypothalamus, which reduces peripheral heat loss but renders the extremity more subject to cold injury. If core temperature is allowed to decrease, cardiac index falls rapidly and peripheral vascular resistance rises markedly, endangering blood supply to all the vital organs.

Classification and Physical Findings

The following is a retrospective classification designed by the United States Army during the Korean War. This classification divides frostbite injury into four degrees:
1. Erythema and swelling with no blister formation.
2. Erythema and swelling with blisters or blebs.
3. Full thickness injury with gangrene but no loss of part.
4. Complete necrosis with loss of part.

This classification is helpful in reporting frostbite injuries; however, a more useful classification is to divide frostbite injuries into superficial and deep, before the injured part has been thawed.

Superficial Frostbite

Superficial frostbite involves only the skin or the tissues immediately beneath it. The injured part is white and frozen on the exterior, but when depressed gently and firmly it is soft and resilient below the surface. After rewarming, the frostbitten area first becomes numb and is a mottled blue or purple color; it then swells, stings, and burns for some time. In more severe cases, blisters occur beneath the epidermis in 24 to 36 hours. These slowly dry up and become hard and black in about two weeks. General swelling of the injured area occurs and subsides in the same period of time. After the swelling disappears, the skin peels and remains red, tender, and extremely sensitive, even to mild cold, and may perspire abnormally for a long time.

Deep Frostbite

In deep unthawed frostbite, a much more serious injury, the injured part is hard and solid and cannot be depressed at all. The damage not only involves the skin and subcutaneous tissues but also goes deep into the tissue beneath and is usually accompanied by the formation of huge blisters. These blisters may require three days to a week to develop. Swelling of the entire hand or foot occurs and lasts up to eight weeks. The blisters eventually dry up, blacken, and slough off, leaving beneath an exceptionally sensitive red, thin layer of new skin which will take months to return to normal.

In extreme cases of deep frostbite, the part, after thawing, turns a lifeless gray and remains cold. If blisters and swelling occur, they will appear along the line of demarcation between the acutely frostbitten area and the remainder of the limb. In a week or two after the injury, the damaged tissue becomes black, dry, and shriveled and eventually will slough. If infection arises in this dead tissue, the tissue will become wet, soft, and inflamed, causing pain and swelling in the remainder of the limb and increasing the extent of tissue loss. Tendons and bone are relatively resistant to frostbite, whereas nerves, muscles, and particularly blood vessels are highly susceptible.

Emergency Treatment of Frostbite

The first and most important principle in treating frostbite is rapid re-warming of the injured part. This can be done either in a large can or in the bathtub. The injured part should be immersed in water which is carefully kept at a temperature between 100 and 110° F. A thermometer should be used to keep a check on the temperature of the water. Re-warming by immersion in water of this temperature usually takes only 20 minutes. Re-warming for a longer period of time is not considered helpful. Using water at higher temperatures than those mentioned may be harmful.

Re-warming is painful and if the patient's condition is otherwise good, he may be given Demerol for the pain; however, if his condition is

PLATE I

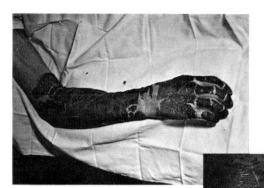

Black or brown leathery char.

Seemingly transparent with visible
network of thrombosed vessels.

Heavy desquamation (broken blisters)
with thin roseate pink beneath.

Char with areas of dead white cadaveric
skin.

Examples of third degree burns.

poor, he should be given only aspirin for the pain. After the injured part is warmed, it should be carefully covered with sterile bandages in order to minimize any friction or trauma to the injured part. It is critically important to protect the injured tissue at this stage. A frozen part should never be rubbed before, during, or after re-warming.

The other measures that can be used if they are available are much the same as those for a patient with a burn injury; that is, the patient should be given a booster shot of tetanus toxoid, he should be placed on penicillin for several days, and he may be given intravenous fluids if they are necessary. The administration of low molecular weight dextran to help improve circulation to the injured part and heparin to prevent further thrombosis of small vessels in the injured area is sometimes carried out and largely depends on the circumstances of the patient. Finally, one should never cut off or debride any tissue, because it is virtually impossible to determine whether the tissue is viable or not in the early stages of a cold injury.

APPENDIX

CHECK LIST FOR THE PHYSICAL EXAMINATION

1. General Appraisal of the Patient

Note the patient's general appearance, facial expression, development, and nutrition. Make an estimate of his mental capacity. Reflect on the possibility of endocrine imbalance. Note his hygiene. Be cognizant of pain, dyspnea, orthopnea, and unusual posture or gait. Scrutinize the skin for pallor, cyanosis, jaundice, pigmentation, or eruption. Record the temperature, pulse, respiration, blood pressure, and weight.

2. Head

Contour, deformity, tumors or abnormal pulsations, condition of the hair and scalp, pediculosis. Rapid cranial nerve tests.

3. Eyes

Pupils—size, equality, regularity, and reaction to light and accommodation. Position and movements of eyeballs. Condition of the conjunctivae and sclerae, jaundice. Gross vision and visual fields. Ophthalmoscopic examination of the media and eyegrounds.

4. Nose

Discharge, deformity, obstruction, perforation of the septum.

5. Mouth

Systematically inspect the lips, the teeth, the alveolar ridges, buccal mucosa, the hard and soft palates, the floor of the mouth, the tongue, the tonsils, and the oral pharynx. Note the condition of the teeth and the presence of dentures. Remove dentures and inspect all surfaces for evidence of irritation or erosion of the mucous membrane. Note tremor or deflection of the protruded tongue. Palpate the tongue, the buccal mucosa, and the floor of the mouth. Palpate any obvious or suspected lesion.

6. Ears

Gross hearing, condition of canal, dermoid cysts, tophi, otoscopic examination.

7. Neck

Symmetry, mobility, sinus tracts, swellings, abnormal pulsations, position of trachea, the size, shape, and consistency of the thyroid gland, thrill or bruit. Size, consistency, position, and character of palpable cervical lymph nodes. Palpate the subclavian artery and the carotid bulb.

8. Thorax

Size, shape, chest expansion, and respirations.

9. Breasts

Size, shape, and symmetry. Note position of nipples, dimpling of skin, retraction of nipples, or excoriation of areola. Palpate for masses, tenderness, and general consistency of breast. Palpate axillary and supraclavicular lymph nodes. Transillumination of masses or questionable masses.

10. Lungs

Inspection. Type of respiration, symmetry of respiratory movements.
Palpation. Estimate of chest expansion, fremitus, and intercostal tenderness.
Percussion. Resonance, position of lung bases, excursion of diaphragm.
Auscultation. Breath sounds, voice and whisper, friction rub or adventitious sounds.

11. Heart

Inspection. Movements of the precordium, position and character of the apex beat.

Palpation.   Apex impulse, thrills, shocks, or abnormal pulsations.
Percussion.   Heart borders, mediastinal dullness.
Auscultation.   Character, rate and rhythm of heart sounds, murmurs or friction rub.

12. Inguinofemoral Regions and Male External Genitalia

Acquire the habit of examining the male external genitalia and the inguinal and femoral canals in both sexes before examining the abdomen. Identify the landmarks. Feel the spermatic cords and the external inguinal ring. Palpate for hernial masses and impulses. If there is a mass, is it reducible, does it transilluminate, are there signs of inflammation? Feel the femoral artery, identify the saphenous canal. Look for hernia, saphenous varix, and enlarged inguinal lymph nodes.

13. External Genitalia, Male

Scars, ulcers, eruptions, urethral discharge. Note deformity of prepuce or meatus. Scrotum and contents, size, consistency, and shape of the testicles. Identify the epididymis. Look for hydrocele, varicocele, or cysts.

14. Abdomen

Inspection.   Contour, symmetry, mobility with respiration, abnormal movements, dilated veins, condition of umbilicus, scars of previous operations, hernia.
Palpation.   Tone of abdominal wall, resistance, or spasticity. If tenderness, one-finger palpation for accurate localization. Are there incisional herniae or abnormal masses?

Organs
Liver—size, tenderness, movements with respirations, edge.
Spleen—palpable, size, splenic notch, mobility.
Kidneys—location, mobility, costovertebral tenderness.
Urinary Bladder—area of dullness, palpable; when did the patient last void?

15. Extremities

Color of skin, development, length, deformity, scars, ulcerations, clubbing of fingers, liver palms, abnormality of vascular tone, tremor, muscular atrophy, muscle tone, or paralysis. Note pulsations of radial, brachial, femoral, popliteal, anterior and posterior tibial, and dorsalis pedis arteries. Study the color of the lower extremities on elevation and dependency.

16. Reflexes

Biceps, triceps, abdominal, cremaster, quadriceps, Achilles, and plantar responses in all cases. Romberg sign and Babinski reflex as indicated.

17. Joints

Limitation of motion, swelling, heat, fluid, crepitation.

18. Spine

Inspection. Gait, posture, curvatures, motions. Special tests—straight leg raising, flexed leg raising, hyperextension of hip and back.

Palpation. Musculature of back, tenderness spasm, areas of thickening, nodules.

Measurements. Chest expansion, circumference of thigh and calf.

19. Female Genitalia; Pelvic Examination

Condition of introitus, urethra, clitoris, labia. Look for cystocele and rectocele. Make cytologic smear prior to palpation of vagina. Bimanual palpation for size, position, shape, and consistency of uterus. Palpation of adnexae. Rectal examination or combined rectovaginal examination for posteriorly placed uterus or masses in the pouch of Douglas. Speculum examination of the vagina and cervix for discharge, bleeding, erosion, chronic cervicitis, or neoplasm.

20. Rectum

Condition of perianal skin, perineum, pilonidal sinus, hemorrhoids, fissures, fistulae, sphincter tone, evidence of prolapse. Size, shape, and consistency of prostate gland. Palpability of seminal vesicles. Inspect examining finger for pus, blood, or feces. Guaiac test for occult blood in feces. Proctosigmoidoscopy.

Summary

Summarize positive physical findings in an orderly fashion.

SUPPLEMENTARY AND ADVANCED READING

Surgical Physiology and Biology

Alexander, J. W., and Good, R. A.: Immunobiology for Surgeons. Philadelphia, W. B. Saunders Co., 1970.

American College of Surgeons Committee on Preoperative and Postoperative Care: Manual of Preoperative and Postoperative Care. 2nd Ed. Philadelphia, W. B. Saunders Co., 1971.

Dunphy, J. E., and Van Winkle, W., Jr.: Repair and Regeneration. New York, McGraw-Hill Book Co., 1969.

Hall, T. E., and Nathanson, L.: The Paraneoplastic Syndromes. *In* Botsford, T. W. (Ed.): Cancer: A Manual for Practitioners. Boston, American Cancer Society (Massachusetts Division), 1968.

Moore, F. D.: Metabolic Care of the Surgical Patient. Philadelphia, W. B. Saunders Co., 1959.

Moore, F. D., et al.: Post-Traumatic Pulmonary Insufficiency. Philadelphia, W. B. Saunders Co., 1969.

Peacock, E. E., Jr., and Van Winkle, W., Jr.: Surgery and Biology of Repair. Philadelphia, W. B. Saunders Co., 1970.

Shires, G. T., et al.: Shock. Vol. XIII in Major Problems in Clinical Surgery. (Dunphy, J. E., Consulting Ed.) Philadelphia, W. B. Saunders Co., 1969.

Wells, C., et al. (Eds.): Scientific Foundations of Surgery. 2nd Ed. Philadelphia, W. B. Saunders Co., 1974.

Zamcheck, N., et al.: Immunologic diagnosis and prognosis of human digestive tract cancer: Carcinoembryonic antigen. N. Engl. J. Med. *281*:83, 1972.

Surgical Pathology

Ackerman, L. V., and Rosai, J.: Surgical Pathology. 5th Ed. St. Louis, C. V. Mosby Co., 1973.

Willis, R. A.: Pathology of Tumors. 4th Ed. London, Butterworth & Co. Ltd., 1968.

Anesthesia

Dripps, R. D., et al.: Introduction to Anesthesia. 4th Ed. Philadelphia, W. B. Saunders Co., 1973.

Burns

Artz, J. A., and Moncrief, J. A.: The Treatment of Burns. 2nd Ed. Philadelphia, W. B. Saunders Co., 1969.
Moore, F. D.: The body weight burn budget. Surg. Clin. North Am. *50*:1249, 1970.

Frostbite

Washburn, B.: Frostbite. N. Engl. J. Med. *266*:974, 1962.

Trauma

American College of Surgeons Committee on Trauma: Early Care of the Injured Patient. Philadelphia, W. B. Saunders Co., 1972.
Madding, C. F., and Kennedy, P. A.: Trauma to the Liver. 2nd Ed. Vol. III in Major Problems in Clinical Surgery. (Dunphy, J. E., Consulting Ed.) Philadelphia, W. B. Saunders Co., 1971.
Martin, J. D., Jr., et al.: Trauma to the Thorax and Abdomen. Springfield, Illinois, Charles C Thomas, 1969.

General Surgical Texts

Dunphy, J. E., and Way, L. W.: Current Surgical Diagnosis and Treatment. Los Altos, California, Lange Medical Publications, 1973.
Sabiston, D. C., Jr. (Ed.): Davis-Christopher Textbook of Surgery. Philadelphia, W. B. Saunders Co., 1972.
Schwartz, S. (Ed.): Principles of Surgery. 2nd Ed. New York, McGraw-Hill Book Co., 1974:

Regarding a Career in Surgery

Davis, L.: A Surgeon's Odyssey. New York, Doubleday & Co., 1973.
Dunphy, J. E.: Surgery. *In* Garland, J., and Stokes, J., III (eds.): The Choice of a Medical Career. Philadelphia, J. B. Lippincott Co., 1961.
Dunphy, J. E.: The role of surgery in the general education of the physician. Am. J. Surg. *110*:100, 1965.
Fulton, J. E.: Harvey Cushing. Springfield, Illinois, Charles C Thomas, 1946.
Hurwitz, A., and Degenshein, G. A.: Milestones in Modern Surgery. New York, Harper and Co., 1958.
MacCallum, W. G.: William Stewart Halsted. Baltimore, Johns Hopkins Press, 1936.

BIBLIOGRAPHY

Adson, A. W., and Coffey, J. R.: Cervical rib; a method of anterior approach for the relief of symptoms by division of the scalenus anticus. Ann. Surg. *85*:839, 1927.

Anson, B. J., and McVay, C. B.: Surgical Anatomy. 5th ed. Philadelphia, W. B. Saunders Co., 1971. (2 vols.).

Artz, C. P., and Hardy, J. D. (Eds.): Management of Surgical Complications. Philadelphia, W. B. Saunders Co., 1975.

Bacon, H. E.: Anus, Rectum, Sigmoid Colon: Diagnosis and Treatment. 2nd Ed. Philadelphia, J. B. Lippincott Co., 1945.

Bailey, H.: Demonstrations of Physical Signs in Clinical Surgery. 15th Ed. Baltimore, Williams & Wilkins Co., 1973.

Beck, C. S.: Wounds of the heart; technic of suture. Arch. Surg., *13*:205, 1926.

Beeson, P. B., and McDermott, W. (Eds.): Cecil-Loeb Textbook of Medicine. 14th Ed. Philadelphia, W. B. Saunders Co., 1975.

Best, C. H., and Taylor, N. B.: The Physiological Basis of Medical Practice. 6th Ed. Baltimore, Williams & Wilkins Co., 1955.

Bill, A. H., Jr.: Cysts and sinuses of the neck of thyroglossal and branchial origin. Surg. Clin. North Am. *36*:1599, 1956.

Botsford, T. W.: Cancer Detection in the Physician's Office. American Cancer Society, Inc. (Massachusetts Division), Boston, Massachusetts, 1955.

Botsford, T. W., and Tucker, M. R.: Application of cytologic smear methods to cancer diagnosis in a general hospital. J.A.M.A. *142*:975, 1950.

Botsford, T. W., and Wilson, R. E.: The Acute Abdomen. Vol. X in Major Problems in clinical Surgery. (Dunphy, J. E., Consulting Ed.) Philadelphia, W. B. Saunders Co., 1969.

Botsford, T. W., and Zollinger, R. M.: Diverticulitis of the colon. Surg. Gynecol. Obstet. *128*:1209, 1969.

Bunnell, S.: Surgery of the Hand. 3rd Ed. Philadelphia, J. B. Lippincott Co., 1956.

Campbell, O. J.: The bleeding nipple. Surgery *19*:40, 1946.

Cave, E. F., and Roberts, S. M.: A method for measuring and recording joint function. J. Bone Joint Surg. *18*:455, 1936.

Codman, E. A.: The Shoulder: Rupture of the Supraspinatus Tendon and Other Lesions in or about the Subacromial Bursa. [N.p., printed by Thomas Todd Co., 14 Beacon Street, Boston,] 1934.

Cope, Z.: The Early Diagnosis of the Acute Abdomen. 14th Ed. New York, Oxford University Press, 1972.

Crane, C.: Deep venous thrombosis in the leg following effort strain. N. Engl. J. Med. *246*:529, 1952.

Crile, G., Jr.: Practical Aspects of Thyroid Disease. Philadelphia, W. B. Saunders Co., 1949.

Dunphy, J. E.: Surgical anatomy of the anal canal. Arch. Surg., 57:791, 1948.

Edwards, E. A.: Nail changes in functional and organic arterial disease. N. Engl. J. Med. 239:362, 1948.

Edwards, E. A.: Thrombosis in Arteriosclerosis of the Lower Extremities. Springfield, Illinois, Charles C Thomas, 1950.

Egan, R. L.: Experience with mammography in a tumor institution. Radiography 75:894, 1960.

Gross, R. E.: The Surgery of Infancy and Childhood. Philadelphia, W. B. Saunders Co., 1953.

Haagensen, C. D.: Diseases of the Breast. 2nd Ed. Philadelphia. W. B. Saunders Co., 1971.

Harrison, J. H.: The treatment of rupture of the urethra, especially when accompanying fractures of pelvic bones. Surg. Gynecol. Obstet. 72:622, 1941.

Harrison, J. H.: Trauma to the kidney; mechanism of injury, diagnosis and management. Northwest Med., 47:337, 1948.

Haymaker, W., and Woodhall, B.: Peripheral Nerve Injuries: Principles of Diagnosis. 2nd Ed. Philadelphia, W. B. Saunders Co., 1953.

Hoerr, S. O., Bliss, W. R., and Kauffman, J.: Clinical evaluation of various tests for occult blood in the feces. J.A.M.A. 141:1213, 1949.

Holman, E.: The art of abdominal percussion in the presence of inflammation. Surg. Gynecol. Obstet. 93:775, 1951.

Homans, J.: Deep quiet venous thrombosis in the lower limbs. Surg. Gynecol. Obstet. 79:70, 1944.

Jeghers, H., McKusick, V. A., and Katz, K. H.: Generalized intestinal polyposis and melanin spots of oral mucosa, lips, and digits; syndrome of diagnostic significance. N. Engl. J. Med. 241:993, 1949.

Jones, P. F.: Emergency Abdominal Surgery. 1st Ed. London, Blackwell Scientific Publications, 1974.

Kendall, H. O., and Kendall, F. P.: Muscles, Testing and Function. Baltimore, Williams & Wilkins Co., 1949.

Lahey, F. H.: A method of palpating the lobes of the thyroid. J.A.M.A. 86:813, 1926.

Lahey, F. H., and Warren, K. W.: A long term appraisal of carotid body tumors with remarks on their removal. Surg. Gynecol. Obstet. 92:481, 1951.

Lawson, J. D., and Weissbein, A. S.: The puddle sign—an aid in the diagnosis of minimal ascites. N. Engl. J. Med. 260:652, 1959.

Leriche, R.: De la résection du carrefour aortico-iliaque avec double sympathectomie lombaire pour thrombose artéritique de l'aorte; le syndrome de l'oblitération termino-aortique pour artérite. Presse Med. 48:601, 1940.

Linton, R. R.: Peripheral vascular disease. N. Engl. J. Med. 240:645, 1949.

Mahorner, H. R., and Ochsner, A.: A new test for evaluating circulation in the venous system of the lower extremity affected by varicosities. Arch. Surg. 33:479, 1936.

Marshall, V. F.: The Diagnosis of Genito-Urinary Neoplasms (Monograph No. 3). New York, American Cancer Society, Inc., 1949.

Martin, H.: Cancer of the Head and Neck (Monograph No. 2). New York, American Cancer Society, Inc., 1949.

Matson, D. D.: The Treatment of Acute Craniocerebral Injuries Due to Missiles. Springfield, Illinois, Charles C Thomas, 1948.

McMurray, T. P.: Practice of Orthopedic Surgery. 3rd Ed. Baltimore, Williams & Wilkins Co., 1949.

Meigs, J. V., and Sturgis, S. H.: Progress in Gynecology. New York, Grune & Stratton, Inc., 1950, Vol. 2.

Milligan, E. T. C., Morgan, C. N., Jones, J. E., and Officer, R.: Surgical anatomy of the anal canal and the operative treatment of hemorrhoids. Lancet 2:1119, 1937.

Moses, W. R.: Early diagnosis of phlebothrombosis. N. Engl. J. Med. 234:288, 1946.

Murphey, F.: Peripheral nerve injuries. In Speed, J. S. (Ed.): Campbell's Operative Orthopedics. 2nd Ed. St. Louis, C. V. Mosby Co., 1949.

Naffziger, H. C., and Grant, W. T.: Neuritis of the brachial plexus mechanical in origin; scalenus syndrome. Surg. Gynecol. Obstet. 67:722, 1938.

Nather, C., and Ochsner, A.: Retroperitoneal operation for subphrenic abscess. Surg. Gynecol. Obstet. 37:665, 1923.

North, J. P.: Clostridial wound infections and gas gangrene; arterial damage as a modifying factor. Surgery *21*:364, 1947.

Ochsner, A., and DeBakey, M.: Subphrenic abscess; collective review and analysis of 3,608 collected and personal cases. Internat. Abstr. Surg. *66*:426, 1938; in Surg. Gynecol. Obstet. May, 1938.

Ochsner, A., and Graves, A. M.: Subphrenic abscess; analysis of 3,372 collected and personal cases. Ann. Surg. *98*:961, 1933.

Papanicolaou, G. N., and Traut, H. F.: Diagnosis of Uterine Cancer by the Vaginal Smear. New York, The Commonwealth Fund, 1943.

Prather, G. C.: Traumatic conditions of the kidney; clinical observations. J.A.M.A. *114*:207, 1940.

Quigley, T. B.: Management of knee injuries incurred in college football. Surg. Gynecol. Obstet. *87*:569, 1948.

Ravitch, M. M.: Pectus excavatum and heart failure. Surgery *30*:178, 1951.

Richards, L. G.: Otolaryngology in General Practice. New York, The MacMillan Co., 1939.

Shumacker, H. B., Jr.: Causalgia; general discussion. Surgery *24*:485, 1948.

Speed, J. S., and Knight, R. A. (Eds.): Campbell's Operative Orthopaedics. 3rd Ed. St. Louis, C. V. Mosby Co., 1956.

Taylor, G. W., and Nathanson, I. R.: Lymph Node Metastases; Incidence and Surgical Treatment in Neoplastic Disease. New York, Oxford University Press, 1942.

Warren, R.: Surgery. Philadelphia, W. B. Saunders Co., 1963.

Warren, R., and Linton, R. R.: The treatment of arterial embolism. N. Engl. J. Med. *238*:421, 1948.

Watson, L. F.: Hernia. St. Louis, C. V. Mosby Co., 1948.

Weed, L. L.: Medical records that guide and teach. N. Engl. J. Med. *278*:593, 1968.

Wharton, L. R.: Gynecology, with a Section on Female Urology. 2nd Ed. Philadelphia, W. B. Saunders Co., 1947.

Index

Note: Page numbers in *italic* indicate illustrations.

Gonococcal infection, of joints, 212
Graham Steell murmur, 112
Granuloma, eosinophilic, of chest wall, 78
Granuloma inguinale, in female, 279
Granuloma venereum, in female, 279
Granulosa cell tumor, of ovary, 282
Graves' disease, 43
Groin, examination of, 121–130
  lymphatics of, 121, *121*
Guaiac test, for occult blood in feces,
  290, *290*
Gynecomastia, *71, 72*

Habitus, body, of surgical cardiac patient,
  93
Hair, examination of, 14
Hallux valgus, 211, *211*
Hammer toe, 211, *211*
Hand, carbuncle of, 200
  collar-button abscess of, 200
  effects of diseases on, 12
  fascial spaces and tendon sheaths of,
    202
  human bite infections of, 200, 203
  in hyperthyroidism, 12, 43
  infections of, 197–204
    signs of, 198–199, 203–204
  injuries to, 368
Hashimoto's struma, 44
Head, examination of, 10, 13, 385
    position of patient in, 13
  infections of, 52
Head injury. See *Injuries, head.*
Hearing, tests of, 14
Heart, auscultation of, 99–105
  contusion of, 340
  dilatation of, 106
  examination of, 386
  functional classification of, 91
  injuries to, 326–340
  murmurs of, 101–105
  rate and rhythm of, 99
Heart disease, congenital, 93
    abdominal examination in, 98
    congestive heart failure and, 105
    corrective surgery in, 107–112
    growth and development and, 93
    inspection in, 93–95
    nutritional status and, 94
    palpation in, 96–98
    physical examination in, 93–105
    precordial pulsations in, 94
    precordium in, 98
    pulse in, 96
    respiration in, 95
    skeletal abnormalities in, 95
    skin color in, 94
Heart failure, congestive, in infancy, 105
  signs of, 106

Heart sounds, auscultation of, 99–105
  intensity of, 99
  normal, 99
Heel, painful, 212
  ulcers of, 259, *259*
Hegar's sign, 281
Hemangiomas, of chest wall, 76
  of palate, *22*
Hematocolpos, 271
Hemoperitoneum, 153
Hemophiliac joints, 212
Hemorrhage. See also *Bleeding.*
  extradural, 322
  in injured patient, control of, 317
  in penetrating abdominal wound, 345
  intra-abdominal, in abdominal wounds,
    345
  intraperitoneal, postoperative, 176
  subdural, 322
Hemorrhagic lung, 82
Hemorrhoids, anal, 286
  external, thrombosed, 295
  internal, 295, *295*
  rectal cancer and, 306
Hemothorax, 331
Hepatomegaly, in congestive heart failure
  in infants, 106
Hernia, abdominal, 122
  components of, 123
  diaphragmatic, congenital posterolateral,
    186
  femoral, 128
    irreducible, *128*
    strangulated, 129
  incarcerated, 122
    reduction of, 126, 127
  inguinal, 122–127
    carcinoma and, 306
    direct, 124, *125*
    in pediatric patients, 186, *187*
      incarcerated, 188
    indirect, 123, *125*
    reduction of, 126, *127*
  inguinal canal and, 122–127
  intra-abdominal, in pediatric patients,
    186
  irreducible, 120, 122
  reducible, 122, 126
  Richter's, 122
  scrotal, 120, 125
    irreducible, 120
  umbilical, in pediatric patients, 185, *186*
Herniated intervertebral disk. See *Disk,
  intervertebral.*
Herpes labialis, 27
High-velocity shells, abdominal wounds
  from, 342
Hip, acute bursitis of, 227
  dislocation of, 369
    congenital, 224
    posterior, 369